DENTAL ANATOMY COLORING BOOK

2nd Edition

Edited by

MARGARET J. FEHRENBACH, RDH, MS

Dental Hygiene Educational Consultant
Dental Science Technical Writer
Seattle, Washington

3251 Riverport Lane
St. Louis, Missouri 63043

DENTAL ANATOMY COLORING BOOK, SECOND EDITION   ISBN: 978-1-4557-4589-0

Notices

Knowledge and best practice in this field are constantly changing. As new research and experience broaden our understanding, changes in research methods, professional practices, or medical treatment may become necessary.

Practitioners and researchers must always rely on their own experience and knowledge in evaluating and using any information, methods, compounds, or experiments described herein. In using such information or methods they should be mindful of their own safety and the safety of others, including parties for whom they have a professional responsibility.

With respect to any drug or pharmaceutical products identified, readers are advised to check the most current information provided (i) on procedures featured or (ii) by the manufacturer of each product to be administered, to verify the recommended dose or formula, the method and duration of administration, and contraindications. It is the responsibility of practitioners, relying on their own experience and knowledge of their patients, to make diagnoses, to determine dosages and the best treatment for each individual patient, and to take all appropriate safety precautions.

To the fullest extent of the law, neither the Publisher nor the authors, contributors, or editors, assume any liability for any injury and/or damage to persons or property as a matter of products liability, negligence or otherwise, or from any use or operation of any methods, products, instructions, or ideas contained in the material herein.

ISBN: 978-1-4557-4589-0

Vice President and Publisher: Linda Duncan
Executive Content Strategist: Kathy Falk
Content Manager: Kristin Hebberd
Content Development Specialist: Joslyn Dumas
Publishing Services Manager: Julie Eddy
Project Manager: Jan Waters
Design Direction: Teresa McBryan

Printed in the United States of America

Last digit is the print number: 9 8 7 6 5 4 3 2 1

A thorough understanding of head and neck anatomy as well as dental anatomy is vital for today's dental professional. The second edition of the *Dental Anatomy Coloring Book* is an ideal companion for anyone studying head and neck anatomy as well as dental anatomy. This new edition has even more structures to color as well as more important details added to previously published structures. It has also been redesigned to not only help you identify differing structures but also to test your knowledge with exciting new features. Knowledge of related facial landmarks, veins, arteries, nerves, bones, and muscles of the head and neck region, as well as dental anatomy, is information that every dental professional needs to have, and this updated resource enhances learning and memory retention in an easy-to-use, FUN format!

The latest edition of the *Dental Anatomy Coloring Book* delivers COMPLETE anatomic coverage for the dental professional, beginning with an overview of body systems, and then moving onto specific areas of the head and neck as well as the oral cavity following the basic anatomic systems, including orofacial anatomy, dental anatomy, as well as the skeletal system, the muscular system, the vascular system, the nervous system, and much more! This fun book will help you to not only visually understand the differing parts of the head and neck as well as the oral cavity but the impact on each other. The final chapter on fasciae and spaces will also give the reader a more regional feel for anatomy of the head and neck. It has been noted that one of the most effective ways medical students, our healthcare allies, learn about the intricacies of the human body is by coloring detailed illustrations of various body parts. It is also a proven method to use in order to increase your memory's retention of important structures.

Studies also show that coloring can reduce stress. Thus, coloring is being used in formal therapeutic settings such as eye-hand coordination development and to help heal victims of trauma. Regardless of your needs, there is so much to be gained by spending some time coloring. Choosing your colors and the gentle, repetitive motion of your hand as you bring color to paper helps quiet your mind, bringing your usual rapid-fire thoughts down to a much slower pace. So take a break from your studies with classroom textbooks and find your creative center!

HOW TO USE THE NEW EDITION

Each page of the new edition describes the body part or system featured and its orientation view, followed by a crisp, easy-to-color illustration(s). Numbered leader lines clearly identify the structures to be colored and correspond to a numbered list. You can create your own "color code" by coloring in the boxed number appearing on the illustration and using the same color to fill in the corresponding numbered box on the list. An example of a completed illustration can be found on the Inside Back Cover. You can be distinctly creative with your "colors" or go the classical route, such as with red for arteries and blue for veins.

For review purposes for classroom or national board examination or certification, the numbered list can easily be covered with a sheet of paper or your hand, allowing self-examination. To help with review even further, basic fill-in-the-blank statements about the figure appear on the opposite page with a list of possible answers that can only be used once; the numbered correct answer appears below inverted on the same page. In addition, textbook references for each figure are noted so the reader can easily obtain more information on each structure presented.

For long-term use, after you are done coloring a page, carefully remove it from the textbook using its perforated edge and place it in a clear plastic, 3-hole cover page. Then add them to your class notebook or purchase a 3-ring binder to keep them in. You can take them with you and study while you're waiting for appointments, waiting for class to start, eating meals, etc. Our hope is that you not only learn the material easily but also have fun doing it!

CONTENTS

CHAPTER 3 Dental Anatomy

v

CONTENTS

CHAPTER 7 Glandular Tissue

CHAPTER 8 Nervous System

CHAPTER 9 Lymphatic System

CHAPTER 10 Fasciae and Spaces

FIGURE 1-1 Body sections and planes (anatomic position)

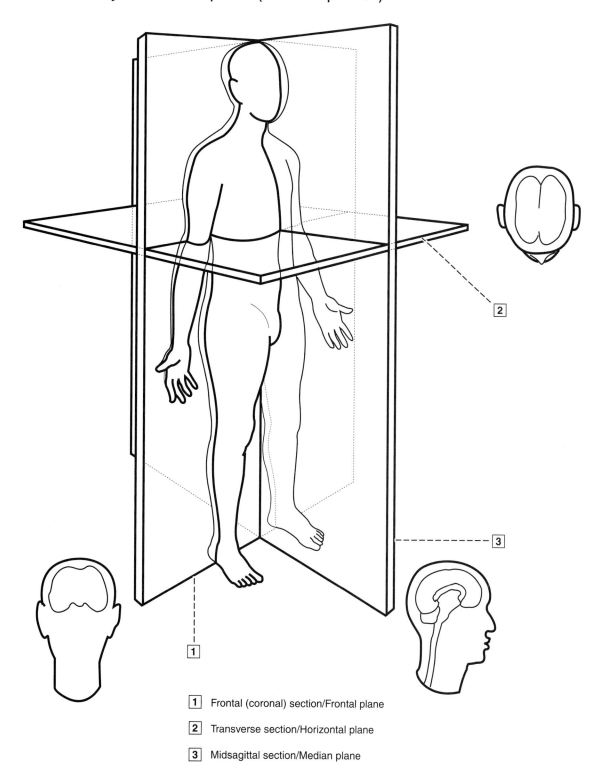

1 Frontal (coronal) section/Frontal plane

2 Transverse section/Horizontal plane

3 Midsagittal section/Median plane

REVIEW QUESTIONS

Fill in the blanks by choosing the appropriate terms from the list below.

1. The _____ used when discussing the body is based on the body being in anatomic position, which is a standard position of the body; when observing a body in the anatomic position, the left of the body is on the clinician's right, and vice versa.

2. In _____, the body is standing erect, with the arms at the sides and the palms and toes directed forward as well as the eyes looking forward.

3. The _____, or *midsagittal section,* is a division through the median plane.

4. The _____, or *frontal section,* is a division through any frontal plane.

5. The _____, or *transverse section,* is a division through a horizontal plane.

6. The _____, or *median plane,* is created by an imaginary line dividing the body into equal right and left halves.

7. An imaginary line dividing the body into anterior and posterior parts at any level creates a(n) _____, or *coronal plane.*

8. A(n) _____ is created by an imaginary line dividing the body at any level into either superior and inferior parts and is always perpendicular to the median plane.

9. A sagittal plane is any plane created by an imaginary plane parallel to the _____.

10. When the body is lying face down in the anatomic position, this is the _____, and when the body is lying face up, this is the supine position.

midsagittal plane	median section	frontal plane
coronal section	horizontal plane	horizontal section
anatomic position	median plane	prone position
anatomic nomenclature		

Reference

Chapter 1, Introduction to head and neck anatomy. In Fehrenbach MJ, Herring SW: *Illustrated anatomy of the head and neck,* ed 4, St. Louis, 2012, Saunders.

FIGURE 1-2 Prenatal development overview

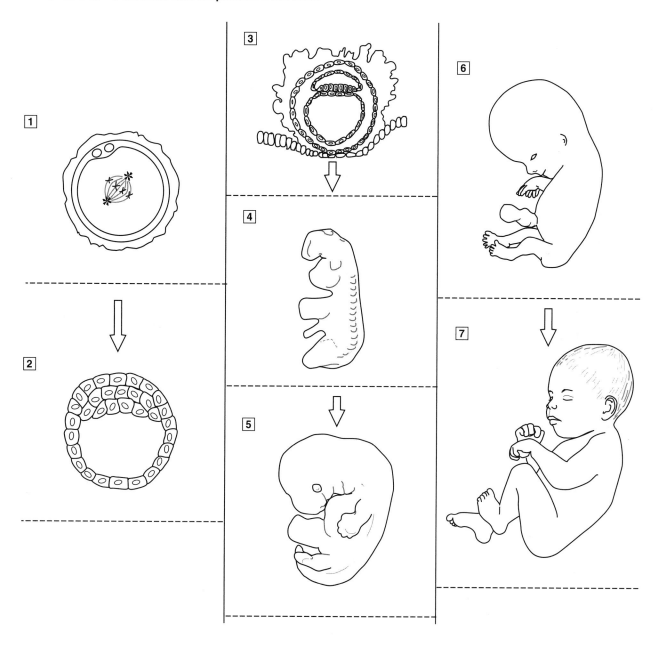

PREIMPLANTATION
PERIOD: 1ST WEEK

EMBRYONIC PERIOD:
2ND-8TH WEEK

FETAL PERIOD:
3RD-9TH MONTH

1 Zygote

2 Blastocyst

3 Blastocyst to disc

4 Disc to embryo

5 Embryo

6 Embryo

7 Fetus

REVIEW QUESTIONS

Fill in the blanks by choosing the appropriate terms from the list below.

1. The process of _prenatal development_ begins with the start of pregnancy and continues until the birth of the child.

2. The nine months of gestation during prenatal development is usually divided into 3-month time spans, or _trimesters_.

3. The study of prenatal development is termed _embryology_.

4. Each of the structures of the face, neck, and oral cavity has a(n) _primordium_, the earliest indication of a tissue type or an organ during prenatal development.

5. At the beginning of the first week, conception takes place, whereby a female's ovum is penetrated by and united with a male's sperm during fertilization; the union of the ovum and sperm subsequently forms a *fertilized egg,* or _zygote_.

6. The first period, the _preimplantation_ of prenatal development, takes place during the first week after conception.

7. Because of the ongoing process of mitosis and secretion of fluid by the cells within the morula, the zygote becomes a vesicle known as a(n) _blastocyst_, or *blastula,* that becomes implanted.

8. During the second week of prenatal development, a(n) _embryonic disk_ eventually develops from the blastocyst, which appears as a flattened, essentially circular plate of bilayered cells.

9. The second period of prenatal development, the embryonic period, extends from the beginning of the second week to the end of the eighth week, with the structure developing further and becoming a(n) _embryo_.

10. The fetal period of prenatal development follows the embryonic period and encompasses the beginning of the ninth week, or third month, to the ninth month, with the maturation of existing structures occurring as the embryo enlarges to become a(n) _fetus_.

embryology	fetus	embryo
prenatal development	embryonic disc	primordium
zygote	blastocyst	preimplantation period
trimesters		

Reference

Chapter 3, Overview of prenatal development. In Bath-Balogh M, Fehrenbach MJ: *Illustrated dental embryology, histology, and anatomy,* ed 3, St. Louis, 2011, Saunders.

ANSWER KEY 1. prenatal development, 2. trimesters, 3. embryology, 4. primordium, 5. zygote, 6. preimplantation period, 7. blastocyst, 8. embryonic disc, 9. embryo, 10. fetus.

FIGURE 1-3 Fertilization during prenatal development

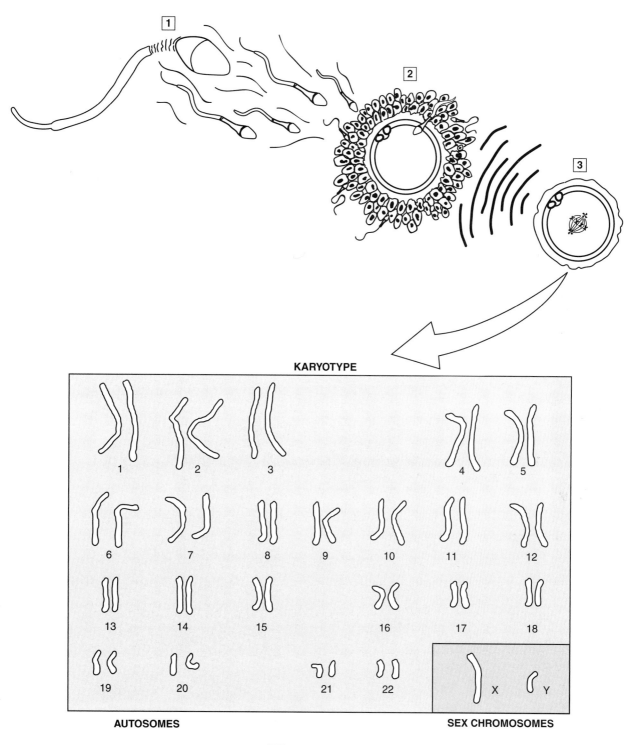

KARYOTYPE

AUTOSOMES

SEX CHROMOSOMES

1 Sperm (enlarged)

2 Ovum

3 Zygote

REVIEW QUESTIONS

Fill in the blanks by choosing the appropriate terms from the list below.

1. At the beginning of the first week of prenatal development __conception__ takes place, whereby a female's ovum is penetrated by and united with a male's sperm during fertilization.

2. The union of the ovum and sperm subsequently forms a(n) __zygote__, or *fertilized egg.*

3. During fertilization, the final stages of the process of __meiosis__ occur in the ovum, resulting in the joining of the ovum's chromosomes with those of the sperm; this joining of chromosomes from both biological parents forms a new individual with "shuffled" chromosomes.

4. The zygote receives half its __chromosomes__ from the female and half from the male, with the resultant genetic material a reflection of both biological parents through the process of meiosis.

5. The photographic analysis or profile of a person's chromosomes is done in an orderly arrangement by size, from largest to smallest, in a(n) __karyotype__; the sex can be demonstrated by the presence of either having XX chromosomes for females or XY chromosomes for males.

zygote	**conception**
karyotype	**chromosomes**
meiosis	

Reference

Chapter 3, Overview of prenatal development. In Bath-Balogh M, Fehrenbach MJ: *Illustrated dental embryology, histology, and anatomy,* ed 3, St. Louis, 2011, Saunders.

FIGURE 1-4 Preimplantation period to implantation during prenatal development

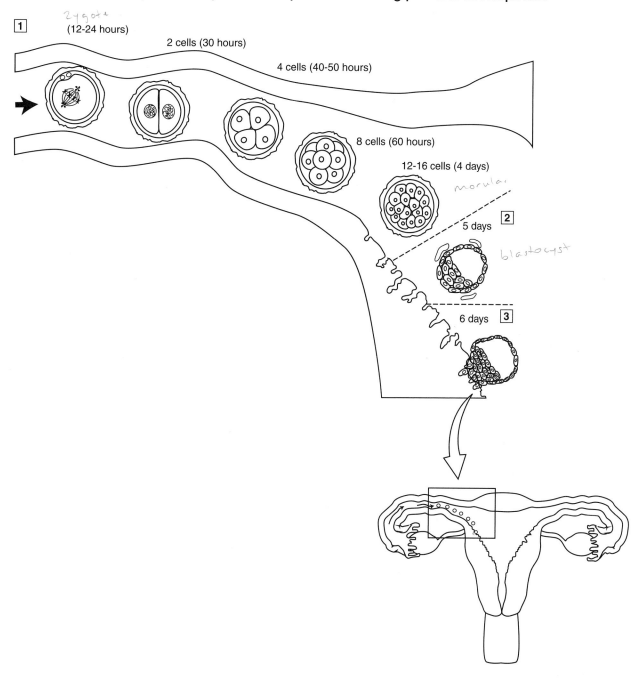

1 *zygote*
(12-24 hours)

2 cells (30 hours)

4 cells (40-50 hours)

8 cells (60 hours)

12-16 cells (4 days)

morula

5 days 2

blastocyst

6 days 3

1 Zygote

2 Blastocyst

3 Implantation

REVIEW QUESTIONS

Fill in the blanks by choosing the appropriate terms from the list below.

1. The first period of prenatal development, the _preimplantation_, takes place during the first week after conception, with the union of the ovum and sperm subsequently forming a fertilized egg, or *zygote*.

2. After fertilization, the zygote then undergoes the process of _mitosis_, or *cell division*, along with cleavage.

3. After initial cleavage, the solid ball of cells is known as a(n) _morula_.

4. Because of the ongoing process of mitosis and secretion of fluid by the cells within the morula, the zygote becomes a vesicle known as a(n) _blastocyst_ or *blastula*.

5. By the end of the first week, the blastocyst stops traveling and undergoes _implantation_ and thus becomes embedded in the prepared endometrium, the innermost lining of the uterus on its back wall.

preimplantation period   implantation

mitosis   morula

blastocyst

Reference

Chapter 3, Overview of prenatal development. In Bath-Balogh M, Fehrenbach MJ: *Illustrated dental embryology, histology, and anatomy,* ed 3, St. Louis, 2011, Saunders.

FIGURE 1-5 Implantation during prenatal development

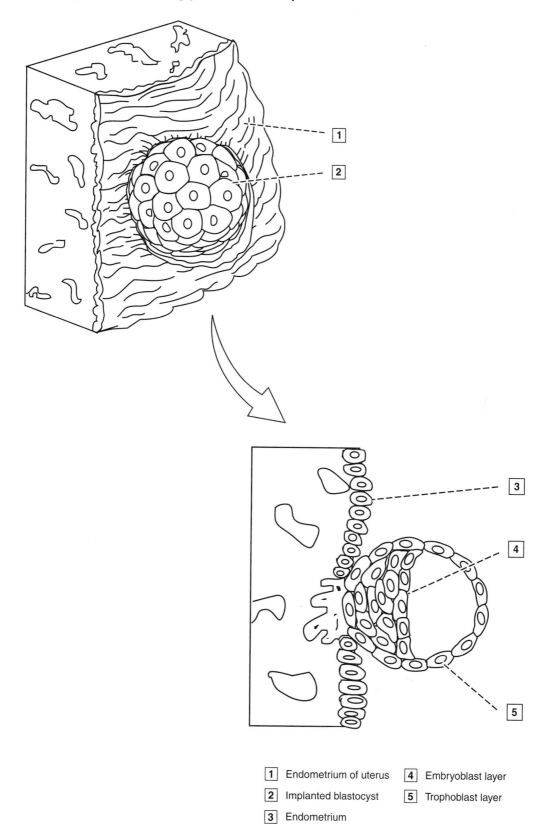

1	Endometrium of uterus	**4**	Embryoblast layer
2	Implanted blastocyst	**5**	Trophoblast layer
3	Endometrium		

REVIEW QUESTIONS

Fill in the blanks by choosing the appropriate terms from the list below.

1. Because of the ongoing process of ___mitosis___ and secretion of fluid by the cells within the morula, the zygote becomes a vesicle known as a blastocyst, or *blastula*.

2. The latter part of the first week of prenatal development is characterized by further mitotic ___cleavage___, in which the blastocyst splits into smaller and more numerous cells as it undergoes successive cell divisions by mitosis.

3. By the end of the first week, the blastocyst stops traveling and undergoes ___implantation___ and thus becomes embedded in the prepared endometrium, the innermost lining of the uterus on its back wall.

4. After a week of cleavage, the blastocyst consists of a layer of peripheral cells, the trophoblast layer, and a small inner mass of embryonic cells, or ___embryoblast layer___

5. The trophoblast layer later gives rise to important prenatal support tissue and the embryoblast layer gives rise to the ___embryo___ during the embryonic period.

embryoblast layer   embryo

implantation   mitosis

cleavage

Reference

Chapter 3, Overview of prenatal development. In Bath-Balogh M, Fehrenbach MJ: *Illustrated dental embryology, histology, and anatomy,* ed 3, St. Louis, 2011, Saunders.

FIGURE 1-6 Second week of prenatal development during embryonic period

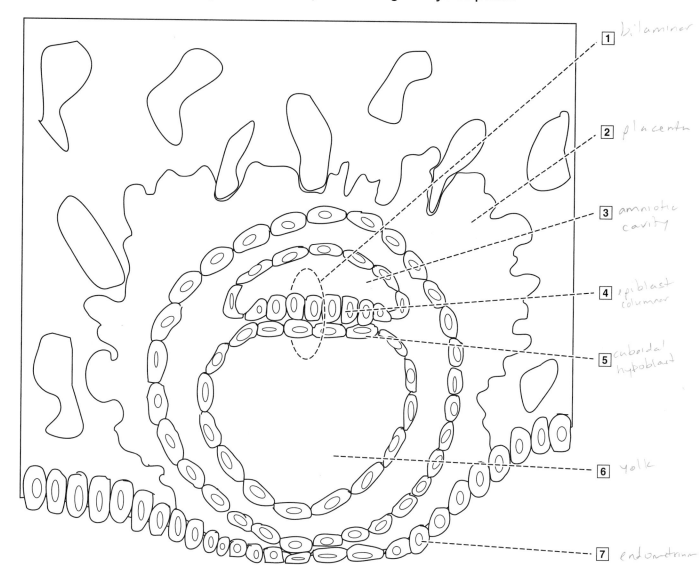

1 — bilaminar
2 — placenta
3 — amniotic cavity
4 — epiblast columnar
5 — cuboidal hypoblast
6 — yolk
7 — endometrium

1	Bilaminar embryonic disc	**5**	Hypoblast layer
2	Placenta	**6**	Yolk sac
3	Amniotic cavity	**7**	Endometrium of uterus
4	Epiblast layer		

REVIEW QUESTIONS

Fill in the blanks by choosing the appropriate terms from the list below.

1. The second period of prenatal development, the _embryonic period_, extends from the beginning of the second week to the end of the eighth week; it includes most of the latter part of the first trimester.

2. Certain physiological processes or spatial and temporal events called *patterning* occur during the embryonic period, which are considered key to the further development during prenatal development; these physiological processes include _induction_, proliferation, differentiation, morphogenesis, and maturation.

3. During the second week of prenatal development, within the embryonic period, the implanted blastocyst grows by increased proliferation of the embryonic cells, with differentiation also occurring resulting in changes in cellular morphogenesis; the increased number of embryonic cells creates the _embryonic cell layers_, or *germ layers,* within the blastocyst.

4. A(n) _bilaminar embryonic disc_ eventually develops from the blastocyst and appears as a flattened, essentially circular plate of bilayered cells.

5. The bilaminar disc has both a superior layer and inferior layer, with the superior _epiblast_ composed of high columnar cells and the inferior hypoblast layer composed of small cuboidal cells.

6. After its creation, the bilaminar embryonic disc is suspended in the uterus's endometrium between two fluid-filled cavities, the _amniotic_, which faces both the epiblast layer and the yolk sac, which faces the hypoblast layer and serves as initial nourishment for the embryonic disc.

7. The bilaminar embryonic disc later develops into the _embryo_ as prenatal development continues during the embryonic period of prenatal development.

8. The _placenta_, a prenatal organ that joins together the pregnant female and developing embryo, develops from the interactions of the trophoblast layer and endometrial tissue.

9. The formation of the placenta and the developing circulation of the _umbilical cord_ permit selective exchange of soluble bloodborne substances between them, which includes oxygen and carbon dioxide as well as nutritional and hormonal substances.

10. During the embryonic period of prenatal development, differentiation occurs at various rates in the embryo affecting cells, tissue types, organs, and systems; it includes different types such as cytodifferentiation and histodifferentiation, as well as _morphodifferentiation_.

embryo	bilaminar embryonic disc	embryonic period
umbilical cord	epiblast layer	amniotic cavity
morphodifferentiation	placenta	embryonic cell layers
induction		

Reference

Chapter 3, Overview of prenatal development. In Bath-Balogh M, Fehrenbach MJ: *Illustrated dental embryology, histology, and anatomy,* ed 3, St. Louis, 2011, Saunders.

ANSWER KEY 1. embryonic period, 2. induction, 3. embryonic cell layers, 4. bilaminar embryonic disc, 5. epiblast layer, 6. amniotic cavity, 7. embryo, 8. placenta, 9. umbilical cord, 10. morphodifferentiation.

FIGURE 1-7 Third week of prenatal development during embryonic period

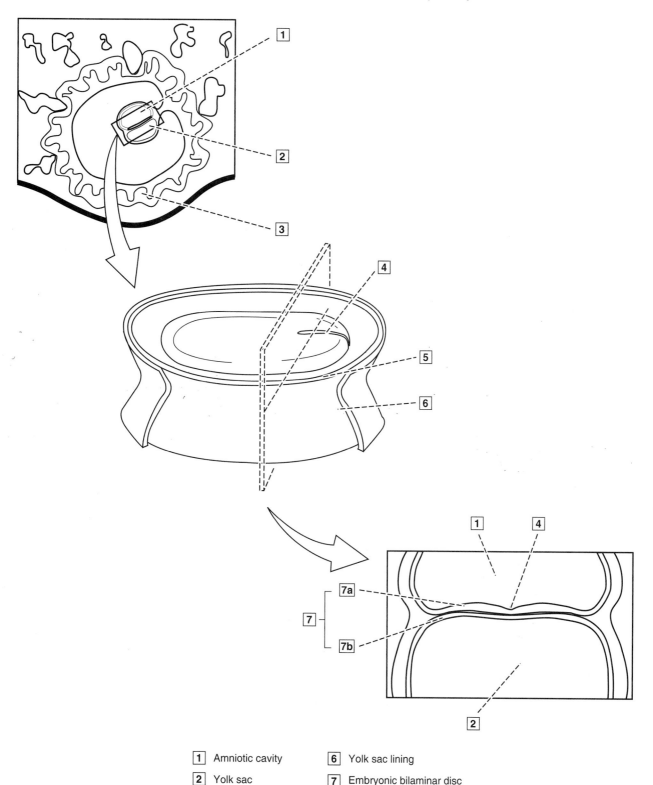

1	Amniotic cavity	**6**	Yolk sac lining
2	Yolk sac	**7**	Embryonic bilaminar disc
3	Placenta	**7a**	Epiblast layer
4	Primitive streak	**7b**	Hypoblast layer
5	Amniotic cavity lining		

REVIEW QUESTIONS

Fill in the blanks by choosing the appropriate terms from the list below.

1. During the beginning of the third week of prenatal development, within the embryonic period, the _primitive streak_ forms within the bilaminar embryonic disc; it is a furrowed, rod-shaped thickening in the middle of the disc that results from an increased proliferation of cells in the midline area.

2. The primitive streak causes the bilaminar embryonic disc to have _bilateral symmetry_, with a right half and left half; most of the further development of each half of the embryo mirrors the other half.

3. During the beginning of the third week, some cells from the _epiblast layer_ move or migrate toward the hypoblast layer only in the area of the primitive streak of the bilaminar embryonic disc.

4. The migratory cells from the epiblast layer into the hypoblast layer of the bilaminar embryonic disc locate in the middle between the two layers and become _mesenchyme_, an embryonic connective tissue.

5. The mesenchymal cells between the epiblast and hypoblast layers have the potential to proliferate and differentiate into diverse types of connective tissue, forming cells (such as fibroblasts, chondroblasts, and osteoblasts); some of this migrated tissue begins to create a new embryonic cell layer, the _mesoderm_.

6. When layers are present, the bilaminar embryonic disc becomes thickened into a(n) _trilaminar_ during the third week of prenatal development.

7. With the creation of a new embryonic cell layer of mesoderm within the trilaminar embryonic disc, the epiblast layer is now considered _ectoderm_, and the hypoblast layer is now endoderm.

8. When the trilaminar embryonic disc undergoes growth during the first three weeks, certain anatomic structures of the disc become apparent and the trilaminar embryonic disc now has a(n) _cephalic_, or *head end.*

9. At the cephalic end of the trilaminar embryonic disc, the _oropharyngeal membrane_ forms; it consists of only ectoderm externally and endoderm internally, without any intermediate mesoderm, which is the location of the future primitive mouth, or *stomodeum,* of the embryo and thus the beginning of the digestive tract.

10. The trilaminar embryonic disc has a(n) _caudal_, or *tail end*; at this end, the cloacal membrane forms, which is the location of the future anus, or terminal end of the digestive tract.

mesoderm	trilaminar embryonic disc	primitive streak
bilateral symmetry	ectoderm	epiblast layer
cephalic end	oropharyngeal membrane	caudal end
mesenchyme		

Reference

Chapter 3, Overview of prenatal development. In Bath-Balogh M, Fehrenbach MJ: *Illustrated dental embryology, histology, and anatomy,* ed 3, St. Louis, 2011, Saunders.

FIGURE 1-8 Central nervous system and muscular system development during embryonic period

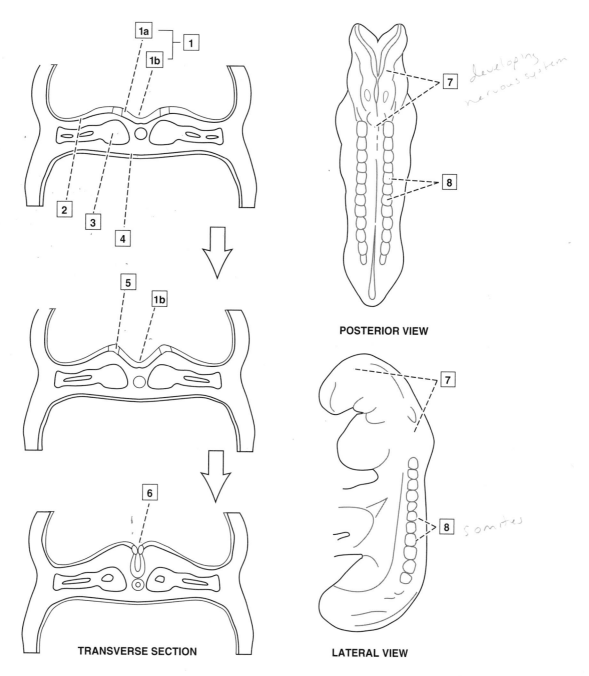

POSTERIOR VIEW

TRANSVERSE SECTION

LATERAL VIEW

1	Neuroectoderm	**4**	Endoderm
1a	Neural plate	**5**	Neural fold
1b	Neural groove	**6**	Neural folds about to fuse to form the neural tube
2	Ectoderm	**7**	Developing nervous system
3	Mesoderm	**8**	Somites

REVIEW QUESTIONS

Fill in the blanks by choosing the appropriate terms from the list below.

1. During the latter part of the third week of prenatal development, the _CNS_ begins to develop in the embryo; in the future this makes up the majority of the nervous system, because it will consist of the brain and the spinal cord.

2. A specialized group of cells differentiates from the ectoderm during the third week of prenatal development and is now considered _neuroectoderm_.

3. The neuroectoderm is localized to the _neural plate_ of the embryo, a central band of cells that extends the length of the embryo, from the cephalic end to the caudal end.

4. The neural plate of the embryo undergoes further growth and thickening within the third week of prenatal development, which cause it to deepen and invaginate inward, forming the _neural groove_.

5. Near the end of the third week of prenatal development, the neural groove deepens further and is surrounded by the _neural fold_.

6. As further growth of the neuroectoderm occurs, the _neural tube_ is formed during the fourth week by the neural folds undergoing fusion at the most superior part; in the future, this structure forms into the spinal cord as well as other neural tissue.

7. During the third week, another specialized group of cells, the _NCCs_, develop from neuroectoderm that migrated from the crests of the neural folds and then dispersed within the mesenchyme to become involved in the development of many face and neck structures, such as the branchial arches, because they differentiate to form most of the connective tissue of the head.

8. The neural crest cells of the embryo are essential in the development of the face and neck, as well as most oral and dental tissue, except the _enamel_ and certain types of cementum.

9. By the end of the third week, the layer of _mesoderm_ additionally differentiates and begins to divide on each side of the tube within the embryo into 38 paired cuboidal segments, forming the somites.

10. The _somites_ appear as distinct elevations on the surface of the sides of the embryo after differentiation of the mesoderm and continue to develop in the following weeks of prenatal development, giving rise to most of the skeletal structures of the head, neck, and trunk, as well as the associated muscles and dermis of the skin.

neural tube	neural groove	central nervous system
enamel	somites	neural folds
mesoderm	neural plate	neuroectoderm
neural crest cells		

Reference

Chapter 3, Overview of prenatal development. In Bath-Balogh M, Fehrenbach MJ: *Illustrated dental embryology, histology, and anatomy,* ed 3, St. Louis, 2011, Saunders.

ANSWER KEY 1. central nervous system, 2. neuroectoderm, 3. neural plate, 4. neural groove, 5. neural folds, 6. neural tube, 7. neural crest cells, 8. enamel, 9. mesoderm, 10. somites.

FIGURE 1-9 Fourth week of prenatal development with embryonic folding and organ development during embryonic period

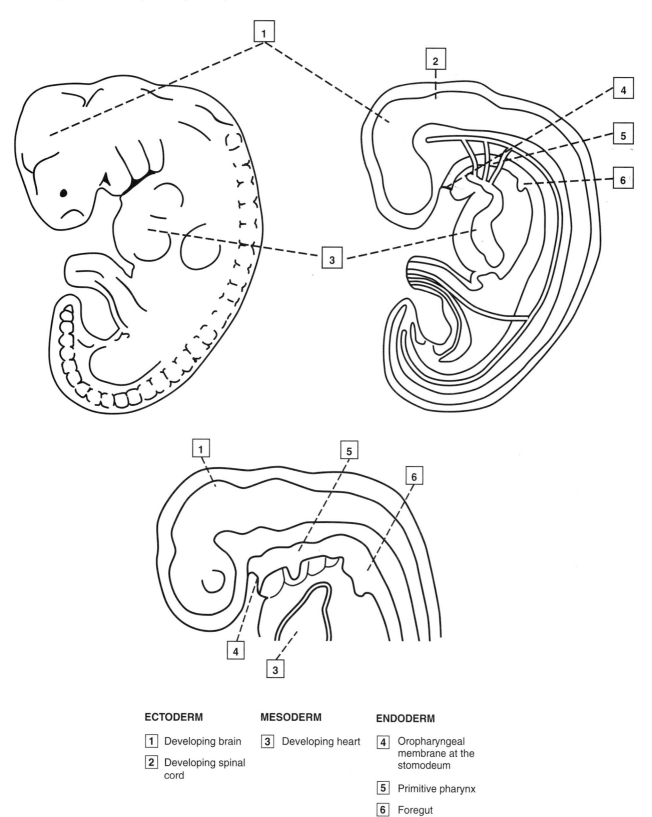

ECTODERM

1 Developing brain

2 Developing spinal cord

MESODERM

3 Developing heart

ENDODERM

4 Oropharyngeal membrane at the stomodeum

5 Primitive pharynx

6 Foregut

REVIEW QUESTIONS

Fill in the blanks by choosing the appropriate terms from the list below.

1. During the fourth week of prenatal development within the embryonic period, the embryonic disc undergoes _embryonic folding_, establishing for the first time the axis, which places forming tissue types into their proper positions for further embryonic development, as well as producing a somewhat tubular embryo.

2. After folding of the embryonic disc into the embryo, the endoderm now lies inside the _ectoderm_, with mesoderm filling in the areas between these two layers, forming one long, hollow tube lined by endoderm from the cephalic end to the caudal end of the embryo; specifically the tube runs from the oropharyngeal membrane to the cloacal membrane.

3. The tube formed during embryonic folding is the future _digestive tract_ and is separated into three major regions: the foregut, midgut, and hindgut.

4. The anterior part of the tube in the embryo when it becomes folded is the foregut, which forms the _primitive pharynx_, or *primitive throat*, and includes a part of the primitive yolk sac as it becomes enclosed with folding; the two more posterior parts, the midgut and hindgut, form the rest of the mature pharynx, as well as the remainder of the digestive tract.

5. During development of the digestive tract, four pairs of _pharyngeal pouches_ form from evaginations on the lateral walls lining the pharynx during the fourth week of prenatal development.

primitive pharynx	digestive tract
pharyngeal pouches	embryonic folding
ectoderm	

Reference

Chapter 3, Overview of prenatal development. In Bath-Balogh M, Fehrenbach MJ: *Illustrated dental embryology, histology, and anatomy,* ed 3, St. Louis, 2011, Saunders.

FIGURE 1-10   Fetal period of prenatal development

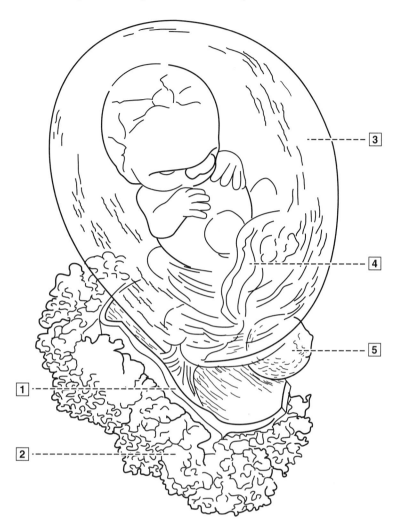

1	Chorion
2	Placenta
3	Amniotic cavity
4	Umbilical cord
5	Yolk sac

ELEVENTH WEEK TO FULL TERM

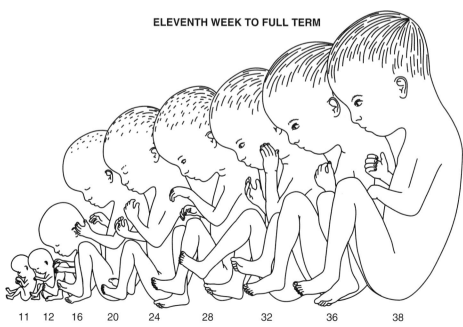

11   12   16   20   24   28   32   36   38

REVIEW QUESTIONS

Fill in the blanks by choosing the appropriate terms from the list below.

1. As the third and final period of prenatal development, the _____ follows the embryonic period.

2. The fetal period of prenatal development encompasses the beginning of the ninth week, or third month, all the way to the ninth month and birth; thus this period includes both the second and third _____.

3. During the fetal period of prenatal development there is maturation of existing structures occurring as the embryo enlarges to become a(n) _____.

4. With the fetal period of prenatal development, the processes involved include not only the physiological process of _____ of the individual tissue types and organs but also further proliferation, differentiation, and morphogenesis, similar to the processes occurring earlier in the embryo.

5. Although developmental changes with the fetus during the fetal period of prenatal development are not as dramatic as those that occurred earlier during the _____, they are important because they allow the newly formed tissue types and organs to function.

embryonic period	maturation
trimesters	fetus
fetal period	

Reference

Chapter 3, Overview of prenatal development. In Bath-Balogh M, Fehrenbach MJ: *Illustrated dental embryology, histology, and anatomy,* ed 3, St. Louis, 2011, Saunders.

FIGURE 1-11   Cell with its cell membrane and organelles

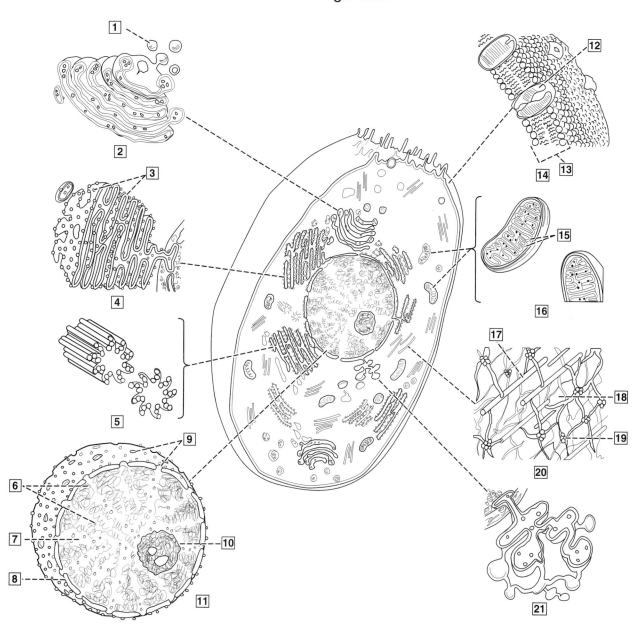

1 Lysosome	**8** Nuclear envelope	**15** Cristae
2 Golgi complex	**9** Nuclear pore	**16** Mitochondria
3 Ribosomes	**10** Nucleolus	**17** Microtubule
4 Rough endoplasmic reticulum	**11** Nucleus	**18** Cytoplasm
5 Centrioles of centrosome	**12** Protein	**19** Microfilament
6 Chromatin	**13** Phospholipid bilayer	**20** Cytoskeleton
7 Nucleoplasm	**14** Cell membrane	**21** Smooth endoplasmic reticulum

REVIEW QUESTIONS

Fill in the blanks by choosing the appropriate terms from the list below.

1. The smallest living unit of organization in the body is the _____ because each is capable of performing any necessary functions without the aid of others; each has a cell membrane, cytoplasm, organelles, and inclusions.

2. The _____, or *plasma membrane,* surrounds the cell; usually it is an intricate bilayer, consisting predominantly of phospholipids and proteins.

3. The _____ of the cell includes the semifluid part contained within the cell membrane boundary, as well as the skeletal system of support or *cytoskeleton.*

4. The _____ are metabolically active specialized structures within the cell that allow each cell to function according to its genetic code; these structures include the nucleus, mitochondria, ribosomes, endoplasmic reticulum, Golgi complex, lysosomes, and cytoskeleton.

5. The _____ is the largest, densest, and most conspicuous organelle in the cell; it is found in all cells of the body except mature red blood cells, and most cells have a single one.

6. The fluid part within the nucleus is the _____, which contains important molecules used in the construction of ribosomes, nucleic acids, and other nuclear materials; the nucleus is also surrounded by the nuclear envelope, a membrane similar to the cell membrane.

7. Contained in the nucleus is the _____, a prominent, rounded nuclear organelle that is centrally placed in the nucleoplasm, mainly producing types of ribonucleic acid.

8. The _____ are the most numerous organelles in the cell and are associated with energy conversion since they are a major source of adenosine triphosphate.

9. The _____ consists of parallel membrane-bound channels that interconnect, forming a system of channels and folds and are continuous with the nuclear envelope so they can modify, store, segregate, and transport proteins; these structures can be classified as either smooth or rough, with classification determined by the absence or presence of ribosomes.

10. Once the endoplasmic reticulum has modified a new protein, it is then transferred to the _____ for subsequent segregation, packaging, and transport of the protein compounds; it is the second largest organelle after the nucleus and is composed of stacks of three to twenty flattened, smooth-membrane vesicular sacs arranged parallel to one another.

nucleus	nucleoplasm	mitochondria
cytoplasm	organelles	nucleolus
Golgi complex	endoplasmic reticulum	cell membrane
cell		

Reference

Chapter 7, Overview of the cell. In Bath-Balogh M, Fehrenbach MJ: *Illustrated dental embryology, histology, and anatomy,* ed 3, St. Louis, 2011, Saunders.

ANSWER KEY 1. cell, 2. cell membrane, 3. cytoplasm, 4. organelles, 5. nucleus, 6. nucleoplasm, 7. nucleolus, 8. mitochondria, 9. endoplasmic reticulum, 10. Golgi complex.

FIGURE 1-12 Cell cycle

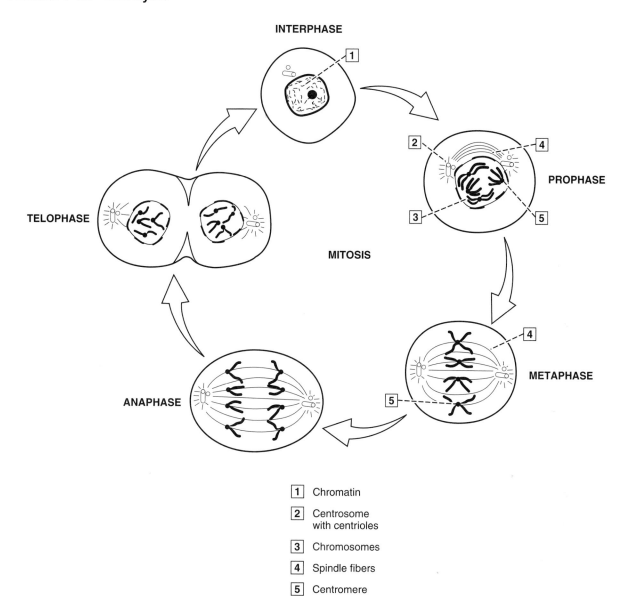

INTERPHASE

PROPHASE

TELOPHASE

MITOSIS

ANAPHASE

METAPHASE

1 Chromatin

2 Centrosome
with centrioles

3 Chromosomes

4 Spindle fibers

5 Centromere

REVIEW QUESTIONS

Fill in the blanks by choosing the appropriate terms from the list below.

1. The chief nucleic acid in the nucleoplasm is _____ in the form of chromatin, which looks like diffuse stippling; in an actively dividing cell, the chromatin condenses into visible, discrete, rodlike chromosomes, with each chromosome having a centromere, or a clear, constricted area near the middle.

2. The _____ become two filamentous, or threadlike, chromatids (daughters) joined by a centromere during cell division; after cell division, these major segments again become uncoiled and dispersed among the other components of the nucleoplasm.

3. The _____ is a dense, somewhat oval-shaped organelle that contains a pair of cylindrical structures, the centrioles, which are always located near the nucleus; there are two centrioles within this organelle, and each is composed of triplets of microtubules arranged in a cartwheel pattern.

4. Before cell division, the cell cycle phase of _____ occurs between cellular divisions so as to engage in cellular growth, metabolism, organelle replacement, and substance production, including chromatin and centrosome replication.

5. The phase of interphase itself has _____ phases: Gap 1, or *G1* (initial resting phase: cell growth and functioning), Synthesis, or *S* (cell deoxyribonucleic acid synthesis by duplication), and Gap 2, or *G2* (second resting phase: resuming cell growth and functioning).

6. The cell division that takes place during mitosis consists of _____ phases: prophase, metaphase, anaphase, and telophase; mitosis is then followed again by interphase so as to continue the cell cycle.

7. During _____ of cell division, the chromatin condenses into chromosomes in cell, replicated centrioles migrate to opposite pole, and nuclear membrane and nucleolus disintegrate.

8. During _____ of cell division, the chromosomes move so that their centromeres are aligned in the equatorial plane and the mitotic spindle forms.

9. During _____ of cell division, the centromeres split, and each chromosome separates into two chromatids and the chromatids migrate to opposite poles by the mitotic spindle.

10. During _____ of cell division, the division into two daughter cells that are identical to the parent cell as well as to each other occurs and the nuclear membrane reappears.

three	chromosomes	telophase
interphase	prophase	anaphase
deoxyribonucleic acid	four	centrosome
metaphase		

Reference

Chapter 7, Overview of the cell. In Bath-Balogh M, Fehrenbach MJ: *Illustrated dental embryology, histology, and anatomy,* ed 3, St. Louis, 2011, Saunders.

ANSWER KEY 1. deoxyribonucleic acid, 2. chromosomes, 3. centrosome, 4. interphase, 5. three, 6. four, 7. prophase, 8. metaphase, 9. anaphase, 10. telophase.

FIGURE 1-13 Major body cavities (midsagittal section)

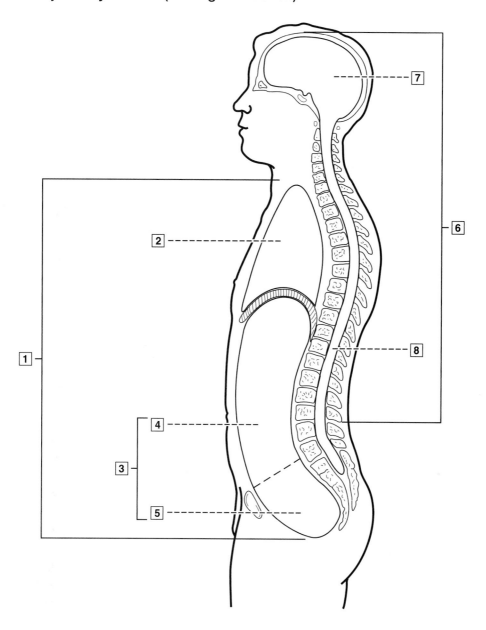

1	Ventral cavity	5	Pelvic cavity
2	Thoracic cavity	6	Dorsal cavity
3	Abdominopelvic cavity	7	Cranial cavity
4	Abdominal cavity	8	Spinal cavity

REVIEW QUESTIONS

Fill in the blanks by choosing the appropriate terms from the list below.

1. A(n) _____ is a space in the body filled with fluid.

2. The _____ is a body cavity in the ventral or anterior aspect of the body; it has two subdivisions: the thoracic cavity and the abdominopelvic cavity.

3. The _____ is a body cavity that is divided into the abdominal cavity and pelvic cavity, but there is no physical barrier between these two subdivisions, only an imaginary line from the pubis up and back to the top of the sacrum dividing them.

4. The _____ is a body cavity that contains digestive organs, spleen, and kidneys, and the pelvic cavity is a body cavity that contains the urinary bladder, internal reproductive organs, and rectum; both of these cavities protected by a layer of the peritoneum.

5. The _____ is body cavity formed by the ribcage; it is divided from the abdomino-pelvic cavity by the diaphragm muscle and is then further divided into the pleural cavity that contains the lungs and the superior mediastinum that includes the pericardial cavity with the heart.

6. The _____ is a body cavity bounded by the pelvic bones that primarily contains reproductive organs, the urinary bladder, the pelvic colon, and the rectum.

7. The _____ is a body cavity in the dorsal or posterior aspect of the body that lies within the skull and vertebral column, with two subdivisions: the cranial cavity and the spinal cavity.

8. The _____, or *intracranial space,* is a body cavity within the cranium that contains the brain, proximal parts of the cranial nerves, blood vessels, and cranial venous sinuses and also has the eyes and ears.

9. The _____, or *spinal canal,* is a body cavity through which the spinal cord passes that is enclosed within the vertebral foramen of the vertebrae.

10. Both the cranial cavity and spinal cavity are lined by the _____.

abdominopelvic cavity	dorsal cavity	cranial cavity
body cavity	spinal cavity	ventral cavity
pelvic cavity	meninges	abdominal cavity
thoracic cavity		

Reference

Various chapters. In Drake R, Vogl AW, Mitchell AWM: *Gray's anatomy for students,* ed 2, Philadelphia, 2010, Churchill Livingstone.

FIGURE 1-14   Major bones (anterior and posterior views)

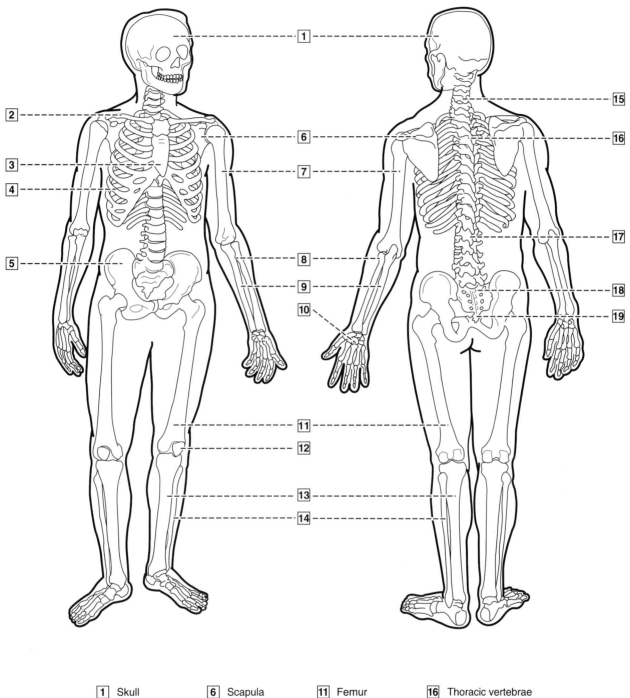

1 Skull	**6** Scapula	**11** Femur	**16** Thoracic vertebrae
2 Clavicle	**7** Humerus	**12** Patella	**17** Lumbar vertebrae
3 Sternum	**8** Radius	**13** Tibia	**18** Sacrum
4 Ribs	**9** Ulna	**14** Fibula	**19** Coccyx
5 Os coxae	**10** Carpals	**15** Vertebral column/ Cervical vertebrae	

REVIEW QUESTIONS

Fill in the blanks by choosing the appropriate terms from the list below.

1. Adults have 206 bones, although at birth there are about 300 bones; however, many of the bones _____ together with growth.

2. The _____ is composed of the cranium and mandible.

3. The _____, or *backbone,* is composed of 24 bones and includes the vertebrae, the sacrum, and the coccyx.

4. The top seven vertebrae, the _____, compose the neck, with the next twelve, the thoracic vertebrae, attaching to the ribs, with the last five vertebrae being the lumbar vertebrae; the sacrum is directly inferior to the lumbar vertebrae and is attached to the pelvic bone, or *hipbone,* and the coccyx or *tailbone* is located further inferior to it, with the os coxa of an adult pelvic girdle formed by the fusion of the ilium, ischium, and pubis.

5. The _____ create a bony cage protecting organs such as the heart, lungs, and liver; although there are usually twelve pairs of ribs, occasionally there is one extra or one missing pair.

6. The superior seven ribs connect to the _____, or *breastbone*; it also attaches to the clavicle, or *collarbone,* and the more inferior thoracic vertebrae hold all twelve ribs in place.

7. The arms each contain one _____, which is the large bone at the superior part of the arm, and two long bones of the forearm, which are the ulna and radius; the carpals are the bones of the wrist.

8. The long bone of the thigh is the _____; the patella, also known as the *kneecap,* articulates with the femur.

9. The two long bones running from the knee to the ankle, the _____ and the fibula, compose the bones of the legs.

10. The bones of the ankle are the _____; the metacarpals and metatarsals are bones of the hand and foot, respectively, and the phalanges are bones of the fingers and toes.

fuse	tibia	skull
cervical vertebrae	femur	humerus
tarsals	sternum	vertebral column
ribs		

Reference

Various chapters. In Drake R, Vogl AW, Mitchell AWM: *Gray's anatomy for students,* ed 2, Philadelphia, 2010, Churchill Livingstone.

FIGURE 1-15 Bone and cartilage anatomy

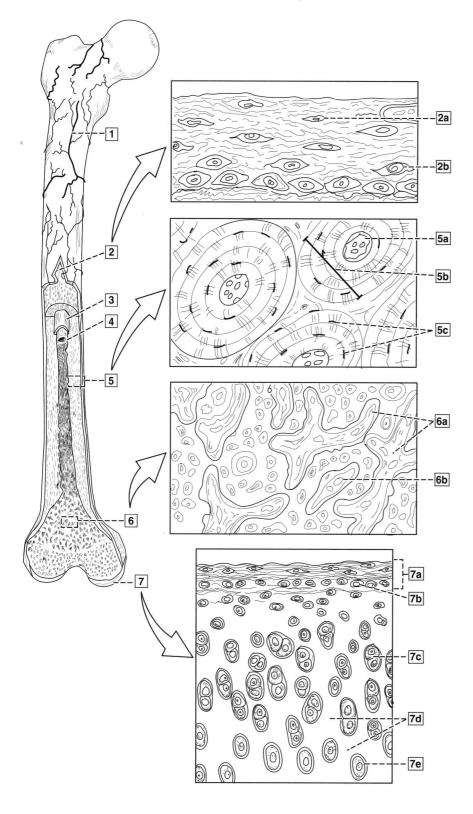

1 Blood vessel
2 Periosteum
2a Fibroblast
2b Osteoblast
3 Endosteum
4 Bone marrow
5 Compact bone
5a Haversian canal
5b Osteon
5c Lamellae

6 Cancellous bone
6a Trabeculae
6b Blood vessel
7 Articular cartilage
7a Perichondrium
7b Chondroblast
7c Daughter chondrocytes
   in lacuna
7d Cartilage matrix
7e Singular chondrocyte
   in lacuna

REVIEW QUESTIONS

Fill in the blanks by choosing the appropriate terms from the list below.

1. The _____ is a rigid connective tissue that constitutes most of the mature skeleton; thus it serves as protective and structural support for soft tissue and as an attachment mechanism.

2. The outer part of bone is covered by the _____, which is a double-layered, dense, connective tissue sheath.

3. The outer layer of periosteum contains blood vessels and nerves, and the inner layer contains a single layer of cells that give rise to bone-forming cells, the _____.

4. Deep to the periosteum is a dense layer of _____, which is that part of a bone composed of densely packed bone tissue; and deep to compact bone is the cancellous bone or *trabecular bone,* which is that part of a bone composed of less dense bone tissue.

5. Lining the medullary cavity of bone on the inside of the layers of compact bone and trabecular bone is the _____, which has the same composition as the periosteum but is thinner; on the innermost part of bone in the medullary cavity is the bone marrow, which is a gelatinous substance where the stem cells of the blood are located, the lymphocytes are created, and B-cells mature.

6. Bone matrix is initially formed as _____, which later undergoes mineralization; this is produced by osteoblasts, cuboidal cells that arise from fibroblasts.

7. The process of _____ involves the formation of osteoid between two dense connective tissue sheets, which then eventually replaces the outer connective tissue; this contrasts with the process of endochondral ossification that involves the formation of the osteoid within a hyaline cartilage model that subsequently becomes mineralized and dies.

8. The _____ is a firm, nonmineralized connective tissue that serves as a skeletal tissue in the body; it can be present at articular surfaces of most freely movable joints such as the temporomandibular joint, or it can serve as a model or template in which certain bones of the body subsequently develop.

9. The connective tissue surrounding most cartilage is the _____, a fibrous connective tissue sheath containing blood vessels.

10. Two types of cells found in cartilage are the immature chondroblasts, which lie internal to the perichondrium and produce cartilage matrix, and the _____, which are mature chondroblasts maintaining the cartilage matrix within their lacunae.

osteoblasts	cartilage	chondrocytes
compact bone	bone	periosteum
endosteum	osteoid	intramembranous ossification
perichondrium		

Reference

Chapter 8, Basic tissue. In Bath-Balogh M, Fehrenbach MJ: *Illustrated dental embryology, histology, and anatomy,* ed 3, St. Louis, 2011, Saunders.

ANSWER KEY 1. bone, 2. periosteum, 3. osteoblasts, 4. compact bone, 5. endosteum, 6. osteoid, 7. intramembranous ossification, 8. cartilage, 9. perichondrium, 10. chondrocytes.

FIGURE 1-16   Bone (transverse section with microanatomic views)

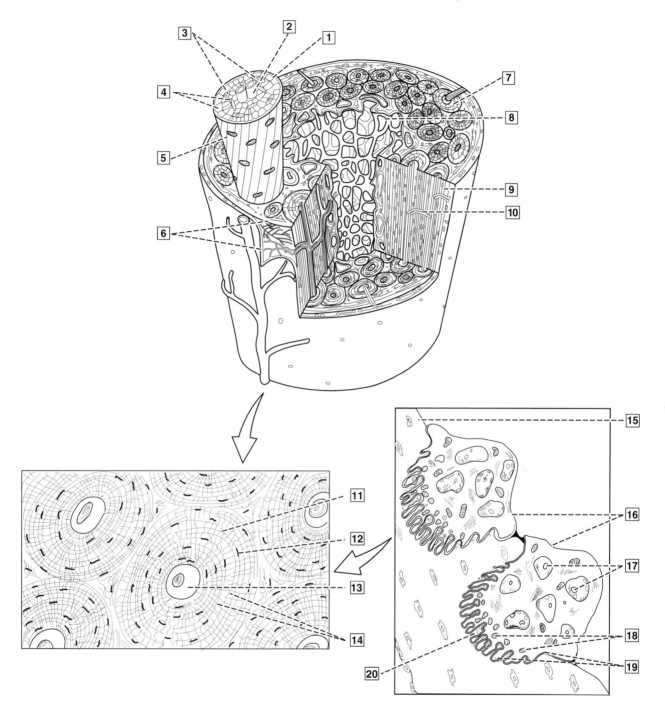

1	Lamellae	6	Periosteum	11	Canaliculi	16	Osteoclasts
2	Haversian canal	7	Osteon of compact bone	12	Osteocyte in lacuna	17	Nuclei
3	Lacunae containing osteocytes	8	Trabeculae of cancellous bone	13	Haversian canal	18	Lysosomes
4	Canaliculi	9	Haversian canal	14	Concentric lamellae	19	Howship lacuna
5	Osteon	10	Volkmann canal	15	Mineralized bone	20	Area of bone resorption

REVIEW QUESTIONS

Fill in the blanks by choosing the appropriate terms from the list below.

1. Bone consists of cells and a partially mineralized matrix that is composed of inorganic material, which is a crystalline formation of mainly _____ that gives bone its hardness.

2. Within fully mineralized bone are _____, which are entrapped mature osteoblasts; similar to the chondrocyte, the cell body is surrounded by bone, except for the space immediately around it, the lacuna.

3. Unlike chondrocytes, _____ never undergo mitosis during tissue formation, and thus only one osteocyte is ever found in its lacuna.

4. The cytoplasmic processes of the osteocyte radiate outward in all directions in the bone and are located in tubular canals of matrix, or _____; these provide for interaction between the osteocytes.

5. Bone matrix in compact bone is formed into closely apposed sheets, or _____; within and between each one is embedded osteocytes with their cytoplasmic processes in the canals.

6. The highly organized arrangement of concentric lamellae in compact bone is the _____.

7. The _____, or *central canal,* is a central vascular canal within each osteon surrounded by the lamellae; it contains longitudinally running blood vessels, nerves, and a small amount of connective tissue and is lined by endosteum.

8. Located on the outer part of the Haversian system in compact bone are _____, which are similar nutrient canals to the Haversian canals.

9. The cell in mature bone that causes resorption of bone is the _____.

10. The osteoclast is a large, multinucleated giant cell located on the surface of secondary bone in a large, shallow pit created by this resorption, the _____.

osteocytes	osteoblasts	lamellae
calcium hydroxyapatite	Haversian system	Haversian canal
Howship lacuna	Volkmann canals	osteoclast
canaliculi		

Reference

Chapter 8, Basic tissue. In Bath-Balogh M, Fehrenbach MJ: *Illustrated dental embryology, histology, and anatomy,* ed 3, St. Louis, 2011, Saunders.

ANSWER KEY 1. calcium hydroxyapatite, 2. osteocytes, 3. osteoblasts, 4. canaliculi, 5. lamellae, 6. Haversian system, 7. Haversian canal, 8. Volkmann canals, 9. osteoclast, 10. Howship lacuna.

FIGURE 1-17   **Joint types**

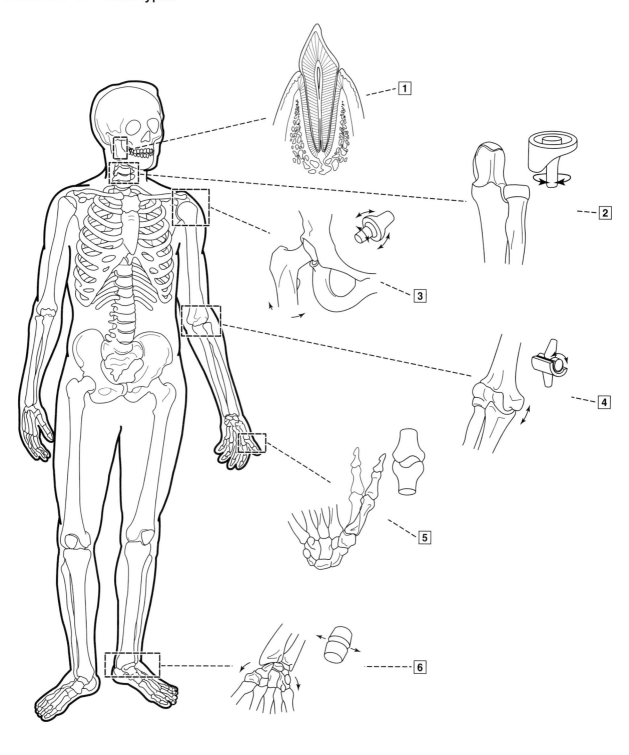

1	Gymphosis	4	Hinge
2	Pivot	5	Saddle
3	Ball-and-socket	6	Gliding

REVIEW QUESTIONS

Fill in the blanks by choosing the appropriate terms from the list below.

1. Joints are areas where usually two _____ elements come together and can be categorized according to function or structure.

2. Joints that do not allow mobility in adults, such as the _____ of the skull are synarthrosis joints, with most being fibrous joints.

3. Other joints that allow slight mobility are amphiarthrosis joints, with most being cartilaginous joints, such as the _____ of the spinal column.

4. Joints that allow a variety of types of mobility are _____ joints, which are the most common type of joint.

5. All diarthrosis joints are _____ joints and include ball-and-socket, hinge, pivot, gliding, or ellipsoidal joints.

6. The _____ joint, such as the shoulder and hip joints, allows backward, forward, sideways, and rotating movements, including flexion, extension, and rotation.

7. The _____ joint, such as in the humeroulnar joint of the elbow, allows only bending and straightening movements, all within one direction.

8. The _____ joint, such as the neck joints including the atlantoaxial joint, allows limited rotating movements as with the head; the gliding or *plane joint* allows sliding movement when one bone moves across the surface of another such as the radioulnar joint.

9. The _____, or *condylar joint*, such as the wrist joint, allows all types of movement except pivotal movements; the saddle joint is noted with the carpometacarpal joint of the thumb when touching the fingers, which allows flexion, extension, abduction, adduction, and circumduction.

10. The gomphosis (plural: *gomphoses*) is a(n) _____ joint involving the root of the tooth to the bony socket (or *dental alveolus*) in either the maxillary bone and mandible that usually allow only slight mobility; the fibrous connection between a tooth and its socket is the periodontal ligament, with the connection made to the bony jaw by way of the cementum of the tooth.

ball-and-socket	hinge	sutures
diarthrosis	pivot	synovial
ellipsoid	skeletal	vertebrae
fibrous		

Reference

Various chapters. In Drake R, Vogl AW, Mitchell AWM: *Gray's anatomy for students,* ed 2, Philadelphia, 2010, Churchill Livingstone.

FIGURE 1-18 Muscle (transverse sections with microanatomic views)

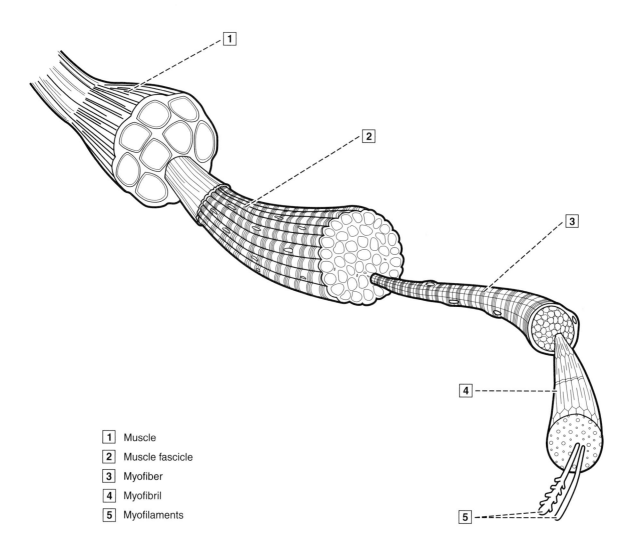

1 Muscle
2 Muscle fascicle
3 Myofiber
4 Myofibril
5 Myofilaments

REVIEW QUESTIONS

Fill in the blanks by choosing the appropriate terms from the list below.

1. The muscle tissue is part of the _____ of the body and similar to connective tissue; the tissue is developmentally derived from somites.

2. Each muscle _____ when it is activated by its neural control, causing soft tissue and bony structures of the body to move.

3. The _____ types of muscle are classified according to structure, function, and innervation, and include skeletal, smooth, and cardiac muscles.

4. The skeletal muscles are considered _____, because they are under voluntary control and involve the somatic nervous system.

5. The skeletal muscles in the head and neck include the muscles of _____, which give the face its expression, as well as the muscles of the tongue, mastication, and pharynx.

6. The skeletal muscles are usually attached to _____ of the skeleton.

7. The skeletal muscles are also considered _____ because the muscle cells appear striped.

8. Each muscle is composed of numerous muscle bundles, or fascicles, which then are composed of numerous muscle cells, or _____.

9. Each myofiber in muscle extends the entire length of the muscle and is composed of smaller _____ surrounded by the other organelles of the cell.

10. Each myofibril in muscle is composed of even smaller _____.

shortens	facial expression	voluntary muscles
muscular system	bones	striated muscles
myofilaments	myofibrils	myofibers
three		

Reference

Chapter 8, Basic tissue. In Bath-Balogh M, Fehrenbach MJ: *Illustrated dental embryology, histology, and anatomy,* ed 3, St. Louis, 2011, Saunders.

FIGURE 1-19 Major body muscles (anterior view)

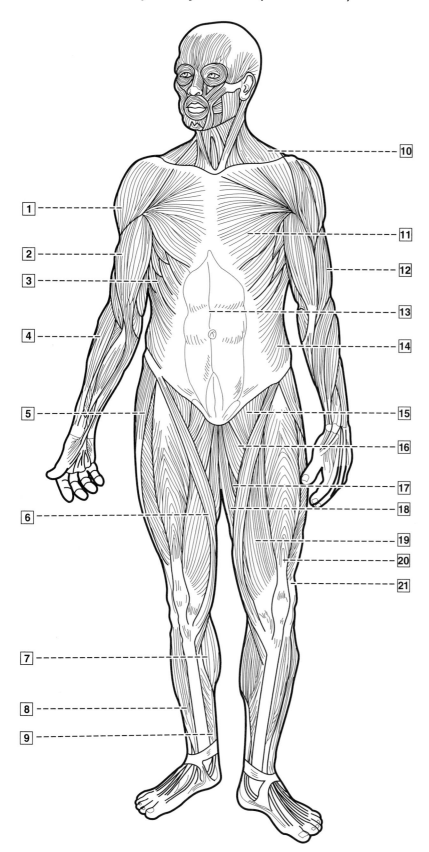

1 Deltoid
2 Biceps brachii
3 Serratus anterior
4 Brachioradialis
5 Tensor fasciae latae

6 Sartorius
7 Gastrocnemius
8 Tibialis anterior
9 Soleus
10 Trapezius

11 Pectoralis major
12 Brachialis
13 Linea alba
14 External abdominal oblique
15 Iliopsoas

16 Adductor longus
17 Adductor magnus
18 Gracilis
19 Vastus medialis
20 Rectus femoris
21 Vastus lateralis

REVIEW QUESTIONS

Fill in the blanks by choosing the appropriate terms from the list below.

1. The _____ enables the arm to draw away from the median axis of the body to direct it toward the anterior and posterior until it is horizontal.

2. The _____ mainly enables the forearm to flex on the arm.

3. The _____ enables the thigh to flex and to rotate outside the median axis; it also allows the leg to flex.

4. The _____ forms the curve of the calf and enables the foot to extend; it also enables the knee to extend.

5. The _____ enables the foot to flex on the leg and to draw near the median axis of the body; the posterior tibial muscle enables the foot to extend.

6. The _____ enables various arm movements, such as drawing the arm near the median axis of the body and rotating it toward the median axis; it also aids in inhalation.

7. The _____ located on the inner thigh mainly enables the knee to extend as it stabilizes the knee; the vastus lateralis muscle in the outer thigh also mainly enables the knee to extend as it stabilizes the knee.

8. The _____ enables the forearm to flex and to rotate outwardly with the palm of the hand toward the anterior; the biceps contracts while the triceps brachii muscle relaxes.

9. The _____ enables the knee to extend and the thigh to flex on the pelvis.

10. The _____ enables thigh to draw near the median axis of the body as well as rotating outside the median axis and to flex.

vastus medialis muscle   biceps brachii muscle   adductor longus muscle

sartorius muscle   pectoralis major muscle   anterior tibialis muscle

deltoid muscle   gastrocnemius muscle   brachioradialis muscle

rectus femoris muscle

Reference

Various chapters. In Drake R, Vogl AW, Mitchell AWM: *Gray's anatomy for students,* ed 2, Philadelphia, 2010, Churchill Livingstone.

ANSWER KEY 1. deltoid muscle, 2. brachioradialis muscle, 3. sartorius muscle, 4. gastrocnemius muscle, 5. anterior tibialis muscle, 6. pectoralis major muscle, 7. vastus medialis muscle, 8. biceps brachii muscle, 9. rectus femoris muscle, 10. adductor longus muscle.

FIGURE 1-20 Major body muscles (posterior view)

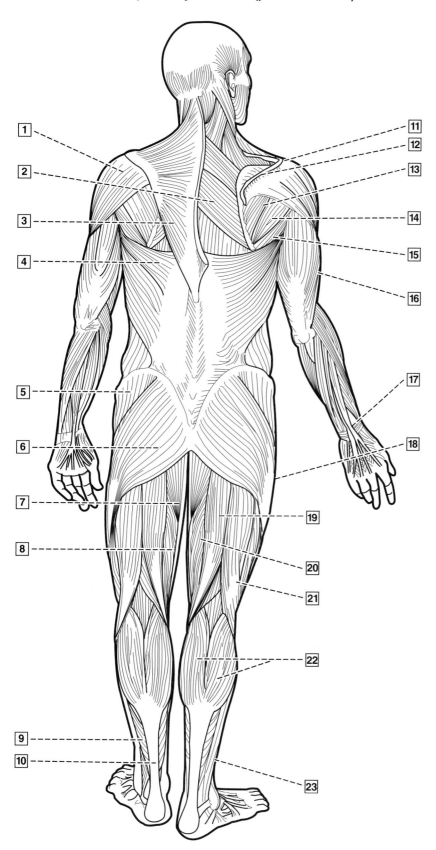

1 Deltoid
2 Rhomboideus major
3 Trapezius
4 Latissimus dorsi
5 Gluteus medius
6 Gluteus maximus

7 Adductor magnus
8 Gracilis
9 Soleus
10 Calcaneal tendon
11 Cut edge of trapezius
12 Supraspinatus

13 Infraspinatus
14 Teres minor
15 Teres major
16 Triceps brachii
17 Extensor digitorum
18 Tensor fasciae latae

19 Semitendinosus
20 Semimembranosus
21 Biceps femoris
22 Gastrocnemius
23 Peroneus longus

REVIEW QUESTIONS

Fill in the blanks by choosing the appropriate terms from the list below.

1. The _____ especially enables the arm to draw near the median axis of the body, to extend, and to rotate inwardly.

2. The _____ enables the hip to extend and to rotate outside the median axis; it also allows the trunk to return to a vertical position.

3. The _____ enables the thigh to draw near the median axis of the body and the leg to flex on the thigh and to rotate toward the median axis.

4. The _____ enables the thigh to draw near the median axis of the body, to rotate outside the median axis, to flex, and to extend.

5. The _____ enables the arm to rotate outside the median axis; it also stabilizes the shoulder joint.

6. The _____ enables the arm to rotate outside the median axis as it stabilizes the shoulder joint; the teres major muscle enables the arm to draw near the median axis of the body and also rotate toward the median axis.

7. The _____ enables the forearm to extend on the arm; it contracts, whereas the biceps brachii muscle relaxes.

8. The _____ especially enables the leg to stretch and the thigh to flex and draw away from the median axis of the body; it also stabilizes the hip and the knee.

9. The _____ enables the thigh to extend on the pelvis, the knee to flex, and the thigh and the leg to rotate toward the median axis.

10. The _____ enables the leg to flex on the thigh and to rotate outside the median axis as well as the thigh to extend on the pelvis.

latissimus dorsi muscle	infraspinatus muscle	gluteus maximus muscle
gracilis muscle	biceps femora muscle	tensor of fascia latae muscle
teres minor muscle	triceps brachii muscle	semimembranosus muscle
adductor magnus muscle		

Reference

Various chapters. In Drake R, Vogl AW, Mitchell AWM: *Gray's anatomy for students,* ed 2, Philadelphia, 2010, Churchill Livingstone.

FIGURE 1-21 **Blood components**

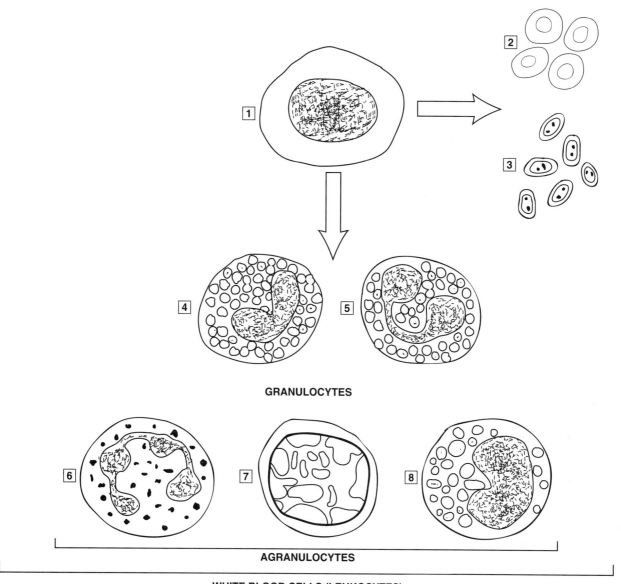

GRANULOCYTES

AGRANULOCYTES

WHITE BLOOD CELLS (LEUKOCYTES)

1	Hemocytoblast	6	Polymorphonuclear leukocyte (Neutrophil)	10a	Buffy coat (white blood cells)
2	Red blood cells (Erythrocytes)	7	Lymphocyte	10b	Red blood cells
3	Platelets (Thrombocytes)	8	Monocyte		
4	Basophil	9	Plasma		
5	Eosinophil	10	Formed elements		

REVIEW QUESTIONS

Fill in the blanks by choosing the appropriate terms from the list below.

1. The most common cell in the blood is the _____, or *red blood cell*, which is a biconcave disc that contains hemoglobin that binds and then transports the oxygen and carbon dioxide; it has no nucleus and does not undergo mitosis because it is formed from bone-marrow stem cells.

2. The blood contains _____, or *platelets*, which are smaller than erythrocytes, disc shaped, and also have no nucleus; however, this is not considered a true blood cell, but instead is a fragment of another blood cell and is found in lesser numbers to function in the clotting mechanism.

3. In lesser numbers in the blood is the _____, or *white blood cell,* and like erythrocyte, it forms from bone-marrow stem cells and later mature in the bone marrow or in various lymphatic organs. It is involved in the defense mechanisms of the body, including the inflammatory and immune responses.

4. The most common leukocytes in the blood are the _____, or *polymorphonuclear leukocyte*s, which are the first cells to appear at an injury site when the inflammatory response is triggered; they have a short life span, contain lysosomal enzymes, are active in phagocytosis, and respond to chemotactic factors.

5. The second most common leukocyte in the blood is the _____, which has three functional types: the B cell, T cell, and NK cell; cytokines are produced by both B cells and T cells and respond to the chemical mediators of the immune response.

6. The B-cell lymphocytes divide during the immune response to form _____, which produce immunoglobulins, or *antibodies,* and have one of five distinct classes: IgA (serum or secretory types), IgE, IgD, IgG, and IgM.

7. The most common leukocyte in the connective tissue proper is the _____, which is considered a monocyte before it migrates from the blood into the tissue; like neutrophils, it contains lysosomal enzymes, is involved in phagocytosis, is actively mobile, and has the ability to respond to chemotactic factors and cytokines; however, unlike neutrophils, it also assists in the immune response, has a longer life span, and has lesser numbers.

8. In some cases, numbers of macrophages may fuse together, forming _____ with multiple nuclei; within bone connective tissue, these are considered *osteoclasts* that will resorb bone.

9. The _____ is normally found only as a small percentage of the leukocyte count, but its percentage is increased during a hypersensitivity response, or *allergy,* and in parasitic diseases because its primary function seems to be the phagocytosis of immune complexes.

10. The _____ is normally found as a very small percentage of the leukocyte count and is involved in the hypersensitivity response, or *allergy.*

thrombocytes	lymphocyte	eosinophil
erythrocyte	leukocyte	basophil
neutrophil	macrophage	plasma cells
giant cells		

Reference

Chapter 8, Basic tissue. In Bath-Balogh M, Fehrenbach MJ: *Illustrated dental embryology, histology, and anatomy,* ed 3, St. Louis, 2011, Saunders.

FIGURE 1-22   Blood vessels (transverse sections with microanatomic views)

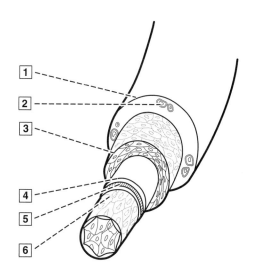

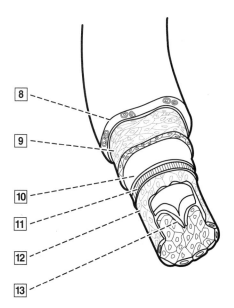

ARTERY

Tunica externa (adventitia)

1 Connective tissue

2 Vasa vasorum

Tunica media

3 Smooth muscle

Tunica intima

4 Elastic fibers

5 Basement membrane

6 Endothelium

CAPILLARY

7 Endothelium

VEIN

Tunica externa

8 Connective tissue

Tunica media

9 Smooth muscle

Tunica intima

10 Elastic fibers

11 Basement membrane

12 Endothelium

13 Venous valve

REVIEW QUESTIONS

Fill in the blanks by choosing the appropriate terms from the list below.

1. The _____ is a blood vessel that carries blood away from the heart; most of the blood in this vessel is normally oxygenated, except for in the pulmonary and umbilical arteries.

2. The outermost layer of the artery is the _____, or *tunica adventitia*, which is composed of connective tissue as well as the vasa vasorum, a network of small blood vessels that supply large blood vessels.

3. Inside the tunica externa of the artery is the _____, which is a layer of smooth muscle cells.

4. The innermost layer of the artery in direct contact with the flow of blood is the _____; it is composed of mainly endothelial cells and elastic fibers.

5. The _____ is the smallest blood vessel and is considered part of the microcirculation, because it forms groups in a capillary bed; at the same time, the arteries branch and narrow into the arterioles and then branch further still into these blood vessels.

6. The _____ is a blood vessel that carries blood towards the heart; most of these vessels carry deoxygenated blood from the tissues back to the heart; it is important to note that the exceptions are the pulmonary and umbilical veins, both of which carry oxygenated blood to the heart.

7. The thick outermost layer of a vein is composed of connective tissue and termed the _____, or *tunica externa*.

8. The inside layer of smooth muscle in a vein is termed the *tunica media,* which is, in general, thin, because veins do not function primarily as a(n) _____ structure.

9. The innermost layer of the vein of the tunica intimae is lined with elastic fibers and _____, as well as a venous valve.

10. The _____ is a very small blood vessel in the microcirculation that allows deoxygenated blood to return from the capillary beds to the larger blood vessels called *veins*.

tunica media	tunica externa	contractile
artery	capillary	tunica intima
tunica adventitia	venule	vein
endothelium		

Reference

Various chapters. In Drake R, Vogl AW, Mitchell AWM: *Gray's anatomy for students,* ed 2, Philadelphia, 2010, Churchill Livingstone.

ANSWER KEY   1. artery, 2. tunica externa, 3. tunica media, 4. tunica intima, 5. capillary, 6. vein, 7. tunica adventitia, 8. contractile, 9. endothelium, 10. venule.

FIGURE 1-23   Major systemic arteries (frontal view)

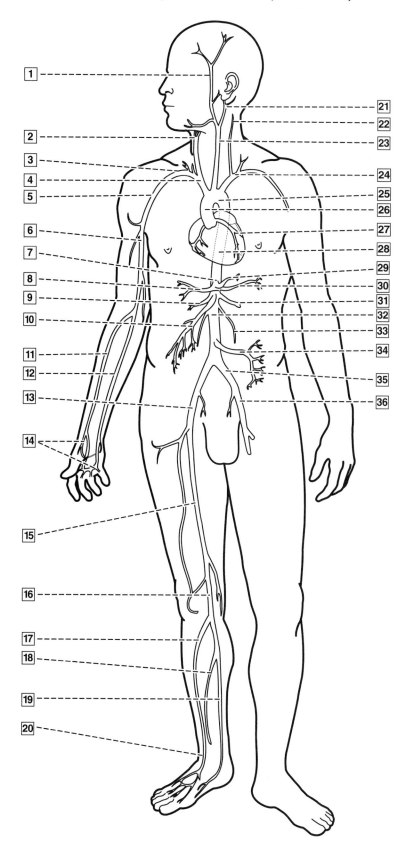

1	External carotid
2	Right common carotid
3	Right subclavian
4	Brachiocephalic
5	Axillary
6	Brachial
7	Celiac
8	Common hepatic
9	Renal
10	Superior mesenteric
11	Radial
12	Ulnar
13	External iliac
14	Palmar arches
15	Femoral
16	Popliteal
17	Anterior tibial
18	Peroneal
19	Posterior tibial
20	Dorsalis pedis
21	Internal carotid
22	Vertebral
23	Left common carotid
24	Left subclavian
25	AORTIC ARCH
26	ASCENDING AORTA
27	Coronary
28	THORACIC AORTA
29	Left gastric
30	Splenic
31	Renal
32	ABDOMINAL AORTA
33	Gonadal
34	Inferior mesenteric
35	Left common iliac
36	Internal iliac

REVIEW QUESTIONS

Fill in the blanks by choosing the appropriate terms from the list below.

1. The _____ are arteries that travel along the neck entering the cranial cavity through the foramen magnum after stemming from the subclavian arteries; these arteries then converge within the cranial cavity forming the basilar artery, which is one of the arteries that supplies the brain.

2. The _____ are the precursors of the internal and external carotid arteries; it is important that the left common carotid artery arises from the aorta and travels along the left side of the neck, whereas the right common carotid artery arises from the brachiocephalic artery, with the right and left common carotid arteries each dividing into an internal carotid artery and an external carotid artery.

3. The _____ is a major artery that is responsible for supplying most of the cerebrum and is also responsible for supplying blood to the eyes; it gives rise to the ophthalmic artery, anterior cerebral artery, and middle cerebral artery.

4. The _____ is a major artery that is responsible for supplying the more superficial structures of the head, with the exception of the eyes; it gives rise to several arteries, including the superior thyroid artery, lingual artery, facial artery, occipital artery, maxillary artery, and superficial temporal artery.

5. The _____ arises from the relatively short brachiocephalic artery (trunk) when it bifurcates into the subclavian and the right common carotid artery, whereas the left subclavian artery arises from the aortic arch.

6. The _____ originates along the first rib bone, stemming from the subclavian artery and gives rise to the brachial artery; the brachial artery is responsible for supplying the muscles of the arm.

7. Originating in the elbow, the _____ arises from the brachial artery; later it follows along the ulnar bone of the forearm and is responsible for supplying the forearm, wrist, and hands; within the elbow, at the same point at which the brachial artery gives rise to this artery, the brachial artery also gives rise to the parallel radial artery, which travels along the radial bone to supply the forearm, wrist, and hand but is smaller than the ulnar artery.

8. The _____ courses along the femoral bone of the lower extremities; it is responsible for supplying the lower extremities and is one of the largest arteries in the body.

9. The _____ extends from the femoral artery and ends near the knee; similar to the femoral artery, the artery is responsible for supplying the leg.

10. The _____ are composed of two arteries; the anterior tibial artery and the posterior tibial artery; these arteries course along the tibial bone of the leg, eventually ending in the foot.

popliteal artery	vertebral arteries	axillary artery
common carotid arteries	external carotid artery	internal carotid artery
right subclavian artery	ulnar artery	tibial arteries
femoral artery		

Reference

Various chapters. In Drake R, Vogl AW, Mitchell AWM: *Gray's anatomy for students,* ed 2, Philadelphia, 2010, Churchill Livingstone.

FIGURE 1-24 Major systemic veins (frontal view)

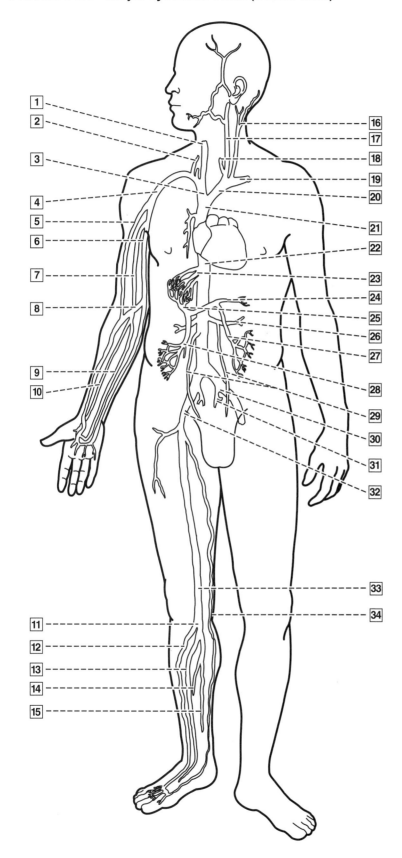

1 Right internal jugular
2 Right external jugular
3 Right brachiocephalic
4 Axillary
5 Cephalic
6 Basilic

7 Brachial
8 Median cubital
9 Ulnar
10 Radial
11 Popliteal
12 Small saphenous

13 Anterior tibial
14 Peroneal
15 Posterior tibial
16 Left external jugular
17 Left internal jugular
18 Vertebral

19 Subclavian
20 Left brachiocephalic
21 Superior vena cava
22 Inferior vena cava
23 Hepatic
24 Splenic

25 Hepatic portal
26 Renal
27 Inferior mesenteric
28 Superior mesenteric
29 Gonadal
30 Common iliac

31 Internal iliac
32 External iliac
33 Femoral
33 Great saphenous

REVIEW QUESTIONS

Fill in the blanks by choosing the appropriate terms from the list below.

1. The _____ is a major vein that travels along the neck and is responsible for draining the more superficial structures of the head and face; it is the more superficial of the two jugular veins and converges with the subclavian vein.

2. The _____ is a major vein that travels along the neck and lies deep to the external jugular vein and is responsible for draining the brain and neck; just as the external jugular vein does, this vein converges with the subclavian vein.

3. The _____ is a vein that lies parallel to the brachial artery along the arm and is responsible for draining the arm.

4. The _____ is a major vein that lies deep to the clavicle bone and is responsible for draining the upper extremities of the body; it has a right and left branch.

5. The _____ is a vein that runs along the axillary artery, and arises from the basilic vein, and which eventually becomes the subclavian vein; it is responsible for draining the axillary division of the body.

6. The _____ is a vein that lies along the ulnar bone, parallel to the ulnar artery, and drains the forearm, wrist and hands; the radial vein lies along the radial bone of the forearm, parallel to the radial artery and it, similar to the ulnar vein, drains the forearm, wrist and hand.

7. The _____ is a vein formed by the convergence of the internal and external iliac veins along the superior portion of the pelvis; the popliteal vein runs parallel to the popliteal artery of the upper leg and is responsible for draining the knee and surrounding tissues.

8. The _____ is a vein that lies parallel to the femoral artery, traveling along the femoral bone of the thigh; it is one of the larger veins and is responsible for draining the lower extremities of the body.

9. The _____ is a vein that lies behind the tibial bone and is responsible for draining the lower leg, ankle, and foot.

10. The _____ is a vein of the leg, running from the foot to the pelvis; it is responsible for draining the lower extremities of the body and delivering it to the femoral vein.

external jugular vein	axillary vein	common iliac vein
brachial vein	femoral vein	posterior tibial vein
internal jugular vein	great saphenous vein	ulnar vein
subclavian vein		

Reference

Various chapters. In Drake, R, Vogl AW, Mitchell AWM: *Gray's anatomy for students,* ed 2, Philadelphia, 2010, Churchill Livingstone.

FIGURE 1-25 Major blood vessels and heart (frontal view)

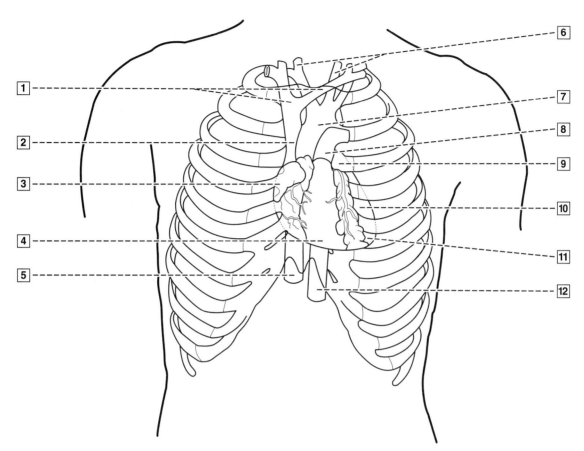

1	Brachiocephalic veins	**7**	Aorta (arch)
2	Superior vena cava	**8**	Pulmonary trunk
3	Right atrium	**9**	Left atrial appendage
4	Right ventricle	**10**	Left ventricle
5	Inferior vena cava	**11**	Apex
6	Common carotid arteries	**12**	Aorta (thoracic)

REVIEW QUESTIONS

Fill in the blanks by choosing the appropriate terms from the list below.

1. The _____ is the largest artery in the body and the artery from which most major arteries branch off; it originates from the left ventricle of the heart and extends down to the abdomen, where it bifurcates into the two smaller common iliac arteries.

2. The _____ (or *brachiocephalic trunk* or *innominate artery*) carries oxygenated blood from the aorta (arch) to the head, neck, and arm regions of the body.

3. The _____ supply oxygenated blood to the head and neck regions of the body.

4. The _____ carry oxygenated blood from the aorta (abdominal) to the legs and feet.

5. The _____ carry deoxygenated blood from the right ventricle to the lungs.

6. The _____ are two large veins that join to form the superior vena cava.

7. The _____ are veins that join to form the inferior vena cava.

8. The _____ transport oxygenated blood from the lungs to the heart.

9. The _____, inferior and superior, transport deoxygenated blood from various regions of the body to the heart.

10. The _____ is a muscular pouch connected to the left atrium of the heart and has a distinct embryologic origin.

common iliac arteries	common iliac veins	pulmonary veins
aorta	brachiocephalic veins	venae cavae
brachiocephalic artery	pulmonary arteries	left atrial appendage
common carotid arteries		

Reference

Various chapters. In Drake R, Vogl AW, Mitchell AWM: *Gray's anatomy for students,* ed 2, Philadelphia, 2010, Churchill Livingstone.

FIGURE 1-26   Heart (internal views)

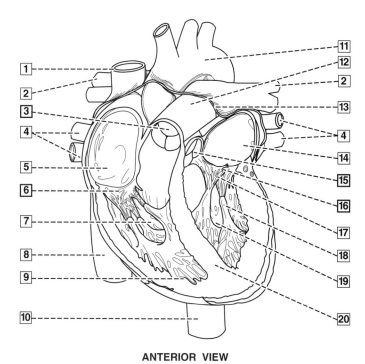

ANTERIOR VIEW

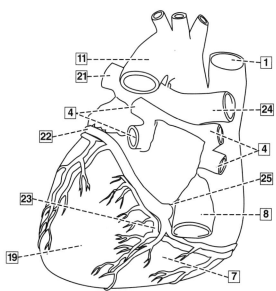

POSTERIOR VIEW

1	Superior vena cava	8	Inferior vena cava	15	**Aortic valve**	22	Coronary vein
2	Pulmonary arteries	9	Trabeculae carneae	16	**Mitral valve**	23	Coronary artery
3	**Pulmonic valve**	10	Aorta (thoracic)	17	Chordae tendineae	24	Right pulmonary artery
4	Pulmonary veins	11	Aorta (arch)	18	Papillary muscle	25	Carotid sinus
5	Right atrium	12	Pulmonary trunk	19	Left ventricle		
6	**Tricuspid valve**	13	Cut edge of pericardium	20	Interventricular septum		
7	Right ventricle	14	Left atrium	21	Left pulmonary artery		

REVIEW QUESTIONS

Fill in the blanks by choosing the appropriate terms from the list below.

1. The heart has _____ main chambers, the two superior atria and the two inferior ventricles and is divided into separate right and left sections by the interventricular septum.

2. The superior _____ are the receiving chambers for the heart; the inferior ventricles are the discharging chambers for the heart.

3. The _____ is a double-walled sac that contains the heart and the roots of the great vessels.

4. Deoxygenated blood flows through the heart in one direction, entering through the _____ and left subclavian artery into the right atrium and is pumped through the tricuspid valve into the right ventricle before being pumped out through the pulmonary valve to the pulmonary arteries into the lungs.

5. The oxygenated blood returns from the lungs through the _____ to the left atrium where it is pumped through the mitral valve into the left ventricle before leaving through the aortic valve to the aorta.

6. The aortic and pulmonic valves are known as the _____, whereas the tricuspid and mitral valves are referred to as the *atrioventricular valves;* all the valves are trileaflet, with the exception of the mitral valve, which has two leaflets.

7. The tricuspid valve separates the right atrium from the right ventricle; the _____, or *pulmonary valve,* separates the right ventricle from the pulmonary artery.

8. The _____, or *bicuspid valve,* separates the left atrium from the left ventricle; the aortic valve separates the left ventricle from the ascending aorta.

9. The _____ are rounded or irregular muscular columns that project from the inner surface of the right and left ventricles of the heart; the chordae tendineae, or *heartstrings,* are cord-like tendons that connect the papillary muscles to the tricuspid valve and the mitral valve in the heart.

10. The aorta is usually divided into _____ segments or sections: the ascending aorta, the arch of aorta, the descending aorta, the thoracic aorta, and the abdominal aorta.

five	**pulmonic valve**	**mitral valve**
pericardium	**trabeculae carneae**	**atria**
pulmonary veins	**semilunar valves**	**superior vena cava**
four		

Reference

Various chapters. In Drake R, Vogl AW, Mitchell AWM: *Gray's anatomy for students,* ed 2, Philadelphia, 2010, Churchill Livingstone.

ANSWER KEY 1. four, 2. atria, 3. pericardium, 4. superior vena cava, 5. pulmonary veins, 6. semilunar valves, 7. pulmonic valve, 8. mitral valve, 9. trabeculae carneae, 10. five.

FIGURE 1-27 Respiratory system (midsagittal section with frontal and microanatomic views)

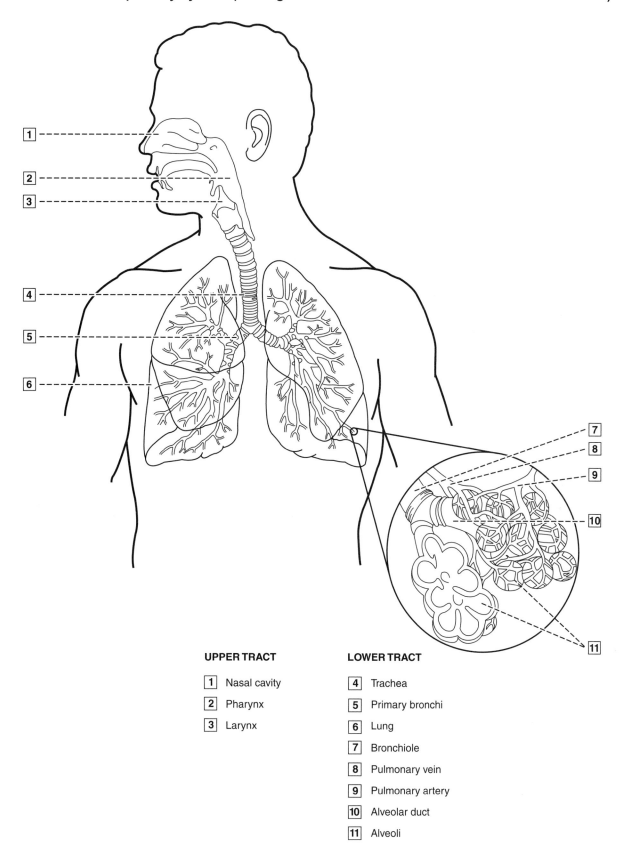

UPPER TRACT

1	Nasal cavity
2	Pharynx
3	Larynx

LOWER TRACT

4	Trachea
5	Primary bronchi
6	Lung
7	Bronchiole
8	Pulmonary vein
9	Pulmonary artery
10	Alveolar duct
11	Alveoli

REVIEW QUESTIONS

Fill in the blanks by choosing the appropriate terms from the list below.

1. The primary function of the _____ is to supply the blood with oxygen via breathing in order for the blood to deliver oxygen to all parts of the body; with breathing, there is mainly the inhaling of oxygen and exhaling of carbon dioxide.

2. The needed oxygen initially enters the respiratory system through the oral cavity and the _____ and then into the pharynx, or *throat.*

3. The oxygen then passes through the _____, or *voice box*, where speech sounds are produced via the vocal folds, or *vocal cords*, and then into the trachea, which filters the air.

4. In the chest cavity, the _____, or *windpipe,* splits into two smaller tubes termed the *primary bronchi,* which enter the roots of the two lungs; the epiglottis covers it so that food does not go down it when eating.

5. The _____ then divide again and again into secondary and tertiary ones, finally forming the bronchioles in the lungs.

6. The _____ terminate in air-filled sacs of the alveoli in the lungs.

7. The inhaled oxygen passes into the very small _____ in the lungs and then diffuses through the surrounding capillaries into the arterial blood; the waste-rich blood from the veins releases its carbon dioxide into them; the carbon dioxide follows the same path out of the lungs when exhaling.

8. The two _____, the main organs of the respiratory system are located in two somewhat similar cavities on either side of the heart; both are separated into lobes by fissures, with three lobes on the right and two on the left, with the lobes further divided into segments and then into lobules; each lobe is surrounded by a pleural cavity.

9. The _____ are two large veins that carry oxygenated blood from the lungs to the left atrium of the heart, which is unusual since almost all other veins of the body carry deoxygenated blood.

10. The _____ are two large arteries that carry deoxygenated blood from the heart to the lungs; they are the only arteries of the body (other than umbilical arteries in the fetus) that carry deoxygenated blood.

lungs	primary bronchi	nasal cavity
pulmonary arteries	bronchioles	respiratory system
alveoli	larynx	pulmonary veins
trachea		

Reference

Various chapters. In Drake R, Vogl AW, Mitchell AWM: *Gray's anatomy for students,* ed 2, Philadelphia, 2010, Churchill Livingstone.

ANSWER KEY 1. respiratory system, 2. nasal cavity, 3. larynx, 4. trachea, 5. primary bronchi, 6. bronchioles, 7. alveoli, 8. lungs, 9. pulmonary veins, 10. pulmonary arteries.

FIGURE 1-28 Endocrine system (midsagittal sections with frontal and posterior views)

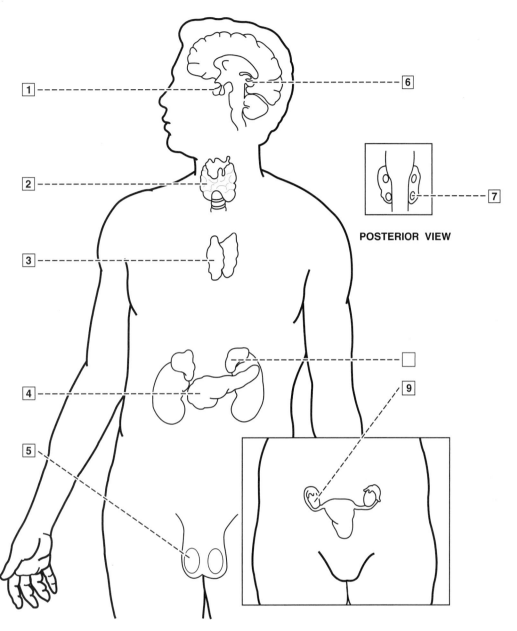

POSTERIOR VIEW

FRONTAL VIEWS

1 Pituitary gland	**6** Pineal gland
2 Thyroid gland	**7** Parathyroid gland (on posterior surface of thyroid gland)
3 Thymus	
4 Pancreas	**8** Adrenal gland
5 Testis	**9** Ovary

REVIEW QUESTIONS

Fill in the blanks by choosing the appropriate terms from the list below.

1. The _____ is the system of glands, each of which secretes a type of hormone directly into the bloodstream to regulate the body; this system is in contrast to the exocrine system, which secretes its chemicals using ducts.

2. The _____ of the endocrine system are the hypothalamus, pituitary, thyroid, parathyroids, adrenals, pineal body, and the reproductive organs (ovaries and testes); the pancreas is also a part of this system, because it has a role in hormone production as well as in digestion.

3. In addition to the specialized endocrine organs that secrete _____, many other organs that are part of other body systems, such as the kidney, liver, and heart, have secondary endocrine functions; for example, the kidney secretes erythropoietin and renin.

4. The _____ belongs to the endocrine system, but it is under the control of the hypothalamus, the true *master gland;* it is important to note that together they secrete a number of hormones, such as those of the female menstrual cycle, pregnancy, and birth; follicle-stimulating hormone, which stimulates development and maturation of a follicle in one of the ovaries; and luteinizing hormone, which causes the bursting of that follicle, or ovulation, and the formation of a corpus luteum from the remains of the follicle.

5. One non–sex hormone secreted by the pituitary gland located at the base of the skull between the optic nerves is the _____, which helps prevent excess water excretion by the kidneys; the same gland releases thyroid-stimulating hormone under influence of hypothalamic thyrotropin-releasing hormone.

6. The _____ can serve both as a ducted exocrine gland, secreting digestive enzymes into the small intestine, as well as a ductless endocrine gland, in that the islets of Langerhans secrete insulin and glucagon to regulate the blood sugar level; they can secrete glucagon, which informs the liver to take carbohydrate out of storage to raise a low blood sugar level, and they can secrete insulin to inform the liver to take excess glucose out of circulation to lower a blood sugar level that is too high.

7. The _____ of the endocrine system that are located superior to the kidneys secrete epinephrine, or *adrenalin,* and other similar hormones in response to stressors such as fright, anger, caffeine, or low blood sugar, as well as cortisone that can be involved in the inflammatory response.

8. The _____, or *sex organs* of the endocrine system, the female ovaries and male testes, also secrete sex hormones through pituitary gland hormones in addition to producing gametes for conception; although both sexes make some of each of the hormones, typically male testes secrete primarily androgens including testosterone and female ovaries make estrogen and progesterone in varying amounts depending on the time of the woman's cycle.

9. The _____ of the endocrine system is located near the center of the brain and is stimulated by nerves from the eyes, which enables it to secrete melatonin to promote sleep; it also affects reproductive functions by depressing the activity of the gonads as well as affecting thyroid and adrenal cortex functions.

10. The endocrine system uses cycles as well as _____ mechanisms to regulate physiological functions; cycles of secretion maintain homeostatic control and can range from hours to months in duration.

gonads	pineal gland	pituitary gland
adrenal glands	antidiuretic hormone	endocrine system
negative feedback	pancreas	major glands
hormones		

Reference

Various chapters. In Drake R, Vogl AW, Mitchell AWM: *Gray's anatomy for students,* ed 2, Philadelphia, 2010, Churchill Livingstone.

FIGURE 1-29   Digestive system (midsagittal section and frontal view)

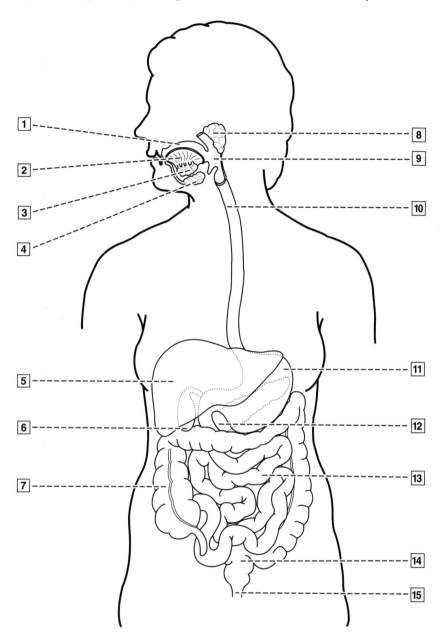

1	Mouth (oral cavity)	**6**	Gallbladder	**11** Stomach
2	Tongue	**7**	Large intestine	**12** Pancreas
3	Sublingual salivary gland	**8**	Parotid salivary gland	**13** Small intestine
4	Submandibular salivary gland	**9**	Pharynx	**14** Rectum
5	Liver	**10**	Esophagus	**15** Anus

REVIEW QUESTIONS

Fill in the blanks by choosing the appropriate terms from the list below.

1. The _____ is composed of the digestive tract, a series of hollow organs joined in a long, twisting tube from the mouth to the anus, as well as other organs that help the body break down and absorb food; the organs that are included along the digestive tract are the oral cavity, esophagus, stomach, small intestine, large intestine, and anus, with parts of the nervous and vascular systems also playing roles.

2. Inside these hollow digestive system organs is a lining of _____; the digestive tract also contains a layer of smooth muscle in the mucosa that helps break down food and move it along the tract.

3. In the oral cavity, stomach, and small intestine, the mucosa contains glands that produce _____ to help digest food; saliva produced by the salivary glands contains amylase that begins to digest the starch from food into smaller molecules, and the stomach has pepsin that begins to digest the protein.

4. In the oral cavity, teeth, jaws, and the tongue begin the mechanical breakdown of food into smaller particles; the mixture of food and saliva, or *bolus,* is pushed into the pharynx, or *throat*, and then through the _____, which is a muscular tube whose muscular contractions of peristalsis propel the bolus to the stomach along with the moisture and lubrication provided by the mucus.

5. The _____ produces not only the enzyme pepsin but also hydrochloric acid for the gastric juice, which does not directly function in digestion but activates the enzyme; the organ also mechanically churns the food into chyme along with mucus.

6. Two of the digestive organs, the _____ and the pancreas, produce bile and pancreatic juice that neutralizes the chyme, respectively; it is important to note that substances reach the intestine through small tubes called *ducts;* the gallbladder stores the bile until it is needed in the intestine.

7. Digestion of carbohydrates, proteins, and fats continues in the _____; starch and glycogen are broken down into maltose by enzymes and proteases, which are enzymes secreted by the pancreas that continue the breakdown of protein into small peptide fragments and amino acids.

8. Most digested molecules of food, as well as water and minerals, are absorbed through the small intestine, because the mucosa contains many folds that are covered with tiny fingerlike projections termed _____, which have their own microscopic projections termed *microvilli.*

9. The _____ produced by the liver dissolve fat into tiny droplets and allow pancreatic and intestinal enzymes to break the large fat molecules into smaller ones such as fatty acids and cholesterol; these then combine with these smaller molecules to help move them into the cells of the mucosa.

10. The _____ is composed of the colon, cecum, appendix, and rectum and is involved in the recovery of water and electrolytes from digested food as well as the formation and storage of feces.

small intestine	large intestine	mucosa
liver	enzymes	esophagus
villi	bile acids	stomach
digestive system		

Reference

Various chapters. In Drake R, Vogl AW, Mitchell AWM: *Gray's anatomy for students,* ed 2, Philadelphia, 2010, Churchill Livingstone.

FIGURE 1-30 **Urinary system (frontal view)**

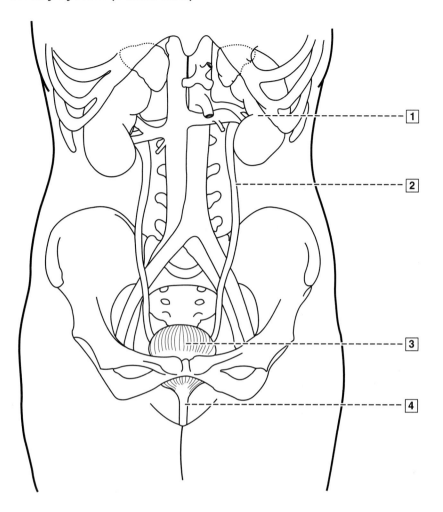

| 1 | Kidney | 3 | Bladder |
| 2 | Ureter | 4 | Urethra |

REVIEW QUESTIONS

Fill in the blanks by choosing the appropriate terms from the list below.

1. The _____, or *urinary tract,* includes two kidneys, two ureters, the bladder, and the urethra that together produce, store, and eliminate urine; this system also eliminates waste products from the body in the urine, as well as maintaining fluid and salt balance (potassium and sodium).

2. The _____ of the urinary system are bean-shaped organs that lie in the abdomen, retroperitoneal to the organs of digestion, around or just inferior to the ribcage and close to the lumbar spine; each organ consists of an outer cortex and medullary pyramid, or *papillae,* and within these two regions are found the components of the structural and functional unit of the organ, the nephron.

3. The _____ has a glomerulus, a tuft of capillaries that produce the glomerular filtrate, housed in the renal corpuscle; this structure is followed by a series of tubules specialized for both excretion and reabsorption.

4. The kidney also includes, besides the glomerulus, the _____, the descending and ascending loop of Henle, and the distal convoluted tubule.

5. Each nephron drains into a collecting tubule, which serves as a duct system to conduct the urine out of the kidney; the urine in the collecting tubules is collected in the renal pelvis and exits the kidney in the _____.

6. The ureter of the urinary system travels to the _____, where the urine can be stored.

7. The bladder of the urinary system is drained by the _____, which leads to the external orifice.

8. The tubule of the nephron functions to reabsorb most of the glomerular filtrate; the cells of the tubule reabsorb vital nutrients and water back into the blood, while retaining the _____ that the body needs to eliminate.

9. The plexus formed by the efferent arteriole from the glomerulus passes closely to the proximal convoluted tubule, allowing direct transfer into the blood; in the _____, the filtrate is further concentrated.

10. The amount of water reabsorbed within the kidney is controlled by the _____ secreted by the pituitary gland, and the amount of salts reabsorbed is controlled by aldosterone secreted by the adrenal gland; these hormones are increased or decreased according to the needs of the body.

bladder	urethra	loop of Henle
proximal convoluted tubule	ureter	kidneys
nephron	antidiuretic hormone	waste products
urinary system		

Reference

Various chapters. In Drake R, Vogl AW, Mitchell AWM: *Gray's anatomy for students,* ed 2, Philadelphia, 2010, Churchill Livingstone.

FIGURE 1-31 Major lymphatics (sagittal section with explanatory view)

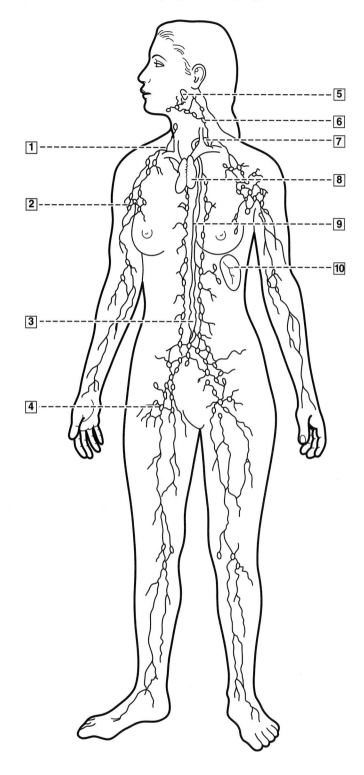

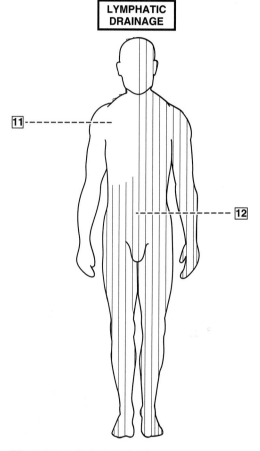

LYMPHATIC DRAINAGE

1 Right lymphatic duct draining into right subclavian vein

2 Axillary nodes

3 Cisterna chyli

4 Inguinal nodes

5 Palatine tonsils

6 Cervical nodes

7 Thoracic duct draining into left subclavian vein

8 Thymus

9 Thoracic duct

10 Spleen

11 Area drained by right lymphatic duct

12 Area drained by thoracic duct

REVIEW QUESTIONS

Fill in the blanks by choosing the appropriate terms from the list below.

1. The _____ is a part of the vascular system, comprising a network of conduits called *lymphatic vessels* that carry a clear fluid called *lymph* unidirectionally toward the heart.

2. The lymphatic organs also play an important part in the _____ that fights disease processes through the immune response and has a considerable overlap with the lymphatic system; lymphoid tissue is found in many organs, particularly the lymph nodes and in the lymphoid follicles associated with the digestive system such as the tonsils.

3. The lymphatic system also includes all the structures dedicated to the circulation and production of the white blood cells, the _____; it is important to note that these structures include the spleen, thymus, bone marrow, and the lymphoid tissue associated with the digestive system.

4. The conducting system carries the clear fluid, the _____, and consists of tubular vessels that include the lymph capillaries, the lymph vessels, and the right and left thoracic ducts.

5. The _____ is the tissue that is primarily involved in the immune response and consists of lymphocytes and other white blood cells enmeshed in connective tissue through which the lymph passes.

6. Both the thymus and the bone marrow constitute the _____ involved in the production and early selection of lymphocytes.

7. The _____ provides the environment for foreign or altered native molecules, the immunogens or *antigens*, to interact with the lymphocytes; it is exemplified by the lymph nodes and the lymphoid follicles in tonsils, Peyer patches, spleen, adenoids, skin, and any area that is associated with the mucosa-associated lymphoid tissue.

8. The regions of the lymphoid tissue that are densely packed with lymphocytes are known as the _____; lymphoid tissue can either be structurally well organized as lymph nodes or may consist of loosely organized tissue such as the mucosa-associated lymphoid tissue.

9. The _____ is a lymphoid organ located in the left side of the abdomen posterior to the stomach, lying between the ninth and eleventh ribs on the left side; it is the primary filtering element for the blood, as well as a storage site for red blood cells, or *erythrocytes,* and platelets, or *thrombocytes.*

10. The _____ consist of masses of lymphoid tissue located in the oral cavity and pharynx, and like lymph nodes, they contain lymphocytes that remove toxins; they are located near airway and food passages to protect the body against disease processes from toxins.

immune system	**lymph**	**secondary lymphoid tissue**
lymphatic system	**tonsils**	**lymphocytes**
primary lymphoid tissue	**lymphoid follicles**	**lymphoid tissue**
spleen		

References

Chapter 10, Lymphatic system. In Fehrenbach MJ, Herring SW: *Illustrated anatomy of the head and neck,* ed 4, St. Louis, 2012, Saunders; and Various chapters. In Drake R, Vogl AW, Mitchell AWM: *Gray's anatomy for students,* ed 2, Philadelphia, 2010, Churchill Livingstone.

FIGURE 1-32   Lymph node (sagittal section)

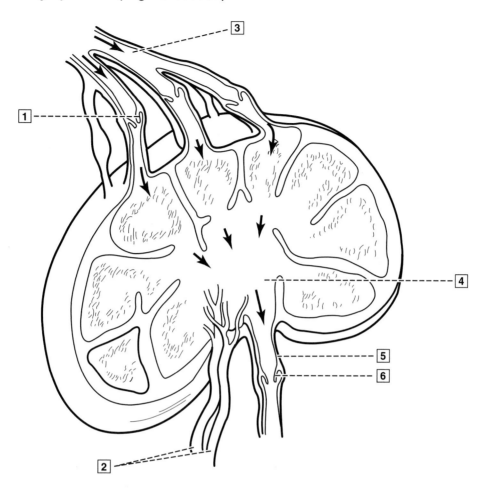

1	Valve	**4**	Hilus
2	Blood vessels	**5**	Efferent lymphatic vessels
3	Afferent lymphatic vessels	**6**	Valve

REVIEW QUESTIONS

Fill in the blanks by choosing the appropriate terms from the list below.

1. The _____ are bean-shaped bodies grouped in clusters along the connecting lymphatic vessels; positioned along the lymphatic vessels, they filter toxic products from the lymph to prevent their entry into the vascular system.

2. The lymph nodes are composed of organized lymphoid tissue and contain _____, white blood cells of the immune system that actively remove toxins to help fight disease processes in the body.

3. The lymph nodes can be superficially located with superficial veins or located deep in the tissue with the deep blood vessels; however, in a healthy situation, they are usually small, soft, and free or mobile in the surrounding tissue, and they are not able to be _____ or palpated by the clinician.

4. The _____ are a system of channels that are parallel to the venous blood vessels yet are more numerous; they are larger and thicker than capillaries, but unlike capillaries they have valves similar to many veins to ensure the one-way flow of lymph.

5. The lymph flows into the lymph node by way of many _____.

6. On one side of the node is a depression or hilus, where the lymph flows out of the node by way of a single _____.

7. The lymph from a particular tissue region drains into a(n) _____, or *regional node*.

8. The primary nodes, in turn, drain into a(n) _____, or *central node*.

9. In the outer tissue of the body, smaller lymphatic vessels containing lymph converge into larger _____, which empty into the venous system of the blood in the chest area.

10. The final drainage endpoint of the lymphatic vessels into the lymphatic ducts depends on which _____ of the body is involved.

lymphatic ducts	primary node	lymphocytes
lymph nodes	secondary node	side
efferent lymphatic vessel	afferent lymphatic vessels	lymphatic vessels
visualized		

Reference

Chapter 10, Lymphatic system. In Fehrenbach MJ, Herring SW: *Illustrated anatomy of the head and neck,* ed 4, St. Louis, 2012, Saunders.

FIGURE 1-33 Central and peripheral nervous systems

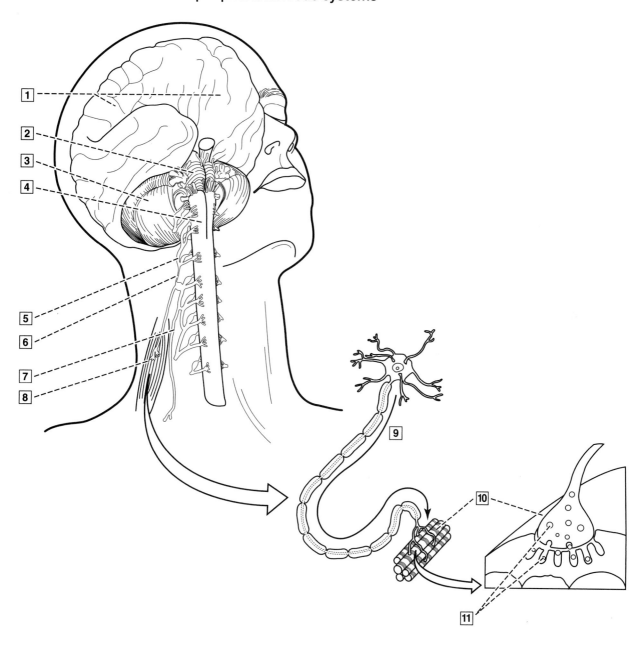

CENTRAL NERVOUS SYSTEM

1 Cerebrum

2 Brainstem

3 Cerebellum

4 Spinal cord

PERIPHERAL NERVOUS SYSTEM

5 Nerve ganglion

6 Nerve

7 Afferent nerve from skin

8 Efferent nerve to muscle

NEURON

9 Action potential (impulse propagation)

10 Muscle fiber

SYNAPSE

10 Muscle fiber

11 Neurotransmitter

REVIEW QUESTIONS

Fill in the blanks by choosing the appropriate terms from the list below.

1. The _____ is an extensive, intricate network of neural structures that activates, coordinates, and controls all functions of the body.

2. One of the major divisions of the nervous system, the _____ includes both the brain and spinal cord.

3. The major divisions of the _____ include the cerebrum, the cerebellum, the brainstem, and the diencephalon.

4. The _____ is the largest division of the brain and consists of two cerebral hemispheres; it coordinates sensory data and motor functions and governs many aspects of intelligence and reasoning, learning, and memory.

5. The _____ is the second largest division of the brain after the cerebrum; it functions to produce muscle coordination and maintains normal muscle tone and posture, as well as coordinating balance.

6. The _____ has a number of divisions including the medulla, pons, and midbrain.

7. A major division of the nervous system, the _____, is composed of all the nerves stretching their pathways among the central nervous system and the receptors, muscles, and glands of the body.

8. The peripheral nervous system is further divided into the _____, or *sensory nervous system*, which carries information from receptors to the brain or spinal cord, and the efferent nervous system, or *motor nervous system*, which carries information from the brain or spinal cord to muscles or glands.

9. The _____ is further subdivided into the somatic nervous system and the autonomic nervous system.

10. The _____ is a subdivision of the efferent nervous system and includes all nerves controlling the muscular system and external sensory receptors.

efferent nervous system	**central nervous system**	**nervous system**
peripheral nervous system	**cerebrum**	**brainstem**
cerebellum	**somatic nervous system**	**afferent nervous system**
brain		

Reference

Chapter 8, Basic tissue. In Bath-Balogh M, Fehrenbach MJ: *Illustrated dental embryology, histology, and anatomy,* ed 3, St. Louis, 2011, Saunders; and Chapter 8, Nervous System. In Fehrenbach MJ, Herring SW: *Illustrated anatomy of the head and neck,* ed 4, St. Louis, 2012, Saunders.

FIGURE 1-34 Neurons with muscular involvement

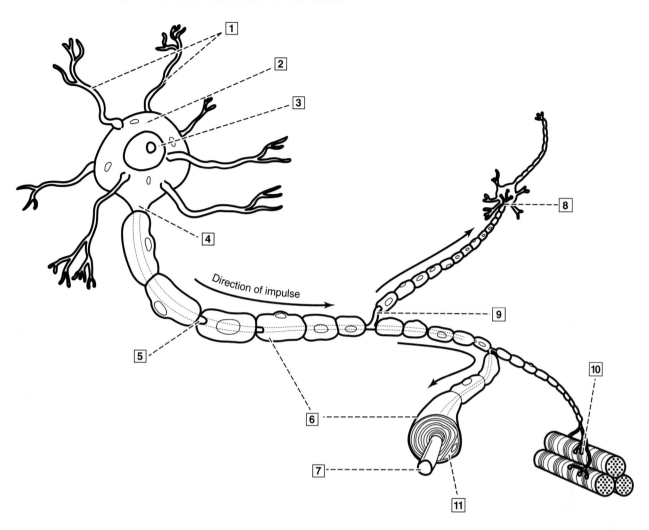

1	Dendrites	7	Axon
2	Cell body	8	Synapse with another neuron
3	Nucleus	9	Collateral branch
4	Axon	10	Synapse with myofibers
5	Node of Ranvier	11	Nucleus of Schwann cell
6	Myelin sheath		

REVIEW QUESTIONS

Fill in the blanks by choosing the appropriate terms from the list below.

1. The _____ is the cellular component of the nervous system and is composed of a cell body and neural processes; a nerve fiber, or *axon,* is a long, slender projection of a neuron that typically conducts electrical impulses away from the cell body.

2. A(n) _____ is a bundle of neural processes outside the central nervous system and in the peripheral nervous system, with an accumulation of neuron cell bodies outside the central nervous system called a *ganglion;* there are two types of these neural processes: afferent and efferent.

3. A(n) _____ is the junction between two neurons or between a neuron and an effector organ, where neural impulses are transmitted; additionally, dendrites are the branched projections of a neuron that act to conduct the electrochemical stimulation received from other neural cells to the cell body.

4. A(n) _____, or *sensory nerve,* carries information from the periphery of the body to the brain or spinal cord.

5. A(n) _____, or *motor nerve,* carries information away from the brain or spinal cord to the periphery of the body.

6. The plasma membrane of a neuron, like all other cells, has an unequal distribution of ions and electric charges between the two sides of the membrane, with the fluid outside of the membrane having a positive charge and the fluid inside having a negative charge; the charge difference is a(n) _____ and is measured in millivolts.

7. The rapid depolarization of the cell membrane results in a(n) _____, which then causes propagation of the nerve impulse along the membrane; this is a temporary reversal of the electric potential along the membrane for a brief period.

8. To have the impulse cross the synapse to another cell requires the actions of certain chemical agents, or _____ from the neuron, which are discharged with the arrival of the action potential; these agents diffuse across the synapse and bind to receptors on the membrane of the other cell.

9. A(n) _____ is a cell of the peripheral nervous system that wraps around a nerve fiber forming the myelin sheath, a sheath that effectively insulates the axon of the neuron.

10. The _____ is a gap occurring at regular intervals between segments of myelin sheath along a nerve axon; here the axonal membrane is uninsulated and therefore capable of generating electrical activity.

resting potential	synapse	neurotransmitters
efferent nerve	action potential	nerve
neuron	Schwann cell	afferent nerve
node of Ranvier		

Reference

Chapter 8, Basic tissue. In Bath-Balogh M, Fehrenbach MJ: *Illustrated dental embryology, histology, and anatomy,* ed 3, St. Louis, 2011, Saunders; and Chapter 8, Nervous System. In Fehrenbach MJ, Herring SW: *Illustrated anatomy of the head and neck,* ed 4, St. Louis, 2012, Saunders.

FIGURE 2-1   Head and neck sections and planes (anatomic position)

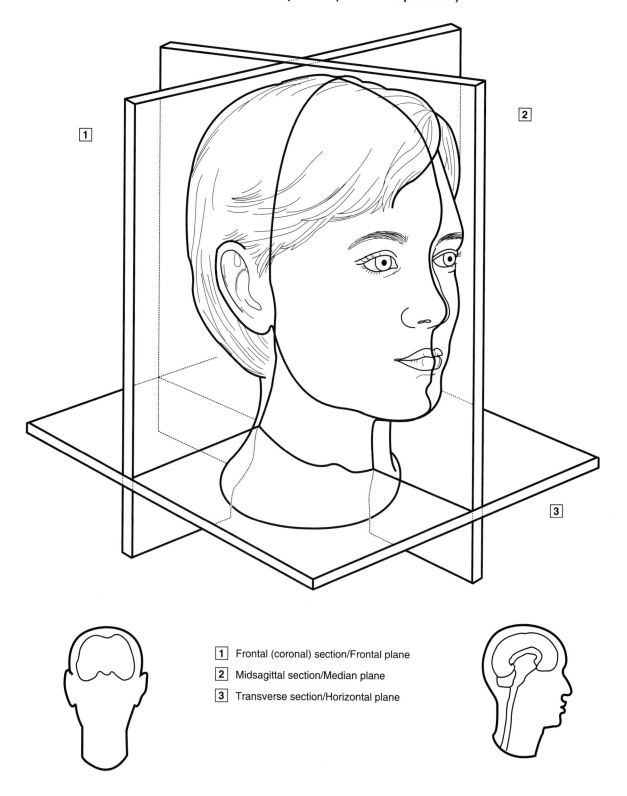

1   Frontal (coronal) section/Frontal plane
2   Midsagittal section/Median plane
3   Transverse section/Horizontal plane

REVIEW QUESTIONS

Fill in the blanks by choosing the appropriate terms from the list below.

1. The _____ is the system of names for anatomic structures used to describe the structure of the human body.

2. The nomenclature of anatomy is based on the body being in _____, a standard position of the body.

3. In anatomic position, the body is standing erect, with the arms at the sides with the palms and toes directed _____ and the eyes looking forward.

4. The midsagittal section or *median section* is a division through the _____.

5. The _____, or *coronal section,* is a division through any frontal plane.

6. The _____, or *transverse section,* is a division through a horizontal plane.

7. The _____, or *median plane,* is created by an imaginary line dividing the body into equal right and left halves.

8. An imaginary line dividing the body into anterior and posterior parts at any level creates the _____, or *frontal plane.*

9. A horizontal plane is created by the _____ dividing the body at any level into superior and inferior parts and is always perpendicular to the median plane.

10. Any place created by an imaginary plane parallel to the median plane is considered the _____.

midsagittal plane	anatomic nomenclature	sagittal plane
forward	median plane	coronal plane
frontal section	imaginary line	horizontal section
anatomic position		

Reference

Chapter 1, Introduction to head and neck anatomy. In Fehrenbach MJ, Herring SW: *Illustrated anatomy of the head and neck,* ed 4, St. Louis, 2012, Saunders.

FIGURE 2-2 Facial development within the third to fourth week of the embryonic period during prenatal development (frontal aspect)

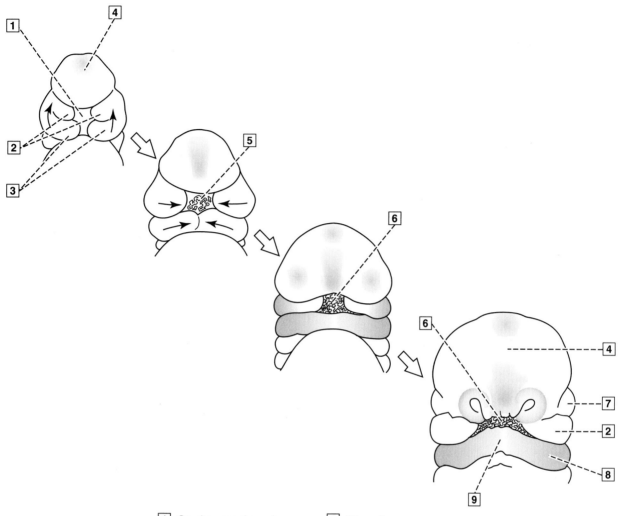

1 Oropharyngeal membrane	6 Stomodeum
2 Maxillary processes	7 Lens placode
3 Mandibular processes	8 Mandibular arch
4 Frontonasal processes	9 Mandibular symphysis
5 Oropharyngeal membrane disintegrating	

REVIEW QUESTIONS

Fill in the blanks by choosing the appropriate terms from the list below.

1. The face and its associated tissue begin to develop within the _____.

2. All three embryonic layers are involved in facial development: ectoderm, mesoderm, and

   _____.

3. The primitive mouth is the _____, which initially appeared as a shallow depression in the embryonic surface ectoderm at the cephalic end before the fourth week of prenatal development.

4. The stomodeum is limited in depth by the _____, which is a temporary membrane consisting of external ectoderm overlying endoderm formed during the third week of prenatal development, which also separates the stomodeum from the primitive pharynx.

5. After formation of the stomodeum but still during the fourth week, two bulges of tissue appear inferior to the primitive mouth: the two _____, which consist of a core of mesenchyme formed in part by neural crest cells that migrate to the facial region, covered externally by ectoderm and internally by endoderm.

6. The paired mandibular processes fuse at the midline to form the _____, the developmental form of the future lower jaw, the mandible.

7. In the midline, on the surface of the mature bony mandible, is the _____, indicating where the mandible is formed by fusion of right and left mandibular processes.

8. During the fourth week, the _____ forms as a bulge of tissue in the upper facial area at the most cephalic end of the embryo and cranial boundary of the stomodeum; in the future, this process gives rise to the upper face, which includes the forehead, bridge of the nose, primary palate, nasal septum, and all structures associated with the medial nasal processes.

9. During the fourth week of prenatal development within the embryonic period, an adjacent swelling from increased growth of the mandibular arch on each side of the stomodeum will form the _____, and each will later grow superiorly and anteriorly around the stomodeum.

10. In the future, the maxillary processes will form the midface, which includes the sides of the upper lip, cheeks, secondary palate, and posterior part of the _____ with its canines, certain posterior teeth, and associated tissue, as well as forming the zygomatic bones and parts of the temporal bones.

mandibular processes	mandibular symphysis	stomodeum
maxilla	frontonasal process	embryonic period
mandibular arch	maxillary process	endoderm
oropharyngeal membrane		

Reference

Chapter 4, Development of the face and neck. In Bath-Balogh M, Fehrenbach MJ: *Illustrated dental embryology, histology, and anatomy,* ed 3, St. Louis, 2011, Saunders.

ANSWER KEY 1. embryonic period, 2. endoderm, 3. stomodeum, 4. oropharyngeal membrane, 5. mandibular processes, 6. mandibular arch, 7. mandibular symphysis, 8. frontonasal process, 9. maxillary process, 10. maxilla.

FIGURE 2-3 Facial development within the fourth week of the embryonic period during prenatal development (frontal and lateral aspects)

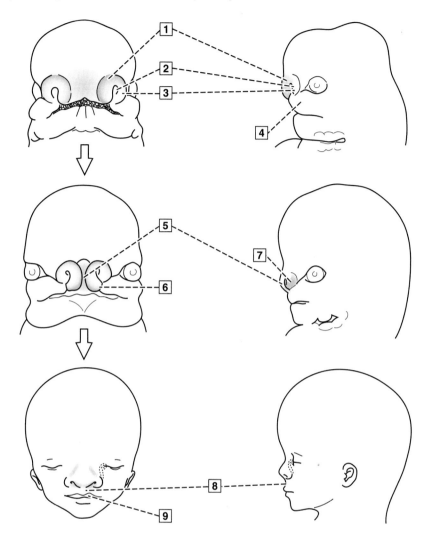

1	Medial nasal process	6	Medial nasal process fusing with maxillary process
2	Nasal pit	7	Lateral nasal process
3	Lateral nasal process	8	Philtrum
4	Maxillary process	9	Upper lip
5	Medial nasal processes fusing with each other		

REVIEW QUESTIONS

Fill in the blanks by choosing the appropriate terms from the list below.

1. The two _nasal placodes_ form in the anterior part of the frontonasal process, just superior to the stomodeum, during the fourth week as button-like structures from bilateral ectodermal thickenings that later develop into olfactory epithelium for the sensation of smell located in the mature nose.

2. During the fourth week, the tissue around the nasal placodes on the frontonasal process undergoes growth, thus starting the development of the nasal region and the nose; later, submerging the placodes by this growth forms a depression in the center of each placode, which is the _nasal pits_ .

3. The middle part of the tissue growing around the nasal placodes appears as two crescent-shaped swellings located between the nasal pits, the _medial nasal processes_.

4. In the future, the medial nasal processes will fuse together externally to form the middle part of the nose from the root of the nose to the apex of the nose, as well as the tubercle of the upper lip and _philtrum_ .

5. On the outer part of the nasal pits are two crescent-shaped swellings, the _lateral nasal processes_

6. In the future, the lateral nasal processes will form the _ala_ of the nose.

7. The fusion of the lateral nasal, maxillary, and medial nasal processes forms the _nares_ .

8. The paired medial nasal processes fuse internally and grow inferiorly on the inside of the stomodeum, forming the _intermaxillary segment_

9. The intermaxillary segment is involved in the formation of certain maxillary teeth (incisors) and associated structures, such as the _primary palate_ and nasal septum.

10. The facial development that starts during the embryonic period will be completed later in the twelfth week, within the _fetal period_ .

fetal period	nasal pits	nasal placodes
nares	primary palate	medial nasal processes
intermaxillary segment	ala	lateral nasal processes
philtrum		

Reference

Chapter 4, Development of the face and neck. In Bath-Balogh M, Fehrenbach MJ: *Illustrated dental embryology, histology, and anatomy,* ed 3, St. Louis, 2011, Saunders.

ANSWER KEY 1. nasal placodes, 2. nasal pits, 3. medial nasal processes, 4. philtrum, 5. lateral nasal processes, 6. ala, 7. nares, 8. intermaxillary segment, 9. primary palate, 10. fetal period.

FIGURE 2-4 Internal development of the head and neck within the fourth week of the embryonic period during prenatal development

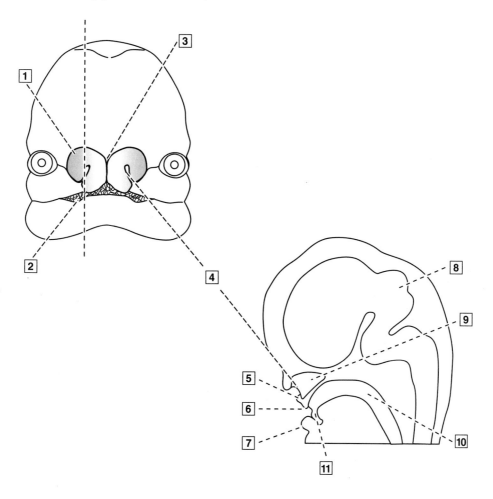

1	Lateral nasal process	7	Developing lower lip
2	Stomodeum	8	Developing brain
3	Fused medial nasal processes	9	Developing nasal cavity
4	Nasal pit	10	Primitive pharynx
5	Intermaxillary segment	11	Primitive mouth
6	Developing upper lip		

REVIEW QUESTIONS

Fill in the blanks by choosing the appropriate terms from the list below.

1. During the third to fourth week, disintegration of the oropharyngeal membrane enlarges the stomodeum of the embryo and allows access between the primitive mouth and the *primitive pharynx*.

2. During the fourth week, the tissue around the *nasal placodes* on the frontonasal process undergoes growth, thus starting the development of the nasal region and the nose by forming a depression in the center of each placode, the nasal pits.

3. The middle part of the tissue growing around the nasal placodes appears as two crescent-shaped swellings located between the nasal pits, the *medial nasal processes*.

4. In the future, the medial nasal processes will fuse together externally to form the middle part of the nose from the root of the nose to the apex of the nose, as well as the tubercle of the *upper lip* and philtrum.

5. The paired medial nasal processes fuse internally and grow inferiorly on the inside of the stomodeum, forming the *intermaxillary segment*.

6. The intermaxillary segment is involved in the formation of certain maxillary teeth (incisors) and associated structures, such as the primary palate and *nasal septum*.

7. On the outer part of the *nasal pit* are two crescent-shaped swellings, the lateral nasal processes.

8. In the future, the *lateral process* form the alae of the nose, and the fusion of the lateral nasal, maxillary, and medial nasal processes forms the nares.

9. Deepening of the nasal pits produces a nasal sac that grows internally toward the developing brain, with the nasal sacs initially separated from the stomodeum by the *oronasal membrane*.

10. The oronasal membrane disintegrates, bringing the *nasal cavity* and oral cavity into communication in the area of the primitive choanae, posterior to the developing primary palate; at the same time, the superior, middle, and inferior nasal conchae are developing on the lateral walls of the developing nasal cavities.

nasal pits	upper lip	nasal cavity
intermaxillary segment	primitive pharynx	nasal septum
oronasal membrane	medial nasal processes	nasal placodes
lateral nasal processes		

Reference

Chapter 4, Development of the face and neck. In Bath-Balogh M, Fehrenbach MJ: *Illustrated dental embryology, histology, and anatomy,* ed 3, St. Louis, 2011, Saunders.

FIGURE 2-5 Development of the neck during prenatal development

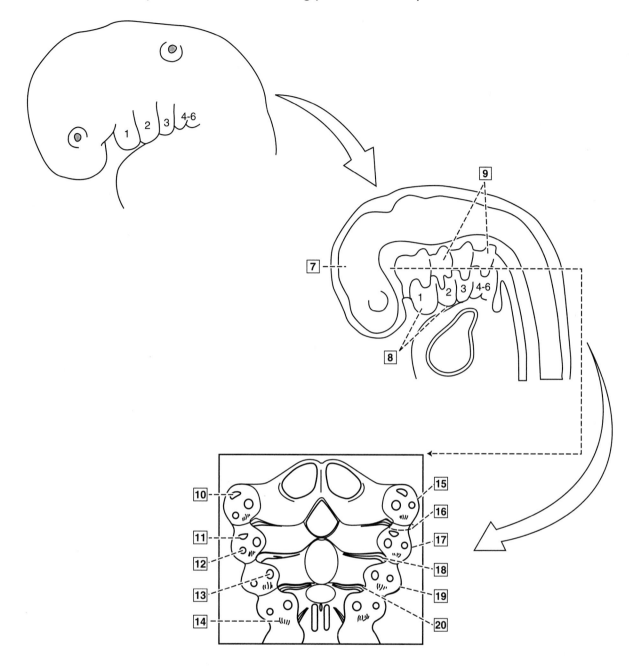

7 Brain	**12** Nerve	**17** Second branchial arch (hyoid arch)
8 Branchial arches	**13** Vessel	
9 Pharyngeal pouches	**14** Muscle	**18** Second branchial pouch
10 Meckel cartilage	**15** First branchial arch (mandibular arch)	**19** Third branchial arch
11 Reichert cartilage	**16** First branchial membrane	**20** Third branchial pouch

REVIEW QUESTIONS

Fill in the blanks by choosing the appropriate terms from the list below.

1.   The development of the _neck_ parallels the development of the face over time, beginning during the fourth week of prenatal development within the embryonic period and completed during the fetal period.

2.   During the fourth week of prenatal development, stacked bilateral swellings of tissue forming the brachial arches appear inferior to the stomodeum and include the _mandibular arch_.

3.   The _branchial arches_ are six pairs of U-shaped bars with a core of mesenchyme formed by neural crest cells that migrate to the neck region and are covered externally by ectoderm, lined internally by endoderm, and support the lateral walls of the primitive pharynx.

4.   The _branchial apparatus_ consists of the branchial arches, branchial grooves and membranes, and pharyngeal pouches.

5.   The endoderm of the pharynx lines the internal parts of the branchial arches and passes into balloon-like areas of the _pharyngeal pouches_.

6.   The first branchial arch, or *mandibular arch,* and its associated tissue include the _Meckel cartilage_.

7.   Forming within the second branchial arch, or *hyoid arch,* is cartilage similar to that of the mandibular arch, the _Reichert_; most of this structure disappears during development; however, parts of it are responsible in the future for a middle ear bone, a process of the temporal bone, and parts of the hyoid bone.

8.   Between neighboring branchial arches, external grooves are noted on each side of the embryo, the _branchial grooves_.

9.   The _palatine tonsil_ are derived from the lining of the second pharyngeal pouches and also from the pharyngeal walls.

10. The parathyroid glands and the _thymus gland_ appear to be derived from the lining of the third and fourth pharyngeal pouches.

mandibular arch	**branchial arches**	**branchial grooves**
thymus gland	**neck**	**branchial apparatus**
pharyngeal pouches	**palatine tonsils**	**Reichert cartilage**
Meckel cartilage		

Reference

Chapter 4, Development of the face and neck. In Bath-Balogh M, Fehrenbach MJ: *Illustrated dental embryology, histology, and anatomy,* ed 3, St. Louis, 2011, Saunders.

FIGURE 2-6   Regions of the head

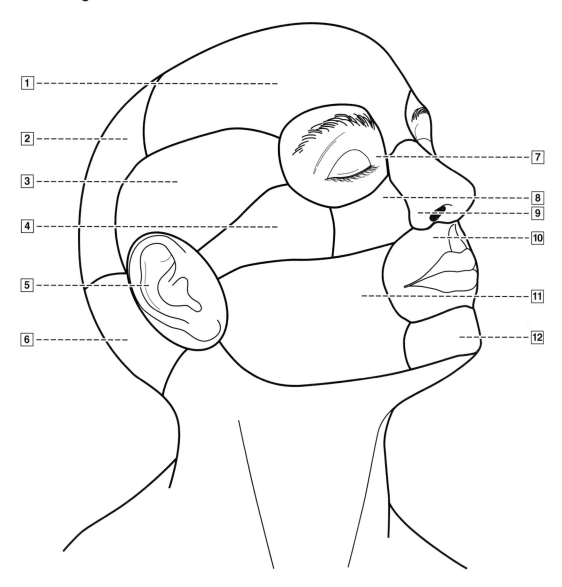

1	Frontal region	7	Orbital region
2	Parietal region	8	Infraorbital region
3	Temporal region	9	Nasal region
4	Zygomatic region	10	Oral region
5	Auricular region	11	Buccal region
6	Occipital region	12	Mental region

REVIEW QUESTIONS

Fill in the blanks by choosing the appropriate terms from the list below.

1. The _Surface anatomy_ represents the external features of the body.

2. The _regions of the head_ include the frontal, parietal, occipital, temporal, auricular, orbital, nasal, infraorbital, zygomatic, buccal, oral, and mental regions.

3. The _frontal_ as a region of the head includes the forehead and the area superior to the eyes.

4. The scalp covers both the parietal region and the _occipital_ of the head, which is the soft tissue envelope of the cranial vault.

5. Within the _temporal_ is the region of the head that has the temple, which is located on the superficial side of the head posterior to each eye.

6. The _auricular_ is a region of each side of the head that has the external ear as a prominent feature.

7. In the _orbital_ is a region of each side of the head with the eyeball and all its supporting structures contained within the bony socket of the orbit.

8. The main feature of the _nasal_ as a region of the head is the external nose, which is the visible part of the human nose that protrudes from the face and bears the nostrils.

9. The infraorbital region, zygomatic region, and _buccal_ on each side of the head are all located on the facial aspect.

10. The _oral_ is a region of the head that has many structures within it such as the lips, oral cavity, palate, tongue, floor of the mouth, and parts of the pharynx.

auricular region	oral region	regions of the head
buccal region	temporal region	nasal region
orbital region	surface anatomy	occipital region
frontal region		

References

Chapter 2, Surface anatomy. In Fehrenbach MJ, Herring SW: *Illustrated anatomy of the head and neck,* ed 4, St. Louis, 2012, Saunders; and Chapter 1, Face and neck regions. In Bath-Balogh M, Fehrenbach MJ: *Illustrated dental embryology, histology, and anatomy,* ed 3, St. Louis, 2011, Saunders.

FIGURE 2-7 Frontal region (including microanatomic view of skin)

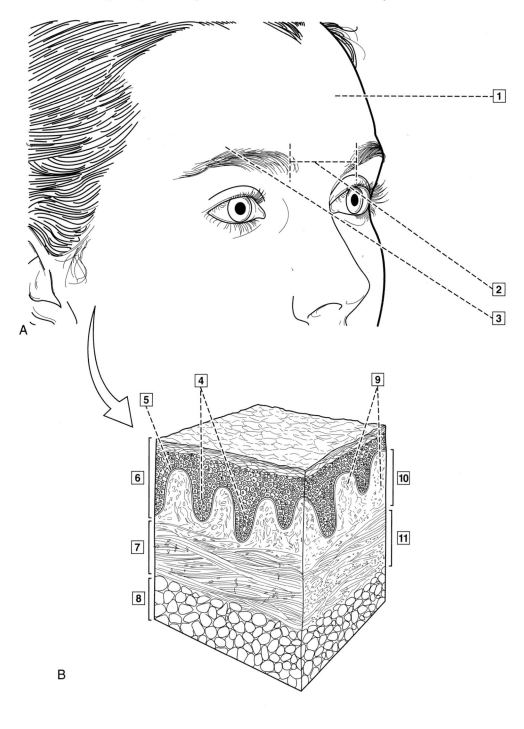

A

B

1	Frontal eminence	**7**	Dermis (connective tissue proper)
2	Glabella	**8**	Hypodermis
3	Supraorbital ridge	**9**	Connective tissue papillae
4	Rete ridges	**10**	Loose connective tissue
5	Basement membrane	**11**	Dense connective tissue
6	Epidermis (epithelium)		

REVIEW QUESTIONS

Fill in the blanks by choosing the appropriate terms from the list below.

1. The _____ of the head includes the forehead and the area superior to the eyes.

2. Just inferior to each eyebrow is the _____, or *superciliary ridge*.

3. The smooth elevated area between the eyebrows is the _____.

4. The prominence of the forehead is the _____.

5. The _____ is the tissue type that covers and lines both the external and internal body surfaces, including vessels and small cavities; it not only serves as a protective covering or lining but is also involved in tissue absorption, secretion, sensory, and other specialized functions.

6. Depending on their classification, epithelial tissue can be derived from any of the _____ embryonic cell layers.

7. Most epithelium in the body is composed of _____, which includes the superficial layer of both the skin and oral mucosa.

8. An example of keratinized stratified squamous epithelium is the _____, which is the superficial layer of the skin that overlies a basement membrane and adjoins the deeper layers of connective tissue, the dermis and the hypodermis, respectively.

9. The connective tissue proper in the skin is considered the _____ and is found deep to the epidermis.

10. Deeper to the dermis in the skin is the _____, which is composed of loose connective tissue and adipose connective tissue, a specialized connective tissue, as well as glandular tissue, large blood vessels, and nerves.

epidermis	stratified squamous epithelium	hypodermis
three	epithelium	frontal region
glabella	dermis	supraorbital ridge
frontal eminence		

References

Chapter 2, Surface anatomy. In Fehrenbach MJ, Herring SW: *Illustrated anatomy of the head and neck,* ed 4, St. Louis, 2012, Saunders; and Chapter 8, Basic tissue. In Bath-Balogh M, Fehrenbach MJ: *Illustrated dental embryology, histology, and anatomy,* ed 3, St. Louis, 2011, Saunders.

FIGURE 2-8 Interface between epithelium and connective tissue such as in skin (microanatomic views)

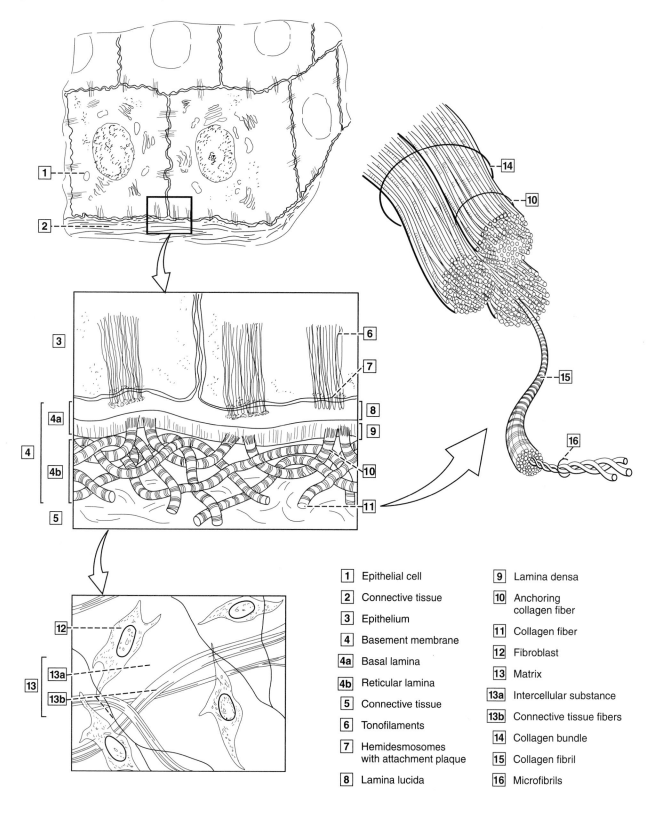

1	Epithelial cell	**9**	Lamina densa
2	Connective tissue	**10**	Anchoring collagen fiber
3	Epithelium	**11**	Collagen fiber
4	Basement membrane	**12**	Fibroblast
4a	Basal lamina	**13**	Matrix
4b	Reticular lamina	**13a**	Intercellular substance
5	Connective tissue	**13b**	Connective tissue fibers
6	Tonofilaments	**14**	Collagen bundle
7	Hemidesmosomes with attachment plaque	**15**	Collagen fibril
8	Lamina lucida	**16**	Microfibrils

REVIEW QUESTIONS

Fill in the blanks by choosing the appropriate terms from the list below.

1. The _____ is a thin, acellular structure located between any form of epithelium and its underlying connective tissue, as noted in both the skin and oral mucosa.

2. The basement membrane consists of two layers: _____ and reticular lamina.

3. The superficial layer of the basement membrane is the basal lamina and is produced by the _____.

4. The basal lamina consists of two sublayers: the lamina lucida that is a clear layer closer to the epithelium, and the _____ that is a dense layer closer to the connective tissue.

5. The deeper layer of the basement membrane is usually the reticular lamina, which consists of collagen fibers and reticular fibers produced and secreted by the underlying _____.

6. Attachment mechanisms are part of the basement membrane and include tonofilaments from the epithelium, hemidesmosomes with the attachment plaque, and the _____ from the connective tissue.

7. The _____ from the epithelium loop through the attachment plaque, whereas the collagen fibers of the reticular lamina loop into the lamina densa of the basal lamina, forming a flexible attachment between the two tissue types.

8. The _____ are the main connective tissue fiber type found in the body and are composed of the protein collagen, including distinct types.

9. The most common distinct type of collagen protein is _____, which is found in the skin dermis, lamina propria, bone, dentitions, tendons, and virtually all other types of connective tissue.

10. Cells responsible for the synthesis of Type I collagen protein include _____, which produce fibers, and osteoblasts, which produce bone, as well as odontoblasts, which produce dentin.

anchoring collagen fibers	tonofilaments	basal lamina
fibroblasts	lamina densa	collagen fibers
Type I	epithelium	basement membrane
connective tissue		

Reference

Chapter 8, Basic tissue. In Bath-Balogh M, Fehrenbach MJ: *Illustrated dental embryology, histology, and anatomy,* ed 3, St. Louis, 2011, Saunders.

ANSWER KEY 1. basement membrane, 2. basal lamina, 3. epithelium, 4. lamina densa, 5. connective tissue, 6. anchoring collagen fibers, 7. tonofilaments, 8. collagen fibers, 9. Type I, 10. fibroblasts.

FIGURE 2-9 Auricular region: external ear (lateral view)

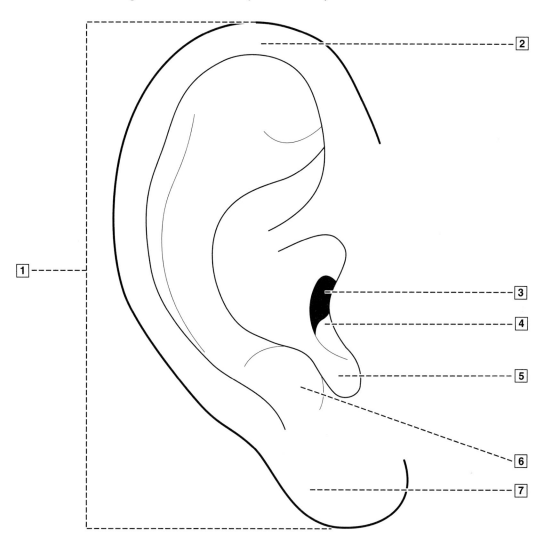

1	Auricle	**5**	Intertragic notch
2	Helix	**6**	Antitragus
3	External acoustic meatus	**7**	Lobule
4	Tragus		

REVIEW QUESTIONS

Fill in the blanks by choosing the appropriate terms from the list below.

1. The _____ is a region on each side of the head that has the external ear as a prominent feature.

2. The first part of the ear consists of the external ear that is attached to the lateral aspect of the head and the canal leading inward to the eardrum, or _____.

3. The _____ is composed of an oval flap, or *auricle,* and the external acoustic meatus.

4. As the visible part of the external ear, the _____ collects sound waves.

5. The _____ is a tube through which sound waves are transmitted to the middle ear within the skull; it is an important landmark to note when taking certain radiographs and administering certain local anesthetic nerve blocks.

6. The posterior free margin of the auricle is the _____.

7. The helix ends inferiorly at the _____, the fleshy protuberance of the earlobe.

8. The _____ is the smaller flap of tissue of the auricle anterior to the external acoustic meatus.

9. The flap of tissue opposite the tragus is the _____, which is an important landmark to note when taking certain radiographs and administering certain local anesthetic nerve blocks.

10. Between the tragus and antitragus is a deep notch, the _____.

intertragic notch	tympanic membrane	external ear
helix	auricular region	antitragus
auricle	external acoustic meatus	lobule
tragus		

References

Chapter 2, Surface anatomy. In Fehrenbach MJ, Herring SW: *Illustrated anatomy of the head and neck,* ed 4, St. Louis, 2012, Saunders; and Chapter 1, Face and neck regions. In Bath-Balogh M, Fehrenbach MJ: *Illustrated dental embryology, histology, and anatomy,* ed 3, St. Louis, 2011, Saunders.

FIGURE 2-10 Auricular region: middle and internal ear (sagittal section)

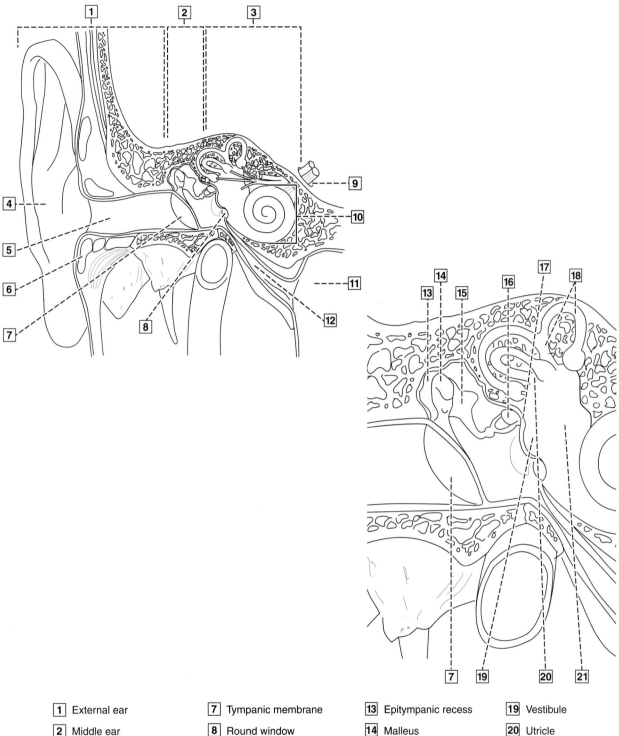

1 External ear	**7** Tympanic membrane	**13** Epitympanic recess	**19** Vestibule
2 Middle ear	**8** Round window	**14** Malleus	**20** Utricle
3 Internal ear	**9** Internal acoustic meatus	**15** Incus	**21** Saccule
4 Auricle	**10** Cochlea	**16** Stapes	
5 External acoustic meatus	**11** Pharynx	**17** Oval window	
6 Cartilage	**12** Pharyngotympanic tube	**18** Semicircular canals	

REVIEW QUESTIONS

Fill in the blanks by choosing the appropriate terms from the list below.

1.   The second part of the ear is the _____, which is a cavity in the petrous part of the temporal bone bounded laterally, and separated from the external canal, by a membrane and connected internally to the pharynx by a narrow tube.

2.   The _____ separates the external acoustic meatus from the middle ear and consists of a connective tissue core lined with skin on the outside and mucous membrane on the inside.

3.   The function of the middle ear is to transmit _____ of the tympanic membrane across the cavity of the middle ear to the internal ear, which it accomplishes through three interconnected but movable bones that bridge the space between the tympanic membrane and the internal ear.

4.   The bones of the middle ear include the _____ (connected to the tympanic membrane), the incus (connected to the malleus by a synovial joint), and the stapes (connected to the incus by a synovial joint and attached to the lateral wall of the internal ear at the oval window).

5.   The third part of the ear is the _____, which consists of a series of cavities within the petrous part of the temporal bone and is located between the laterally placed middle ear and the medially placed internal acoustic meatus.

6.   The internal ear consists of the _____ (a series of bony cavities) and the membranous labyrinth (membranous ducts and sacs) within these cavities.

7.   The bony labyrinth consists of the _____, three semicircular canals, and the cochlea that contain a clear fluid, the perilymph.

8.   Suspended within the perilymph but not filling all spaces of the bony labyrinth is the _____, which consists of the semicircular ducts, the cochlear duct, and two sacs (the utricle and the saccule) that are filled with endolymph.

9.   The vestibule contains the _____ in its lateral wall, which is the central part of the bony labyrinth that communicates anteriorly with the cochlea and posterosuperiorly with the semicircular canals.

10.   Projecting in an anterior direction from the vestibule is the _____, which is a bony structure that twists on itself around a central column of bone.

internal ear	**middle ear**	**tympanic membrane**
oval window	**malleus**	**vibrations**
vestibule	**cochlea**	**bony labyrinth**
membranous labyrinth		

Reference

Chapter 8, Head and neck. In Drake R, Vogl AW, Mitchell AWM: *Gray's anatomy for students,* ed 2, Philadelphia, 2010, Churchill Livingstone.

ANSWER KEY   1. middle ear, 2. tympanic membrane, 3. vibrations, 4. malleus, 5. internal ear, 6. bony labyrinth, 7. vestibule, 8. membranous labyrinth, 9. oval window, 10. cochlea.

FIGURE 2-11 Orbital region (frontal and internal view)

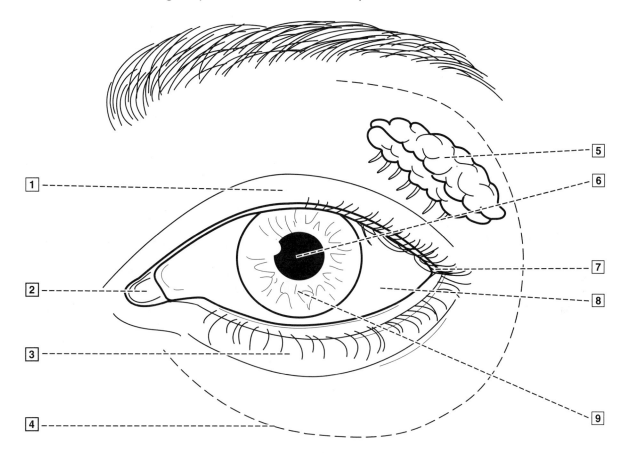

1 Upper eyelid		**7** Lateral canthus
2 Medial canthus		**8** Sclera (covered by conjunctiva)
3 Lower eyelid		**9** Iris
4 Orbit (outlined)		
5 Lacrimal gland (deep)		
6 Pupil		

REVIEW QUESTIONS

Fill in the blanks by choosing the appropriate terms from the list below.

1. In the orbital region of each side of the head, the eyeball and all its supporting structures are contained within the _____, a bony socket of the skull.

2. The orbits are a pair of conical or four-sided pyramidal cavities, which open into the midline of the face and point back into the head, with each having a(n) _____, an apex, and four walls.

3. On the eyeball is the _____, the white area of the eye.

4. The sclera has a central area of coloration, the circular _____.

5. The opening in the center of the iris is the _____, which appears black and changes size as the iris responds to changing light conditions.

6. Two movable eyelids, upper and lower, cover and protect each _____.

7. Behind each upper eyelid and deep within the orbit are the _____, which produce lacrimal fluid, or tears.

8. The _____ is the delicate and thin membrane lining the inside of the eyelids and the front of the eyeball.

9. The outer corner where the upper and lower eyelids meet is the _____, or *outer canthus;* the canthi are important landmarks when taking extraoral radiographs.

10. The inner angle of the eye is the _____, or *inner canthus;* the canthi are important landmarks when taking extraoral radiographs.

eyeball	conjunctiva	orbit
pupil	lateral canthus	medial canthus
lacrimal glands	base	sclera
iris		

References

Chapter 2, Surface anatomy. In Fehrenbach MJ, Herring SW: *Illustrated anatomy of the head and neck,* ed 4, St. Louis, 2012, Saunders; and Chapter 1, Face and neck regions. In Bath-Balogh M, Fehrenbach MJ: *Illustrated dental embryology, histology, and anatomy,* ed 3, St. Louis, 2011, Saunders.

FIGURE 2-12   Orbital region: eye (sagittal section)

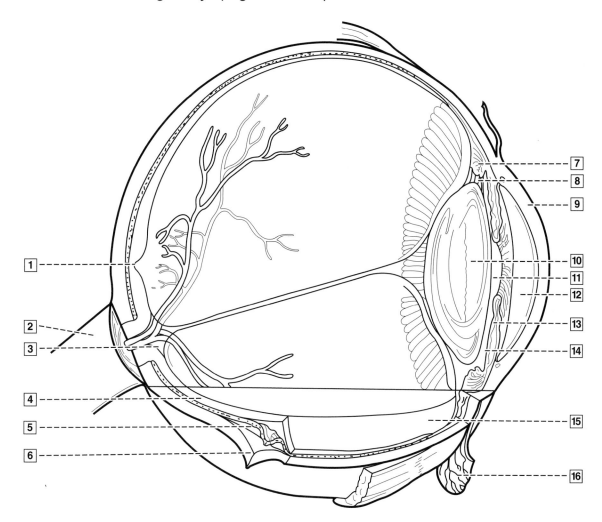

1 Fovea centralis	**6** Sclera	**11** Pupil
2 Optic nerve	**7** Ciliary body	**12** Anterior chamber filled with aqueous humor
3 Optic disk	**8** Suspensory ligament	**13** Iris
4 Retina	**9** Cornea	**14** Posterior chamber
5 Choroid	**10** Lens	**15** Postremal chamber filled with vitreous humor
		16 Conjunctiva

REVIEW QUESTIONS

Fill in the blanks by choosing the appropriate terms from the list below.

1. The _____ is the area directly posterior to the cornea and anterior to the colored part of the eye, the iris; the central opening in the iris is the pupil; and posterior to the iris and anterior to the lens is the smaller posterior chamber.

2. The anterior and posterior chambers are continuous with each other through the pupillary opening and filled with a fluid, _____, which is secreted into the posterior chamber and flows into the anterior chamber through the pupil.

3. The _____ is a transparent, biconvex elastic disc attached circumferentially to muscles associated with the outer wall of the eyeball, and whose lateral attachment provides it with the ability to change its refractive ability to maintain visual acuity.

4. The posterior part of the eyeball, from the lens to the retina, is filled with a gelatinous substance, the _____.

5. The _____ is an opaque layer of dense connective tissue that can be seen anteriorly through its covering of conjunctiva; it is pierced by numerous vessels and nerves, including the optic nerve posteriorly, and provides attachment for the various muscles involved in eyeball movements.

6. Continuous with the sclera anteriorly is the transparent _____, which covers the anterior surface of the eyeball and allows light to enter the eyeball.

7. The _____ is a posterior part of the eyeball and consists of a thin, highly vascular, pigmented layer with smaller vessels adjacent to the retina and larger vessels more peripherally; it is firmly attached to the retina internally and loosely attached to the sclera externally.

8. Extending from the anterior border of the choroid is the _____, which is a triangular-shaped structure located between the choroid and the iris, forming a complete ring around the eyeball.

9. The inner layer of the eyeball is the _____, which consists of two parts: posteriorly and laterally is the optic part, which is sensitive to light, and anteriorly is the nonvisual part, which covers the internal surface of the ciliary body and the iris.

10. The optic disc is where the optic nerve leaves the retina (its "blind spot"), and lateral to the optic disc a small area with a hint of yellowish coloration is the macula lutea with its central depression, the _____, which is the thinnest and most sensitive part.

sclera	aqueous humor	anterior chamber
choroid	lens	vitreous humor
retina	cornea	fovea centralis
ciliary body		

Reference

Chapter 8, Head and neck. In Drake R, Vogl AW, Mitchell AWM: *Gray's anatomy for students,* ed 2, Philadelphia, 2010, Churchill Livingstone.

FIGURE 2-13 Nasal region: external nose (frontal view)

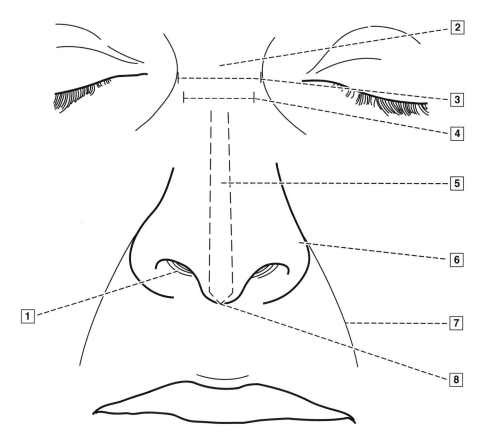

1	Naris	**5**	Nasal septum (outlined)
2	Position of nasion	**6**	Ala
3	Root of nose	**7**	Nasolabial sulcus
4	Bridge of nose	**8**	Apex

REVIEW QUESTIONS

Fill in the blanks by choosing the appropriate terms from the list below.

1. The main feature of the nasal region of the head is the _____.

2. The _____ is located between the eyes in the nasal region.

3. Inferior to the glabella is a midpoint landmark of the nasal region that corresponds with the junction between the underlying bones, the _____, which is an important landmark when taking extraoral radiographs.

4. Inferior to the nasion is the bony structure that forms the _____.

5. The _____, or *tip,* is flexible because it is formed from cartilage.

6. Inferior to the apex on each side of the nose is a(n) _____, or *nostril.*

7. The nares are separated by the midline _____.

8. The nares are bounded laterally on each side by a winglike cartilaginous structure, the _____ of the nose, which is an important landmark when taking extraoral radiographs.

9. The nose is a protuberance on the face, which admits and expels air for respiration in conjunction with the _____.

10. Behind the nose are the _____ and the paranasal sinuses.

oral cavity	bridge of the nose	ala
olfactory mucosa	nasion	root of the nose
naris	external nose	nasal septum
apex of the nose		

Reference

Chapter 2, Surface anatomy. In Fehrenbach MJ, Herring SW: *Illustrated anatomy of the head and neck,* ed 4, St. Louis, 2012, Saunders; and Chapter 1, Face and neck regions. In Bath-Balogh M, Fehrenbach MJ: *Illustrated dental embryology, histology, and anatomy,* ed 3, St. Louis, 2011, Saunders.

ANSWER KEY   1. external nose, 2. root of the nose, 3. nasion, 4. bridge of the nose, 5. apex of the nose, 6. naris, 7. nasal septum, 8. ala, 9. oral cavity, 10. olfactory mucosa.

FIGURE 2-14   Nasal region: nasal cavity (sagittal section with microanatomic view)

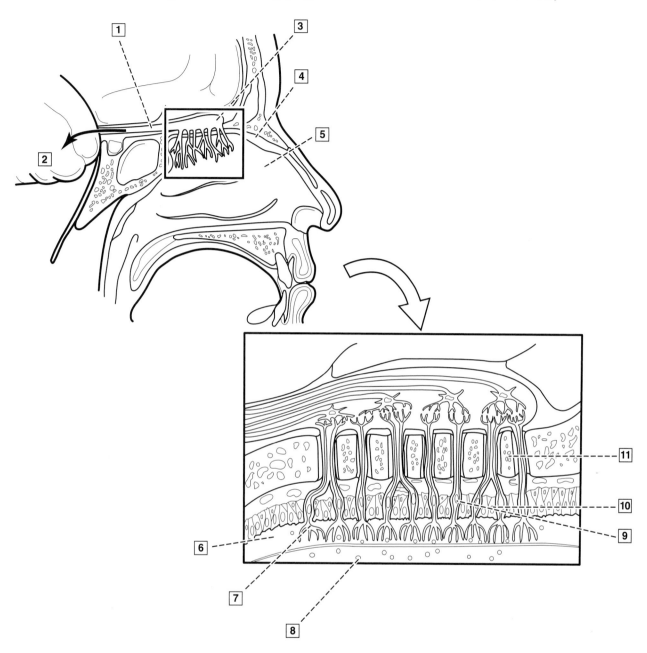

1	Olfactory tract	**6**	Mucous layer
2	Olfactory cortex	**7**	Cilia of receptor cell
3	Olfactory bulb	**8**	Odor molecule
4	Olfactory epithelium	**9**	Cell body of olfactory neuron
5	Nasal cavity	**10**	Supporting cells
		11	Cribriform plate of ethmoid bone

REVIEW QUESTIONS

Fill in the blanks by choosing the appropriate terms from the list below.

1.   Each _____ consists of three general regions: the nasal vestibule, respiratory region, and olfactory region, with each having a floor, roof, medial wall, and lateral wall.

2.   The nasal vestibule is just internal to each _____ of the nasal cavity and is lined by skin that contains hair follicles.

3.   The _____ is the largest general region of the nasal cavity, and is lined by respiratory epithelium composed mainly of ciliated and mucous cells.

4.   The olfactory region at the apex of each nasal cavity is lined by _____, and contains the olfactory receptors.

5.   In addition to functioning for the sense of smell, the nasal cavities adjust the temperature and humidity; these cavities also filter the air through hair in the vestibule and capture foreign material in the _____, which is moved posteriorly by cilia on epithelial cells in the nasal cavities to the digestive tract.

6.   The lateral wall is characterized by three curved shelves of bone, the _____, which are one above the other and project medially and inferiorly across the nasal cavity, dividing each nasal cavity into four air channels to also increase the surface area.

7.   The openings of the _____, air-filled spaces in the bones of the skull, are located on the lateral wall and roof of the nasal cavities.

8.   The lateral wall of the nasal cavity contains the opening of the _____, which drains tears or lacrimal fluid from the lacrimal gland of the eye into the nasal cavity.

9.   The _____ of the ethmoid bone is at the apex of the nasal cavities and separates the nasal cavities below from the cranial cavity above; there are small perforations in the bone that allow the fibers of the first cranial nerve or olfactory nerve to pass between the two regions.

10. The _____, which transmits the sense of smell from the nose to the brain, is supported and protected by the cribriform plate of the ethmoid bone, which separates it from the olfactory epithelium, and which is perforated by olfactory nerve axons.

naris	mucus	respiratory region
nasolacrimal duct	conchae	olfactory epithelium
paranasal sinuses	nasal cavity	cribriform plate
olfactory bulb		

Reference

Chapter 8, Head and neck. In Drake R, Vogl AW, Mitchell AWM: *Gray's anatomy for students,* ed 2, Philadelphia, 2010, Churchill Livingstone.

ANSWER KEY   1. nasal cavity, 2. naris, 3. respiratory region, 4. olfactory epithelium, 5. mucus, 6. conchae, 7. paranasal sinuses, 8. nasolacrimal duct, 9. cribriform plate, 10. olfactory bulb.

FIGURE 2-15 Zygomatic, infraorbital, buccal, oral, and mental regions (lateral, frontal, and internal views)

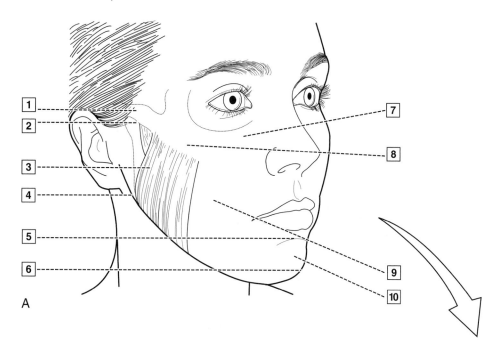

A

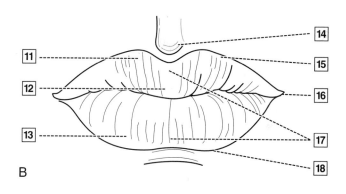

B

1	Zygomatic arch (deep)	11	Upper lip
2	Temporomandibular joint	12	Tubercle
3	Masseter muscle (deep)	13	Lower lip
4	Angle of mandible	14	Philtrum
5	Labiomental groove	15	Vermilion border
6	Mental protuberance	16	Labial commissure
7	Infraorbital region	17	Vermilion border
8	Zygomatic region	18	Mucocutaneous junction
9	Buccal region		
10	Mental region		

REVIEW QUESTIONS

Fill in the blanks by choosing the appropriate terms from the list below.

1. The _____ of the head is located inferior to the orbital region and lateral to the nasal region.

2. Further lateral to the infraorbital region is the _____, which overlies the zygomatic arch, or *cheekbone*.

3. With the zygomatic region is the _____, which extends from just inferior to the lateral margin of the eye toward the middle part of the ear.

4. Inferior to the zygomatic arch, and just anterior to the ear, is the _____, where the upper skull forms a joint with the lower jaw.

5. The _____ of the head is composed of the soft tissue of the cheek.

6. One of the muscles within the cheek is the strong _____, which is noticeable when a patient clenches the teeth together.

7. The sharp angle of the lower jaw inferior to the lobule of the ear is the _____.

8. The lips are the gateway of the oral region and each lip has a(n) _____.

9. Superior to the midline of the upper lip, extending downward from the nasal septum, is a vertical groove on the skin, the _____; inferior to this is the midline of the upper lip, which terminates in a thicker area or tubercle of the upper lip.

10. The _____ is the prominence of the chin, which is inferior to the labiomental groove, a horizontal groove between the lower lip and the chin.

zygomatic arch	temporomandibular joint	masseter muscle
buccal region	mental protuberance	vermilion border
infraorbital region	angle of the mandible	philtrum
zygomatic region		

References

Chapter 2, Surface anatomy. In Fehrenbach MJ, Herring SW: *Illustrated anatomy of the head and neck,* ed 4, St. Louis, 2012, Saunders; and Chapter 2, Oral cavity and pharynx. In Bath-Balogh M, Fehrenbach MJ: *Illustrated dental embryology, histology, and anatomy,* ed 3, St. Louis, 2011, Saunders.

FIGURE 2-16 Oral region: oral cavity (oral view)

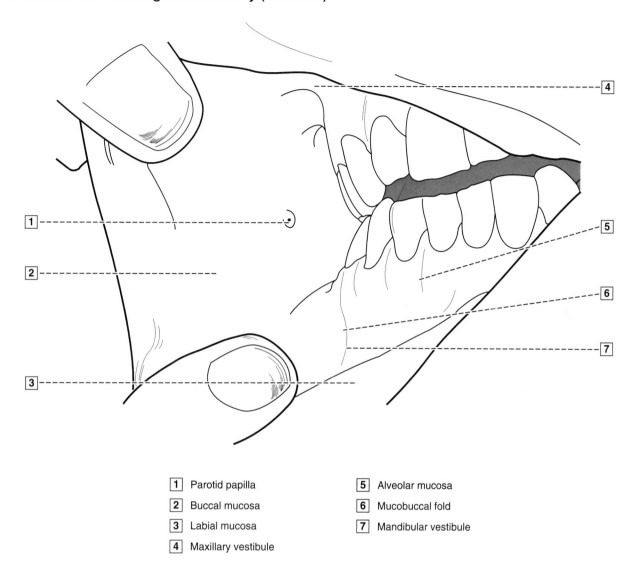

1	Parotid papilla	5	Alveolar mucosa
2	Buccal mucosa	6	Mucobuccal fold
3	Labial mucosa	7	Mandibular vestibule
4	Maxillary vestibule		

REVIEW QUESTIONS

Fill in the blanks by choosing the appropriate terms from the list below.

1. The inside of the mouth is known as the _____.

2. Underlying the upper lip is the _____, or *upper jaw*.

3. The bone underlying the lower lip is the _____, or *lower jaw*.

4. The oral cavity is lined by a mucous membrane, the _____.

5. The inner parts of the lips are lined by a pink and thick _____.

6. The labial mucosa is continuous with the equally pink and thick _____ that lines the inner cheek.

7. The upper and lower horseshoe-shaped spaces in the oral cavity between the lips and cheeks anteriorly and laterally and the teeth and their soft tissue medially and posteriorly are considered the maxillary and mandibular _____.

8. Deep within each vestibule is the vestibular fornix, where the pink and thick labial or buccal mucosa meets the redder and thinner _____ at the mucobuccal fold.

9. On the inner part of the buccal mucosa, just opposite the maxillary second molar, is the _____, a small elevation of tissue that protects the duct opening from the parotid salivary gland.

10. The _____ is a fold of tissue located at the midline between the labial mucosa and the alveolar mucosa on both the maxilla and mandible.

alveolar mucosa	vestibules	oral cavity
labial mucosa	parotid papilla	maxillae
buccal mucosa	mandible	labial frenum
oral mucosa		

References

Chapter 2, Surface anatomy. In Fehrenbach MJ, Herring SW: *Illustrated anatomy of the head and neck,* ed 4, St. Louis, 2012, Saunders; and Chapter 2, Oral cavity and pharynx. In Bath-Balogh M, Fehrenbach MJ: *Illustrated dental embryology, histology, and anatomy,* ed 3, St. Louis, 2011, Saunders.

FIGURE 2-17 Oral region: gingiva (frontal views)

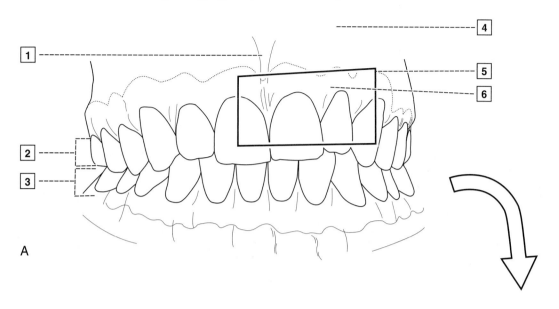

A

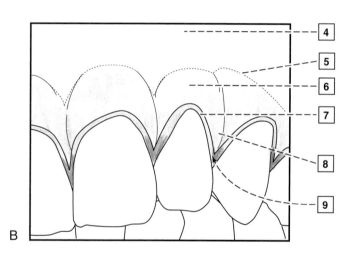

B

1 Labial frenum	**6** Attached gingiva
2 Maxillary teeth	**7** Marginal gingiva
3 Mandibular teeth	**8** Interdental gingiva
4 Alveolar mucosa	**9** Sulcus (inside)
5 Mucogingival junction (outlined)	

REVIEW QUESTIONS

Fill in the blanks by choosing the appropriate terms from the list below.

1. The teeth of the maxillae are the _____, and the teeth of the mandible are the mandibular teeth.

2. Surrounding both the maxillary and mandibular teeth are the gums, or _____.

3. The type of gingiva that tightly adheres to the bone around the roots of the teeth is the _____, and it may have areas of pigmentation.

4. The line of demarcation between the firmer and pinker attached gingiva and the movable and redder alveolar mucosa is the scallop-shaped _____.

5. At the gingival margin of each tooth is the nonattached gingiva, or _____ or *free gingiva*.

6. The inner surface of the marginal gingiva faces a space, or _____.

7. The _____, or *interdental papilla*, is an extension of attached gingiva between the teeth.

8. The labial frenum is a fold of tissue located at the _____ between the labial mucosa and the alveolar mucosa on both the maxilla and mandible.

9. The maxillary anterior teeth should overlap the _____, and posteriorly the maxillary buccal cusps should overlap the mandibular buccal cusps.

10. Both dental arches in the adult have _____ that include the incisors, canines, premolars, and molars.

permanent teeth	**attached gingiva**	**gingiva**
mandibular anterior teeth	**maxillary teeth**	**mucogingival junction**
gingival sulcus	**interdental gingiva**	**midline**
marginal		

References

Chapter 2, Surface anatomy. In Fehrenbach MJ, Herring SW: *Illustrated anatomy of the head and neck,* ed 4, St. Louis, 2012, Saunders; and Chapter 2, Oral cavity and pharynx. In Bath-Balogh M, Fehrenbach MJ: *Illustrated dental embryology, histology, and anatomy,* ed 3, St. Louis, 2011, Saunders.

FIGURE 2-18   Oral region: oral vestibule and gingiva (frontal view and microanatomic view)

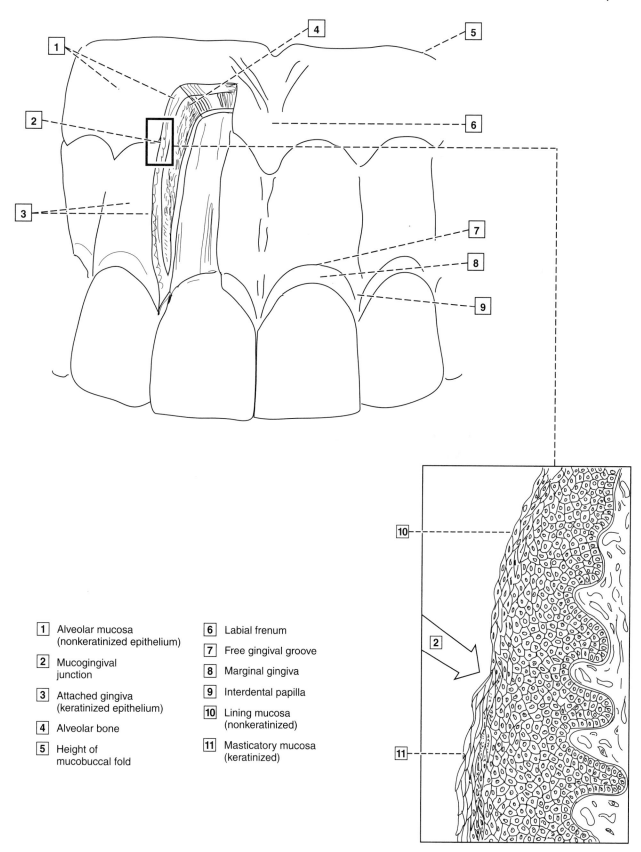

1	Alveolar mucosa (nonkeratinized epithelium)	6	Labial frenum
2	Mucogingival junction	7	Free gingival groove
3	Attached gingiva (keratinized epithelium)	8	Marginal gingiva
4	Alveolar bone	9	Interdental papilla
5	Height of mucobuccal fold	10	Lining mucosa (nonkeratinized)
		11	Masticatory mucosa (keratinized)

REVIEW QUESTIONS

Fill in the blanks by choosing the appropriate terms from the list below.

1. The _____ is a reddish-pink tissue with blue vascular areas that is shiny, moist, and extremely mobile as it lines the vestibules of the oral cavity.

2. Alveolar mucosa is classified as a(n) _____.

3. The epithelium of the alveolar mucosa is extremely thin, _____ stratified squamous epithelium that overlies, but does not obscure, an extensive vascular supply in the lamina propria, making the mucosa redder than the labial mucosa or buccal mucosa.

4. The connective tissue papillae in the alveolar mucosa are sometimes absent, and numerous elastic fibers are present in the _____, thus allowing mobility of the tissue.

5. The _____ is a sharply defined scalloped junction between the pinker attached gingiva and the redder alveolar mucosa.

6. The _____ has a thick layer of mainly parakeratinized stratified squamous epithelium that obscures the extensive vascular supply in the lamina propria, making the tissue appear opaque and pinkish as it covers the alveolar bone of the dental arches.

7. The lamina propria of the attached gingiva has tall, narrow _____.

8. The attached gingiva that covers the _____ of the dental arches is classified as a masticatory mucosa.

9. The lamina propria of the attached gingiva acts as a periosteum to the underlying bony jaws, and thus is termed a(n) _____.

10. The mucogingival junction can be seen as a dividing zone between the keratinized attached gingiva and the nonkeratinized alveolar mucosa, and thus is also considered as being between a(n) _____ and a lining mucosa.

masticatory mucosa	nonkeratinized	lamina propria
mucoperiosteum	alveolar bone	attached gingiva
connective tissue papillae	alveolar mucosa	lining mucosa
mucogingival junction		

Reference

Chapter 9, Oral mucosa. In Bath-Balogh M, Fehrenbach MJ: *Illustrated dental embryology, histology, and anatomy,* ed 3, St. Louis, 2011, Saunders.

FIGURE 2-19 Oral region: oral mucosa (microanatomic view)

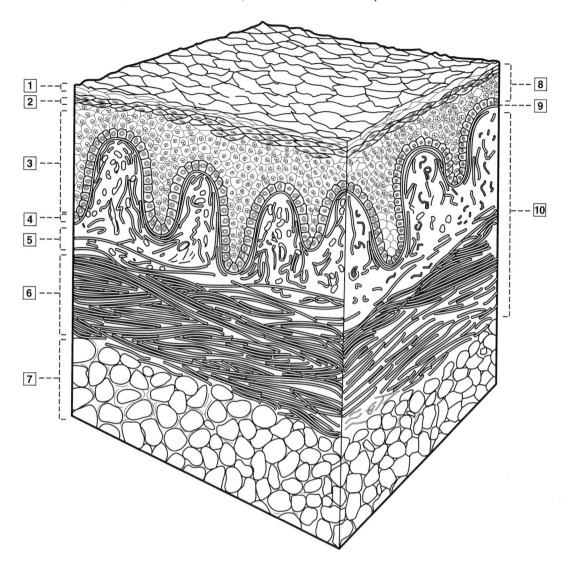

1	Keratin layer	6	Dense fibrous layer
2	Granular layer	7	Submucosa
3	Prickle layer	8	Oral epithelium
4	Basal layer	9	Basement membrane
5	Papillary layer	10	Lamina propria

REVIEW QUESTIONS

Fill in the blanks by choosing the appropriate terms from the list below.

1. The _____ almost continuously lines the oral cavity.

2. The oral mucosa is composed of _____ overlying a connective tissue proper, or lamina propria, with possibly a deeper submucosa present.

3. A(n) _____ lies between the epithelium and connective tissue in the oral mucosa.

4. There are _____ main types of oral mucosa are found in the oral cavity: lining, masticatory, and specialized mucosa; the classification of mucosa is based on the general features of the tissue.

5. The lining mucosa is a type of oral mucosa that is associated with _____ stratified squamous epithelium and includes the buccal mucosa, labial mucosa, alveolar mucosa, as well as the mucosa lining the ventral surface of the tongue, floor of the mouth, and soft palate.

6. The _____ is a type of oral mucosa associated with orthokeratinized stratified squamous epithelium, as well as parakeratinized stratified squamous epithelium, and includes the hard palate, attached gingiva, and dorsal surface of the tongue.

7. The _____, or *stratum basale,* is the deepest layer of the oral mucosa and consists of a single layer of cuboidal epithelial cells overlying the basement membrane, which in turn is situated superior to the lamina propria.

8. Superficial to the basal layer in oral mucosa is the _____, or *stratum spinosum,* in which a spiky look results when the individual dehydrated epithelial cells are shrinking when fixed for study but still joined at their outer edges.

9. In keratinized oral mucosa, superficial to the prickle layer is the _____, or *stratum granulosum,* with its epithelial cells having prominent keratohyaline granules, which stain as dark spots.

10. In keratinized oral mucosa, the most superficial layer is the _____, or *stratum corneum,* which has keratin-filled epithelial cells.

basal layer	nonkeratinized	basement membrane
prickle layer	keratin layer	stratified squamous epithelium
granular layer	three	oral mucosa
masticatory mucosa		

Reference

Chapter 9, Oral mucosa. In Bath-Balogh M, Fehrenbach MJ: *Illustrated dental embryology, histology, and anatomy,* ed 3, St. Louis, 2011, Saunders.

FIGURE 2-20   Oral region: gingival tissue (microanatomic views)

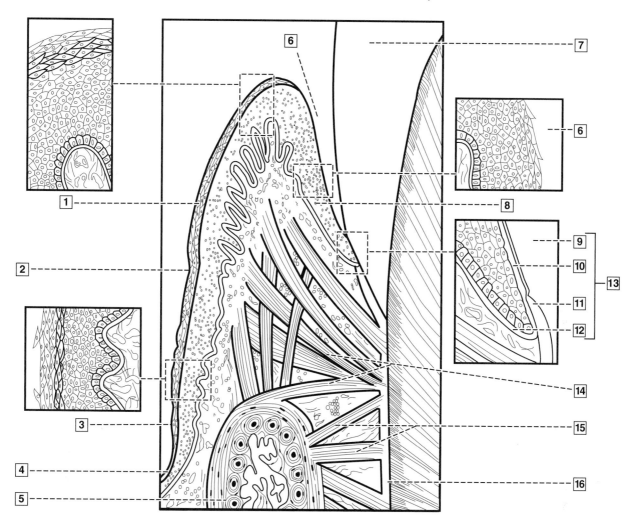

1	Marginal gingiva	9	Enamel
2	Free gingival groove	10	Internal basal lamina
3	Attached gingiva	11	Cementum
4	Alveolar mucosa	12	External basal lamina
5	Alveolar bone	13	Junctional epithelium
6	Gingival sulcus	14	Gingival fiber group
7	Tooth surface	15	Periodontal ligament
8	Sulcular epithelium	16	Cementum

REVIEW QUESTIONS

Fill in the blanks by choosing the appropriate terms from the list below.

1. Surrounding the maxillary and mandibular teeth in the alveoli and covering the alveolar processes is the _____, or *gums*.

2. The gingival tissue that tightly adheres to the bone around the roots of the teeth is the _____.

3. At the gingival margin of each tooth is the _____, or *free gingiva*, which is continuous with the attached gingiva.

4. The _____, or *gingival margin*, is at the most superficial part of the marginal gingiva.

5. The _____ separates the attached gingiva from the marginal gingiva on the superficial surface of gingival tissue.

6. Together the sulcular epithelium and junctional epithelium form the _____.

7. The _____, or *crevicular epithelium*, stands away from the tooth, creating a gingival sulcus, or space that is filled with gingival crevicular fluid.

8. A deeper extension of the sulcular epithelium is the _____, which lines the floor of the gingival sulcus and is attached to the tooth surface.

9. The junctional epithelium is attached to the tooth surface by way of a(n) _____, which attaches this tissue to the tooth surface of either enamel, cementum, or dentin.

10. The deeper interface between the thin junctional epithelium and the underlying _____ is relatively smooth, without rete ridges or connective tissue papillae; the epithelial cells are loosely packed, with fewer intercellular junctions with desmosomes between cells and more intercellular spaces.

sulcular epithelium	epithelial attachment	free gingival crest
free gingival groove	attached gingiva	junctional epithelium
dentogingival junctional tissue	gingival tissue	lamina propria
marginal gingiva		

Reference

Chapter 10, Gingival and dentogingival junctional tissue. In Bath-Balogh M, Fehrenbach MJ:
Illustrated dental embryology, histology, and anatomy, ed 3, St. Louis, 2011, Saunders.

ANSWER KEY 1. gingival tissue, 2. attached gingiva, 3. marginal gingiva, 4. free gingival crest, 5. free gingival groove, 6. dentogingival junctional tissue, 7. sulcular epithelium, 8. junctional epithelium, 9. epithelial attachment, 10. lamina propria.

FIGURE 2-21   Oral region: dentogingival junction (microanatomic view)

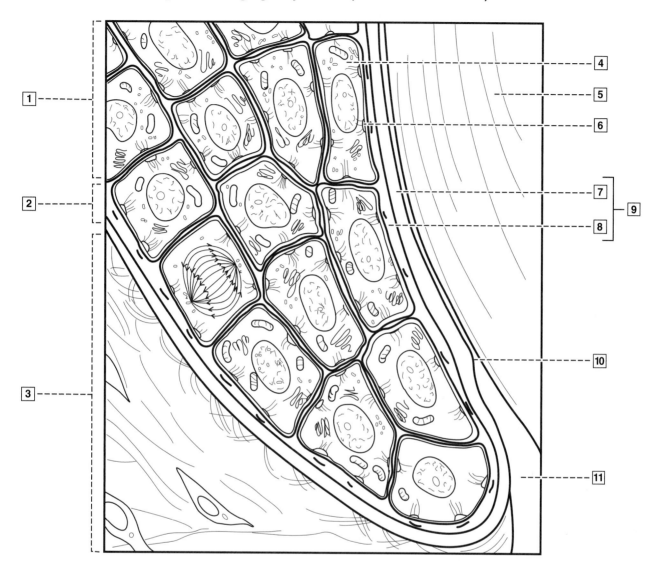

1	Basal layer	**7**	Lamina densa
2	External basal lamina	**8**	Lamina lucida
3	Lamina propria	**9**	Internal basal lamina
4	Junctional epithelial cell	**10**	Cementoenamel junction
5	Enamel	**11**	Cementum
6	Hemidesmosome		

REVIEW QUESTIONS

Fill in the blanks by choosing the appropriate terms from the list below.

1. The superficial epithelial cells of the junctional epithelium provide the hemidesmosomes and an internal basal lamina that create the _____, a cell-to-noncellular type of intercellular junction.

2. The structure of the epithelial attachment is similar to that of the junction between the epithelium and subadjacent connective tissue, because the internal basal lamina consists of a(n) _____ and lamina densa.

3. The internal basal lamina of the epithelial attachment is continuous with the external basal lamina between the junctional epithelium and the _____ at the apical extent of the junctional epithelium.

4. The deepest layer of the _____, its basal layer, undergoes constant and rapid cell division or mitosis, which allows a constant coronal migration as the cells die and are shed into the gingival sulcus.

5. The junctional epithelium cells do not _____, forming into a granular layer, or intermediate layer, as do other gingival tissue.

6. Before the eruption of the tooth and after enamel maturation, the enamel-producing _____ secrete a basal lamina on the tooth surface that serves as a part of the primary epithelial attachment.

7. As the tooth actively erupts, the coronal part of the fused _____ and surrounding epithelium peel back off the crown serving as the primary epithelial attachment, which is later replaced by a definitive junctional epithelium as the root is formed.

8. The position of the epithelial attachment on the tooth surface is initially on the cervical half of the _____ when the tooth first becomes functional after eruption.

9. The _____ seeps between the epithelial cells and into the gingival sulcus, allowing the components of the blood to reach the tooth surface through the junctional epithelium from the blood vessels of the adjacent lamina propria.

10. A calibrated periodontal probe measures the probing depth of the healthy _____; after the probe is gently inserted, it slides by the sulcular epithelium, and is stopped by the epithelial attachment between the junctional epithelium and the tooth surface.

gingival sulcus	epithelial attachment	reduced enamel epithelium
gingival crevicular fluid	lamina lucida	junctional epithelium
anatomic crown	lamina propria	ameloblasts
mature		

Reference

Chapter 10, Gingival and dentogingival junctional tissue. In Bath-Balogh M, Fehrenbach MJ: *Illustrated dental embryology, histology, and anatomy,* ed 3, St. Louis, 2011, Saunders.

FIGURE 2-22 **Palate (inferior view)**

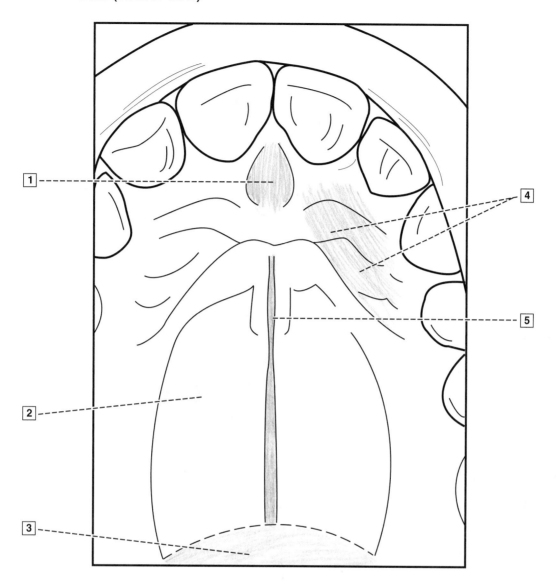

1 Incisive papilla
2 Hard palate
3 Soft palate
4 Palatine rugae
5 Median palatine raphe

REVIEW QUESTIONS

Fill in the blanks by choosing the appropriate terms from the list below.

1. At the anterior part of the inferior surface of the skull is the _____, which is bordered by the alveolar process of the maxilla with its maxillary teeth.

2. The hard palate is formed by the two palatine processes of the maxillae anteriorly and the two horizontal plates of the _____ posteriorly.

3. The articulation between the maxillae and palatine bones on the hard palate is noted by the prominent _____.

4. The median palatine suture is clinically noted as the _____.

5. The transverse palatine suture is an articulation between the two palatine processes of the _____ and the two horizontal plates of the palatine bones.

6. The hard palate forms the floor of the _____ as well as the roof of the mouth.

7. The posterior edge of the hard palate forms the inferior border of two funnel-shaped cavities, the _____, or *choanae,* which are the posterior openings of the nasal cavity.

8. The superior border of each posterior nasal aperture is formed by the vomer and the _____.

9. The posterior edge of the _____ forms the medial border of the posterior nasal apertures.

10. Near the superior border of each posterior nasal aperture is a small canal, the _____, which extends to open into the pterygopalatine fossa and carries the pterygoid nerve and blood vessels.

palatine bones	posterior nasal apertures	maxillae
pterygoid canal	hard palate	nasal cavity
vomer	median palatine raphe	sphenoid bone
median palatine suture		

Reference

Chapter 3, Skeletal system. In Fehrenbach MJ, Herring SW: *Illustrated anatomy of the head and neck,* ed 4, St. Louis, 2012, Saunders.

FIGURE 2-23 Palatal and nasal cavity development during prenatal development (sagittal sections)

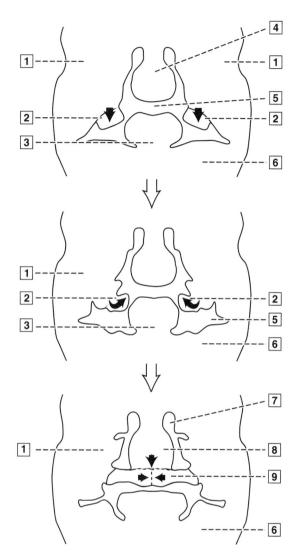

1 Maxillary process
2 Palatal shelf
3 Developing tongue
4 Developing nasal septum
5 Stomodeum

6 Developing mandible
7 Developing nasal cavity
8 Nasal septum
9 Fusing palate

REVIEW QUESTIONS

Fill in the blanks by choosing the appropriate terms from the list below.

1. The formation of the palate, initially in the embryo and later in the fetus, takes place over several weeks of _____.

2. During the _____ week of prenatal development, still within the embryonic period, the intermaxillary segment is formed.

3. The intermaxillary segment arises as a result of fusion of the two _____ within the embryo.

4. The _____ is an internal wedge-shaped mass that extends inferiorly and deep to the nasal pits on the inside of the stomodeum.

5. The intermaxillary segment will develop into the floor of the _____ and the nasal septum.

6. The intermaxillary segment gives rise to the _____, or *primitive palate*.

7. The primary palate serves only as a partial separation between the developing _____ and nasal cavity.

8. In the future, the primary palate will form the premaxillary part of the _____, which is the anterior one third of the final palate.

9. The premaxillary part of the maxilla is a small part of the _____, which is anterior to the incisive foramen and will contain certain maxillary teeth, the incisors.

10. The formation of the primary palate completes the _____ stage of palate development.

oral cavity proper	prenatal development	primary palate
fifth	intermaxillary segment	first
nasal cavity	medial nasal processes	hard palate
maxilla		

Reference

Chapter 5, Development of orofacial structures. In Bath-Balogh M, Fehrenbach MJ: *Illustrated dental embryology, histology, and anatomy,* ed 3, St. Louis, 2011, Saunders.

FIGURE 2-24 Palatal and nasal cavity development during prenatal development (inferior views)

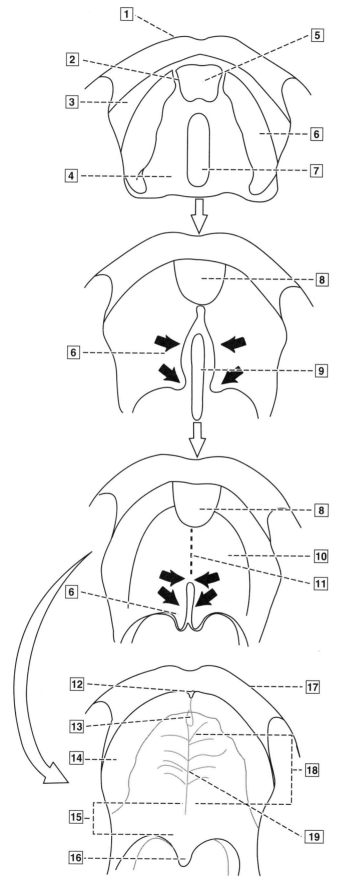

1	Developing upper lip
2	Site of future fusion
3	Developing maxillary alveolar process
4	Developing nasal cavity
5	Intermaxillary segment
6	Palatal shelf
7	Developing nasal septum
8	Primary palate
9	Nasal septum
10	Secondary palate
11	Median palatine suture
12	Labial frenum
13	Incisive papilla
14	Gingiva covering maxillary process
15	Soft palate
16	Uvula
17	Upper lip
18	Hard palate
19	Median palatine raphe

REVIEW QUESTIONS

Fill in the blanks by choosing the appropriate terms from the list below.

1.   The completion of the final palate involves the _____ of swellings, which involve tissue from different surfaces of the embryo meeting and joining, similar to that of the neural tube.

2.   During the sixth week of prenatal development, within the embryonic period, the bilateral maxillary processes give rise to two _____.

3.   The palatal shelves grow inferiorly and deep on the inside of the stomodeum in a vertical direction, along both sides of the developing _____, which will later move anteriorly and inferiorly out of the way of the growing palatal shelves.

4.   The palatal shelves will later move into a horizontal position, now superior to the developing tongue and then the two palatal shelves elongate and move medially toward each other, meeting and joining, and fusing to form the _____; the formation of this structure completes the second stage of palatal development.

5.   The secondary palate will give rise to the posterior two thirds of the hard palate, which contains certain _____ anterior teeth (canines) and posterior teeth, posterior to the incisive foramen, as well as the soft palate and its uvula.

6.   The _____ within the mucosa and the deeper median palatine suture on the adult bone of the hard palate indicate the fusion of the palatal shelves.

7.   To complete the final stage of palatal development, the posterior part of the primary palate meets the secondary palate, and these structures gradually fuse in an anterior to posterior direction; the three processes completely fuse, forming the final palate, having both hard and soft parts, during the _____ of prenatal development.

8.   The future nasal septum of the nasal cavity is also developing when the palate is forming from a growth from the fused _____, similar to the primary palate.

9.   The tissue types that form the nasal septum will grow inferiorly and deep to the medial nasal processes and superior to the _____.

10.   The vertical nasal septum fuses with the horizontally oriented final palate after it forms; this fusion begins in the _____ week and is completed by the twelfth week resulting in the paired nasal cavity and the single oral cavity in the fetus becoming completely separate.

median palatine raphe	stomodeum	tongue
maxillary	fusion	medial nasal processes
secondary palate	twelfth week	ninth
palatal shelves		

Reference

Chapter 5, Development of orofacial structures. In Bath-Balogh M, Fehrenbach MJ: *Illustrated dental embryology, histology, and anatomy,* ed 3, St. Louis, 2011, Saunders.

ANSWER KEY   1. fusion, 2. palatal shelves, 3. tongue, 4. secondary palate, 5. maxillary, 6. median palatine raphe, 7. twelfth week, 8. medial nasal processes, 9. stomodeum, 10. ninth.

FIGURE 2-25   Oral region: tongue (lateral view)

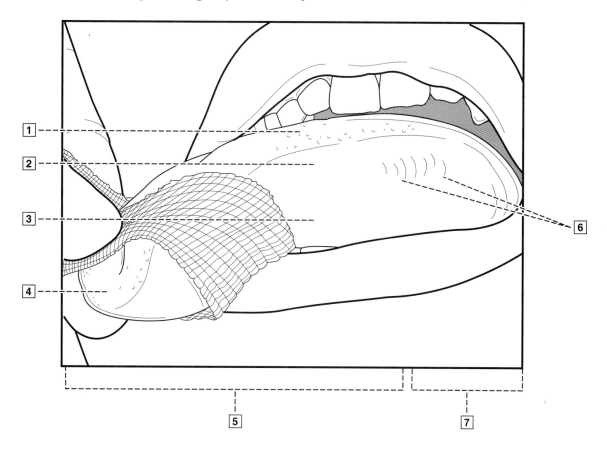

1 Dorsal surface	**5** Body
2 Lateral surface	**6** Foliate lingual papillae
3 Ventral surface	**7** Base
4 Apex	

REVIEW QUESTIONS

Fill in the blanks by choosing the appropriate terms from the list below.

1. The _____ is a prominent feature of the oral region, with its posterior third considered its base or pharyngeal part.

2. The _____ attaches to the floor of the mouth.

3. The base of the tongue does not lie within the oral cavity but within the oral part of the _____.

4. The anterior two thirds of the tongue is termed the _____.

5. The body of the tongue is considered its oral part since it lies within the _____.

6. The tip of the tongue is the _____.

7. Certain surfaces of the tongue have small elevated structures of specialized mucosa, the _____, some of which are associated with taste buds; they consist of small, discrete structures or appendages of keratinized epithelium, with both orthokeratinized and parakeratinized epithelium present overlying a lamina propria core.

8. The side or lateral surface of the tongue is noted for its vertical ridges, the _____, which consist of leaf-shaped structures of orthokeratinized or parakeratinized epithelium that contain taste buds overlying a lamina propria core.

9. The top surface of the tongue is considered the _____.

10. The underside of the tongue is considered the _____.

oral cavity	base of the tongue	apex of the tongue
pharynx	tongue	lingual papillae
ventral surface	body of the tongue	dorsal surface
foliate lingual papillae		

References

Chapter 2, Surface anatomy. In Fehrenbach MJ, Herring SW: *Illustrated anatomy of the head and neck,* ed 4, St. Louis, 2012, Saunders; and Chapter 2, Oral cavity and pharynx. In Bath-Balogh M, Fehrenbach MJ: *Illustrated dental embryology, histology, and anatomy,* ed 3, St. Louis, 2011, Saunders.

FIGURE 2-26 Oral region: tongue (dorsal surface and microanatomic views)

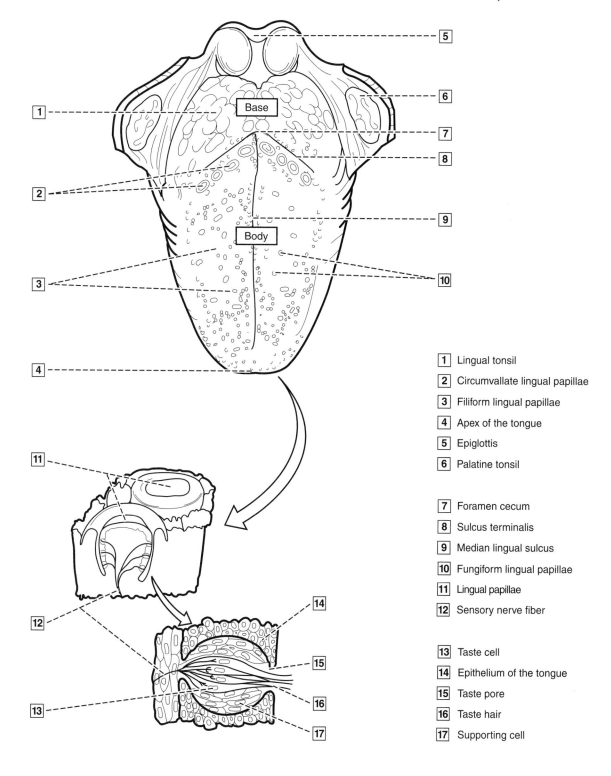

1	Lingual tonsil
2	Circumvallate lingual papillae
3	Filiform lingual papillae
4	Apex of the tongue
5	Epiglottis
6	Palatine tonsil
7	Foramen cecum
8	Sulcus terminalis
9	Median lingual sulcus
10	Fungiform lingual papillae
11	Lingual papillae
12	Sensory nerve fiber
13	Taste cell
14	Epithelium of the tongue
15	Taste pore
16	Taste hair
17	Supporting cell

REVIEW QUESTIONS

Fill in the blanks by choosing the appropriate terms from the list below.

1. The dorsal surface of the tongue has a midline depression, the _____, corresponding with the position of a midline fibrous structure deep within the tongue, the median septum.

2. The slender, threadlike lingual papillae shaped like fine-pointed cones are the _____, which give the dorsal surface of the tongue its velvety texture; they consist of thick orthokeratinized or parakeratinized epithelium overlying a lamina propria core, with an increased amount of keratin on the surface.

3. The slightly raised, red, mushroom-shaped dots are the _____, which are more numerous on the apex; they consist of thin orthokeratinized or parakeratinized epithelium with taste buds overlying a highly vascularized lamina propria core.

4. Posteriorly on the dorsal surface of the tongue is a V-shaped groove, the _____, which separates the base of the tongue from the body of the tongue, and where a small, pitlike depression, the foramen cecum, is located.

5. The _____ line up along the anterior side of the sulcus terminalis; these large, mushroom-shaped structures consist of orthokeratinized or parakeratinized epithelium with hundreds of taste buds that overlie a lamina propria core and are surrounded by a circular trough.

6. The _____ are present in the submucosa deep to the lamina propria of the circumvallate lingual papillae; these minor serous salivary glands flush the trough surrounding the circumvallate lingual papillae.

7. The _____ are barrel-shaped organs of taste derived from the epithelium and composed of spindle-shaped cells that extend from the basement membrane to the epithelial surface of the lingual papilla.

8. The supporting cells support the taste bud and are usually located on the outer part of the taste bud; in contrast, the _____ are usually located in the central part of the taste bud.

9. The taste cells have superficial taste receptors that are responsible for making contact with dissolved molecules of food at the _____ and producing a taste sensation.

10. At the most posterior surface of the tongue base on each side is an irregular mass of lymphoid tissue, the _____.

fungiform lingual papillae	**circumvallate lingual papillae**	**taste buds**
lingual tonsil	**median lingual sulcus**	**taste cells**
sulcus terminalis	**filiform lingual papillae**	**taste pore**
von Ebner salivary glands		

References

Chapter 2, Surface anatomy. In Fehrenbach MJ, Herring SW: *Illustrated anatomy of the head and neck,* ed 4, St. Louis, 2012, Saunders; and Chapter 9, Oral mucosa. In Bath-Balogh M, Fehrenbach MJ: *Illustrated dental embryology, histology, and anatomy,* ed 3, St. Louis, 2011, Saunders.

FIGURE 2-27 Tongue development during prenatal development

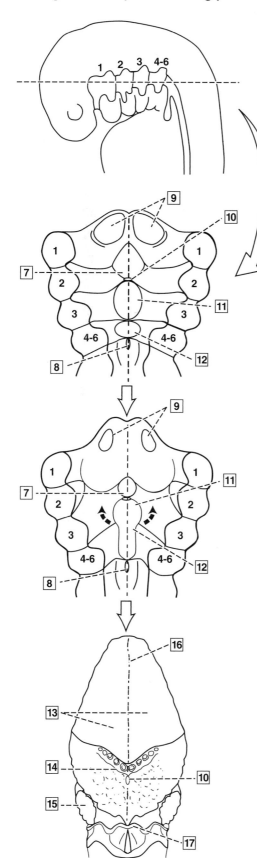

7   Tuberculum impar

8   Laryngeal orifice

9   Lateral lingual swellings

10   Foramen cecum

11   Copula

12   Epiglottic swelling

13   Body of the tongue

14   Sulcus terminalis

15   Palatine tonsil

16   Median lingual sulcus

17   Epiglottis

REVIEW QUESTIONS

Fill in the blanks by choosing the appropriate terms from the list below.

1. The tongue develops during the fourth to eighth weeks of prenatal development from independent swellings located internally on the floor of the primitive pharynx, formed from the first four

   _____.

2. The _____ develops from the first branchial arch, and the base of the tongue originates later from the second, third, and fourth branchial arches.

3. During the fourth week of prenatal development, within the embryonic period, the tongue begins its development as a triangular median swelling, the _____, which is located in the midline on the floor of the primitive pharynx, within the conjoined nasal and oral cavities of the embryo.

4. Later, two oval _____ develop and merge with each other on each side of the tuberculum impar, which are from the growth of the first branchial arch, or *mandibular arch*.

5. Then, the two fused lateral lingual swellings overgrow and encompass the disappearing tuberculum impar to form the anterior two thirds, or body, of the tongue, which lies within the oral cavity proper; the _____ is a superficial demarcation of the fusion of lateral lingual swellings.

6. Around the lingual swellings, the cells degenerate, forming a sulcus, which frees the body of the tongue from the floor of the mouth, except for the attachment of the midline _____.

7. Immediately posterior to these fused anterior swellings, a pair of swellings, the _____, is formed from the fusion of mainly the third and parts of the fourth branchial arch; it gradually overgrows the second branchial arch, or *hyoid arch,* to form the base of the tongue, or posterior one third.

8. Even farther posterior to the copula is the projection of a third median swelling, the _____, which develops from the fourth branchial arches.

9. As the tongue develops still further, the copula of the tongue base, after overgrowing the second branchial arch, merges with the anterior swellings of the first branchial arch of the tongue body during the eighth week of prenatal development, which has its fusion superficially demarcated by the

   _____.

10. The sulcus terminalis points backward toward the oropharynx at a small pitlike depression, the _____, which is the beginning of the thyroglossal duct, where the origin of the thyroid gland is located as well as its pathway showing the migration of the thyroid gland into the neck region.

copula	sulcus terminalis	branchial arches
median lingual sulcus	tuberculum impar	epiglottic swelling
lingual frenum	lateral lingual swellings	foramen cecum
body of the tongue		

Reference

Chapter 5, Development of orofacial structures. In Bath-Balogh M, Fehrenbach MJ: *Illustrated dental embryology, histology, and anatomy,* ed 3, St. Louis, 2011, Saunders.

FIGURE 2-28 Oral region: tongue (ventral surface)

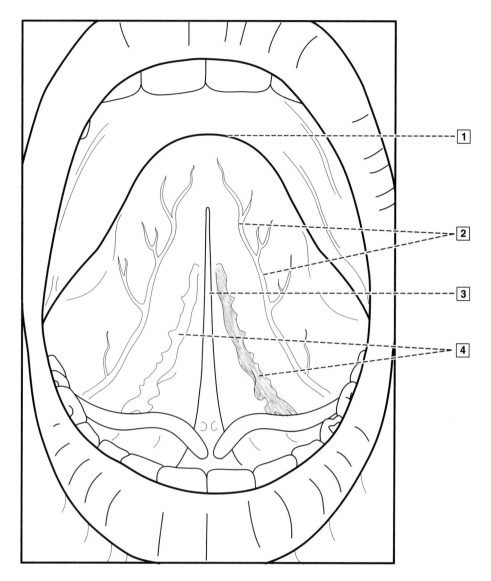

1 Apex

2 Deep lingual veins

3 Lingual frenum

4 Plicae fimbriatae

REVIEW QUESTIONS

Fill in the blanks by choosing the appropriate terms from the list below.

1.   The underside of the tongue is considered the ___ventral surface___

2.   The ventral surface of the tongue is noted for its visibly large blood vessels, the deeper ___lingual vein___, running close to the surface.

3.   Lateral to the deep lingual veins on each side of the tongue is the ___plica fimbriata___, a fold with fringelike projections.

4.   Having the patient slightly lift the ___apex of the tongue___ allows visualization of the ventral surface of the tongue.

5.   The patient should gently touch the surface of the ___hard palate___ with the apex of the tongue, to visualize fully the underside of the tongue.

<table>
<tr><td>hard palate</td><td>lingual veins</td></tr>
<tr><td>apex of the tongue</td><td>ventral surface of the tongue</td></tr>
<tr><td>plica fimbriata</td><td></td></tr>
</table>

References

Chapter 2, Surface anatomy. In Fehrenbach MJ, Herring SW: *Illustrated anatomy of the head and neck,* ed 4, St. Louis, 2012, Saunders; and Chapter 2, Oral cavity and pharynx. In Bath-Balogh M, Fehrenbach MJ: *Illustrated dental embryology, histology, and anatomy,* ed 3, St. Louis, 2011, Saunders.

FIGURE 2-29   Oral region: floor of the mouth (superior view)

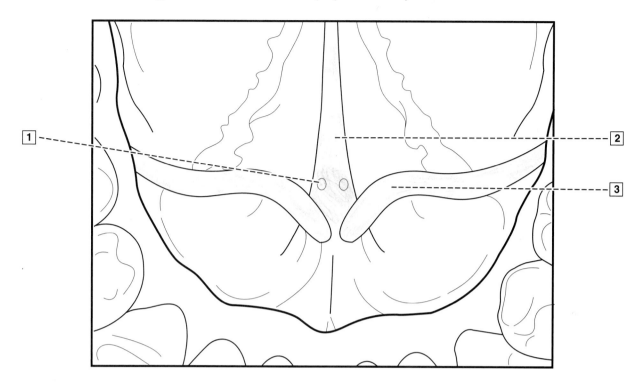

1 Sublingual caruncle
2 Lingual frenum
3 Sublingual fold

REVIEW QUESTIONS

Fill in the blanks by choosing the appropriate terms from the list below.

1. The _____ is located inferior to the ventral surface of the tongue.

2. The _____ is a midline fold of tissue between the ventral surface of the tongue and the floor of the mouth.

3. A ridge of tissue exists on each side of the floor of the mouth, the _____, which contains duct openings from the sublingual salivary gland.

4. Together the sublingual folds are arranged in a V-shaped configuration from the lingual frenum to the _____.

5. The small papilla, the _____, at the anterior end of each sublingual fold contains the duct openings from both the submandibular and sublingual salivary glands.

base of the tongue	lingual frenum
sublingual caruncle	floor of the mouth
sublingual fold	

References

Chapter 2, Surface anatomy. In Fehrenbach MJ, Herring SW: *Illustrated anatomy of the head and neck,* ed 4, St. Louis, 2012, Saunders; and Chapter 2, Oral cavity and pharynx. In Bath-Balogh M, Fehrenbach MJ: *Illustrated dental embryology, histology, and anatomy,* ed 3, St. Louis, 2011, Saunders.

FIGURE 2-30 Pharynx and associated anatomy (midsagittal section)

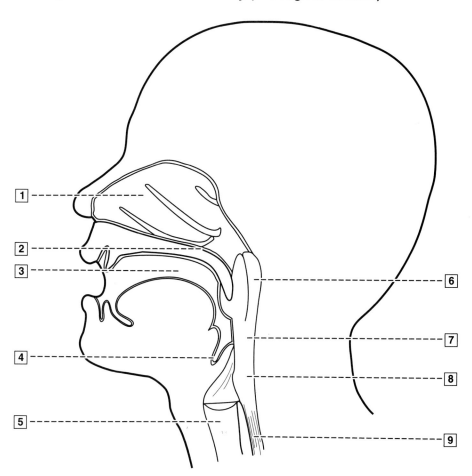

1	Nasal cavity	**6**	Nasopharynx
2	Soft palate	**7**	Oropharynx
3	Oral cavity	**8**	Laryngopharynx
4	Epiglottis	**9**	Esophagus
5	Larynx		

REVIEW QUESTIONS

Fill in the blanks by choosing the appropriate terms from the list below.

1. The oral cavity also provides the entrance into the _____, or *throat*.

2. The pharynx is a muscular tube that serves both the respiratory and digestive systems and consists of _____ parts: the nasopharynx, oropharynx, and laryngopharynx.

3. The _____ is the part of the pharynx that located more inferior than the other parts as well as being close to the laryngeal opening.

4. The part of the pharynx that is superior to the level of the soft palate is the _____, which is also continuous with the nasal cavity.

5. The part of the pharynx that is between the soft palate and the opening of the larynx is the _____.

nasopharynx	**oropharynx**
laryngopharynx	**pharynx**
three	

References

Chapter 2, Surface anatomy. In Fehrenbach MJ, Herring SW: *Illustrated anatomy of the head and neck,* ed 4, St. Louis, 2012, Saunders; and Chapter 2, Oral cavity and pharynx. In Bath-Balogh M, Fehrenbach MJ: *Illustrated dental embryology, histology, and anatomy,* ed 3, St. Louis, 2011, Saunders.

FIGURE 2-31 Oropharynx and associated anatomy (frontal view)

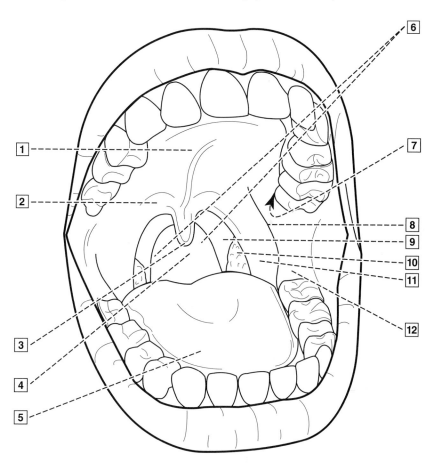

1	Hard palate	7	Maxillary tuberosity
2	Soft palate	8	Pterygomandibular fold
3	Uvula	9	Posterior faucial pillar
4	Posterior wall of pharynx	10	Palatine tonsil
5	Dorsal surface of tongue	11	Anterior faucial pillar
6	Fauces	12	Retromandibular pad

REVIEW QUESTIONS

Fill in the blanks by choosing the appropriate terms from the list below.

1. The part of the pharynx that is between the soft palate and the opening of the larynx is the

   _____.

2. Behind the base of the tongue and in front of the oropharynx is the _____, a flap of cartilage, which at rest is upright and allows air to pass through the larynx and into the rest of the respiratory system; during swallowing, it folds back to cover the entrance to the larynx, preventing food and liquid from entering the trachea and then entering the lungs.

3. The opening from the oral region into the oropharynx is the _____.

4. The fauces are formed laterally on each side of the oral cavity by both the _____ and the posterior faucial pillar.

5. The tonsillar tissue, the _____, is located between each set of faucial pillars or folds of tissue created by underlying muscles.

oropharynx	fauces
anterior faucial pillar	epiglottis
palatine tonsils	

References

Chapter 2, Surface anatomy. In Fehrenbach MJ, Herring SW: *Illustrated anatomy of the head and neck,* ed 4, St. Louis, 2012, Saunders; and Chapter 2, Oral cavity and pharynx. In Bath-Balogh M, Fehrenbach MJ: *Illustrated dental embryology, histology, and anatomy,* ed 3, St. Louis, 2011, Saunders.

FIGURE 2-32 Regions of neck: landmarks and triangles

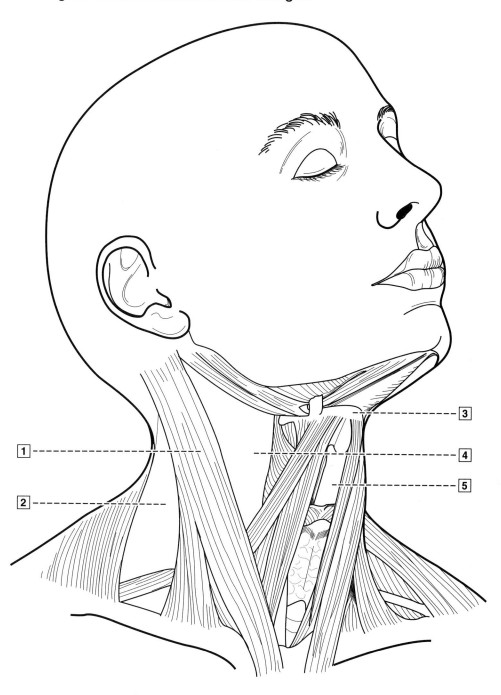

1 Sternocleidomastoid muscle

2 Posterior cervical triangle

3 Hyoid bone

4 Anterior cervical triangle

5 Thyroid cartilage

REVIEW QUESTIONS

Fill in the blanks by choosing the appropriate terms from the list below.

1. The _____ extends from the skull and mandible down to the clavicles and sternum.

2. The large strap muscle, the _____, divides each side of the neck diagonally into an anterior cervical triangle and posterior cervical triangle.

3. The anterior region of the neck corresponds with the two _____, which are separated by a midline; major structures that pass between the head and thorax can be accessed through this triangle.

4. The lateral region of the neck, posterior to the sternocleidomastoid muscle, is considered the _____ on each side.

5. At the anterior midline, the largest of the larynx's cartilages, the _____, is visible as the laryngeal prominence, or *Adam's apple*.

6. The thyroid cartilage is superior to the _____.

7. The _____ of the thyroid cartilage is just superior to the laryngeal prominence.

8. The vocal cords, or ligaments of the _____ or voice box, are attached to the posterior surface of the thyroid cartilage.

9. The _____ is located in the anterior midline and suspended in the neck, superior to the thyroid cartilage.

10. Many _____ attach to the hyoid bone, which controls the position of the base of the tongue.

larynx	hyoid bone	posterior cervical triangle
thyroid cartilage	superior thyroid notch	neck
anterior cervical triangles	thyroid gland	muscles
sternocleidomastoid muscle		

References

Chapter 2, Surface anatomy. In Fehrenbach MJ, Herring SW: *Illustrated anatomy of the head and neck,* ed 4, St. Louis, 2012, Saunders; and Chapter 1, Face and neck regions. In Bath-Balogh M, Fehrenbach MJ: *Illustrated dental embryology, histology, and anatomy,* ed 3, St. Louis, 2011, Saunders.

FIGURE 2-33 Regions of neck: anterior cervical triangle landmarks

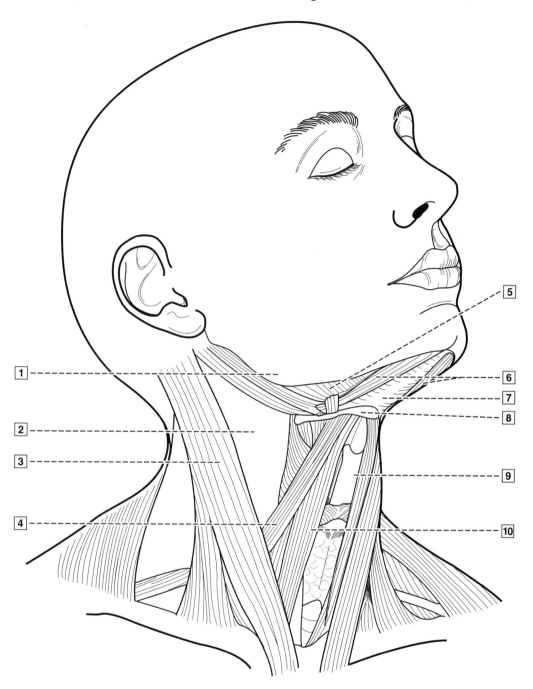

1	Mandible	**6**	Digastric muscles
2	Carotid triangle	**7**	Submental triangle
3	Sternocleidomastoid muscle	**8**	Hyoid bone
4	Omohyoid muscle	**9**	Thyroid cartilage
5	Submandibular triangle	**10**	Muscular triangle

REVIEW QUESTIONS

Fill in the blanks by choosing the appropriate terms from the list below.

1. The _____ is a region of the neck on each side can be further subdivided into smaller triangular regions by muscles in the area but that are not as prominent as those of the sternocleidomastoid muscle.

2. The superior part of each anterior cervical triangle is demarcated by the main parts of both the bellies: the digastric muscle and the mandible, forming the _____ as a region of the neck.

3. The inferior part of each anterior cervical triangle is further subdivided by the omohyoid muscle into the _____, a region of the neck that is superior to the muscle.

4. The inferior part of each anterior cervical triangle is further subdivided by the omohyoid muscle into the _____, a region of the neck that is inferior to the muscle.

5. A midline triangle, the _____, a region of the neck is formed by the two main parts of the digastric muscle (its right and left anterior bellies) and the hyoid bone.

submandibular triangle

anterior cervical triangle

submental triangle

carotid triangle

muscular triangle

References

Chapter 2, Surface anatomy. In Fehrenbach MJ, Herring SW: *Illustrated anatomy of the head and neck,* ed 4, St. Louis, 2012, Saunders; and Chapter 1, Face and neck regions. In Bath-Balogh M, Fehrenbach MJ: *Illustrated dental embryology, histology, and anatomy,* ed 3, St. Louis, 2011, Saunders.

FIGURE 2-34 Regions of neck: posterior cervical triangle landmarks

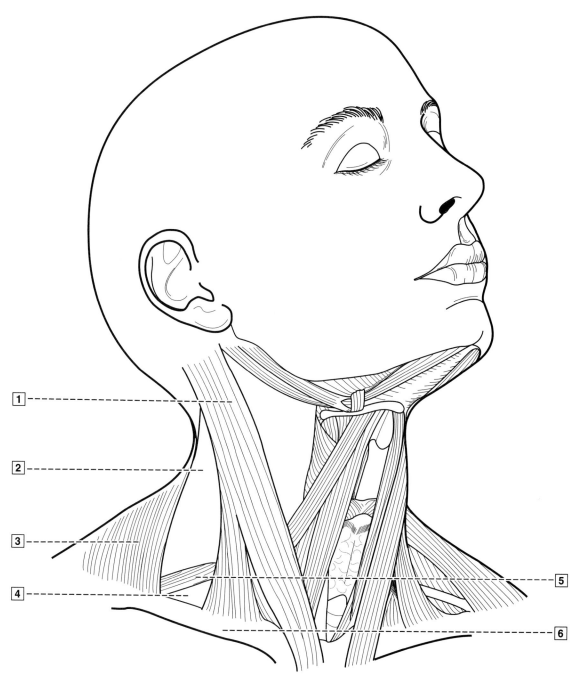

| 1 | Sternocleidomastoid muscle | 3 | Trapezius muscle | 5 | Omohyoid muscle |
| 2 | Occipital triangle | 4 | Subclavian triangle | 6 | Clavicle |

REVIEW QUESTIONS

Fill in the blanks by choosing the appropriate terms from the list below.

1. Each _____ is a region of the neck that can be further subdivided into smaller triangular regions on each side by muscles in the area.

2. The omohyoid muscle divides the posterior cervical triangle into the _____, a region of the neck that is superior to the muscle on each side.

3. The omohyoid muscle divides the posterior cervical triangle into the _____, a region of the neck that is inferior to the muscle on each side but superior to the clavicle.

4. The _____ is a region of the neck that adjoins the medial aspect of the occipital triangle.

5. The _____ is a region of the neck that adjoins the lateral aspect of the occipital triangle.

occipital triangle   posterior cervical triangle

sternocleidomastoid muscle   subclavian triangle

trapezius muscle

Reference

Chapter 2, Surface anatomy. In Fehrenbach MJ, Herring SW: *Illustrated anatomy of the head and neck,* ed 4, St. Louis, 2012, Saunders; and Chapter 1, Face and neck regions. In Bath-Balogh M, Fehrenbach MJ: *Illustrated dental embryology, histology, and anatomy,* ed 3, St. Louis, 2011, Saunders.

FIGURE 3-1 Stages of tooth development

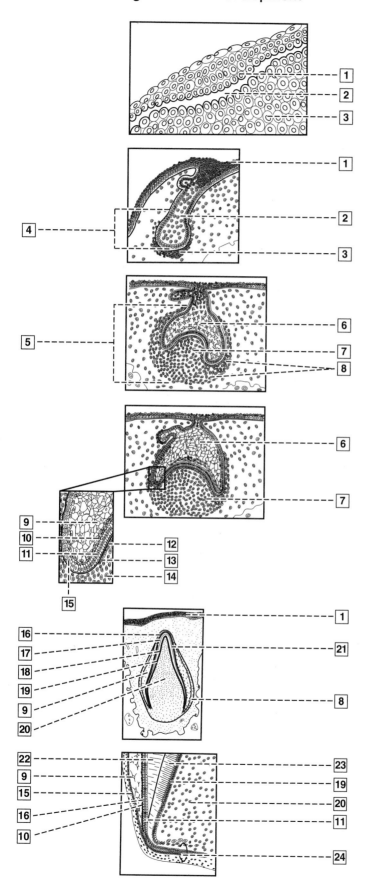

Initiation and bud stages

1 Oral epithelium

2 Dental lamina

3 Ectomesenchyme

4 Tooth bud

Cap stage

5 Tooth germ

6 Enamel organ

7 Dental papilla

8 Dental sac

Bell stage

9 Stellate reticulum

10 Stratum intermedium

11 Inner enamel epithelium

12 Basement membrane

13 Outer cells of the dental papilla

14 Central cells of the dental papilla

15 Outer enamel epithelium

Apposition stage

16 Ameloblasts

17 Enamel matrix

18 Dentin matrix

19 Odontoblasts

20 Pulp

21 Dentinoenamel junction

Maturation stage

22 Enamel

23 Dentin

24 Hertwig's epithelial root sheath

REVIEW QUESTIONS

Fill in the blanks by choosing the appropriate terms from the list below.

1. The first stage of tooth development is the _____ stage that begins for the primary dentition between the sixth and seventh week of prenatal development.

2. During the second stage of tooth development that occurs during at the beginning of the eighth week of prenatal development for the primary dentition, there is extensive proliferation of the dental lamina into a(n) _____, one for each of the 20 primary teeth.

3. During the third stage of tooth development that occurs during the ninth and tenth week of prenatal development for the primary dentition, formation of the tooth germ occurs with the enamel organ creating a(n) _____ shape around the dental papilla as well as beneath the dental sac.

4. The _____ stage of tooth development occurs between the eleventh and twelfth week of prenatal development for the primary dentition.

5. During the fourth stage of tooth development, the enamel organ differentiates into many layers, one of which is the _____ that will later become enamel-secreting cells or ameloblasts.

6. Within the concavity of the differentiating enamel organ, the _____ undergoes extensive differentiation during the fourth week of prenatal development to later become dentin-secreting cells, or odontoblasts.

7. Each hard dental tissue of the mature tooth is initially secreted as a partially mineralized matrix during the stage of _____, thus serving as a framework that will later undergo maturation when each tissue is mineralized to its fullest extent.

8. The first cells to undergo repolarization near the basement membrane in the developing tooth germ are the _____, which then will induce the outer cells of the dental papilla to become odontoblasts.

9. The first cells to start their secretory activity near the basement membrane after repolarization to produce predentin are the _____, thus obtaining a thicker layer of predentin than enamel matrix at any location during the apposition stage of tooth development.

10. The cervical loop, composed only of inner and outer enamel epithelium, begins to grow deeper after forming, moving away from the newly completed crown area to enclose more of the dental papilla so as to produce the _____, which functions to shape the root(s) by inducing dentin formation.

apposition	bell	cap
inner enamel epithelium	Hertwig epithelial root sheath	preameloblasts
initiation	outer cells of the dental papilla	bud
odontoblasts		

Reference

Chapter 6, Tooth development and eruption. In Bath-Balogh M, Fehrenbach MJ: *Illustrated dental embryology, histology, and anatomy,* ed 3, St. Louis, 2011, Saunders.

ANSWER KEY 1. initiation, 2. bud, 3. cap, 4. bell, 5. inner enamel epithelium, 6. outer cells of the dental papilla, 7. apposition, 8. preameloblasts, 9. odontoblasts, 10. Hertwig epithelial root sheath.

FIGURE 3-2 Primary and adult crown, root(s), and clinical view (anterior teeth: labial view; posterior teeth: mesial view)

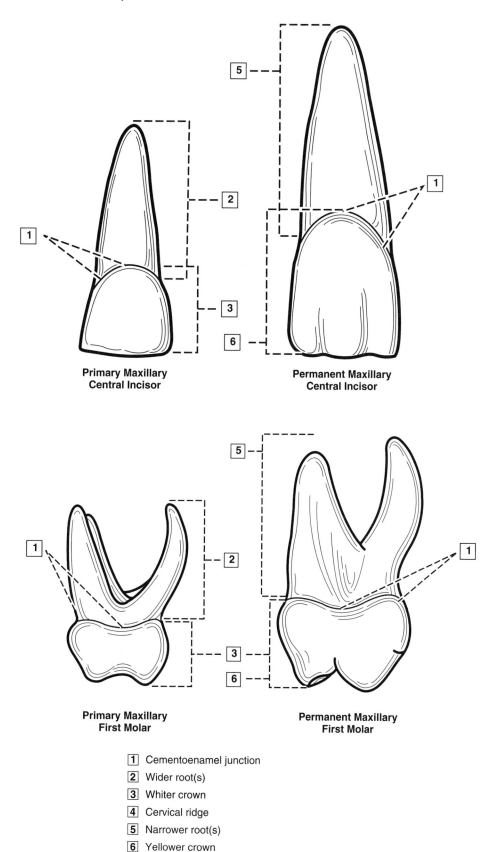

Primary Maxillary Central Incisor

Permanent Maxillary Central Incisor

Primary Maxillary First Molar

Permanent Maxillary First Molar

1 Cementoenamel junction
2 Wider root(s)
3 Whiter crown
4 Cervical ridge
5 Narrower root(s)
6 Yellower crown

REVIEW QUESTIONS

Fill in the blanks by choosing the appropriate terms from the list below.

1. Primary teeth have a whiter color of the _____ that can be noted clinically, with permanent teeth being more yellow in that part of the tooth because of increased opacity of the enamel that covers the underlying yellow dentin.

2. Primary teeth have an overall smaller _____, with permanent teeth being larger; however, this does not mean the primary teeth are less important to overall oral health than permanent teeth.

3. The crowns of primary teeth are more constricted, or narrower, at the _____, making them appear bulbous in comparison to the thinness of the necks of the teeth.

4. Primary teeth have a prominent _____ that is present on both the labial and lingual surfaces of anterior teeth and on the buccal surfaces of molars, even more so than any similar structure on the even larger permanent molars.

5. Primary teeth have narrower _____, which are longer than the crown length, with partial resorption possibly noted radiographically as the teeth begin to shed or exfoliate.

6. Each crown-to-root _____ of primary teeth is smaller than those of their permanent dentition counterparts.

7. The cavity of the _____ on primary teeth shows that the chambers and horns are relatively large in proportion to those of the permanent teeth, especially the mesial pulpal horns of the molars.

8. Overall, the thickness of the _____ between the pulp chambers and the enamel is increased in primary teeth, especially in the primary mandibular second molar.

9. The _____ is relatively thin in primary teeth in comparison to the permanent counterparts, but it still has a consistent thickness overlying the dentin of the crown.

10. Within the primary dentition, certain _____ are present in the dentition of most children that allow for the proper alignment of the coming permanent dentition; these are mainly present between the primary maxillary lateral incisor and canine and also between the primary mandibular canine and first molar.

ratio	cementoenamel junction	crown
primate spaces	enamel	size
dentin	pulp	cervical ridge
roots		

Reference

Chapter 18, Primary dentition. In Bath-Balogh M, Fehrenbach MJ: *Illustrated dental embryology, histology, and anatomy,* ed 3, St. Louis, 2011, Saunders.

ANSWER KEY 1. crown, 2. size, 3. cementoenamel junction, 4. cervical ridge, 5. roots, 6. ratio, 7. pulp, 8. dentin, 9. enamel, 10. primate spaces.

FIGURE 3-3 Primary dentition eruption and shedding timeline

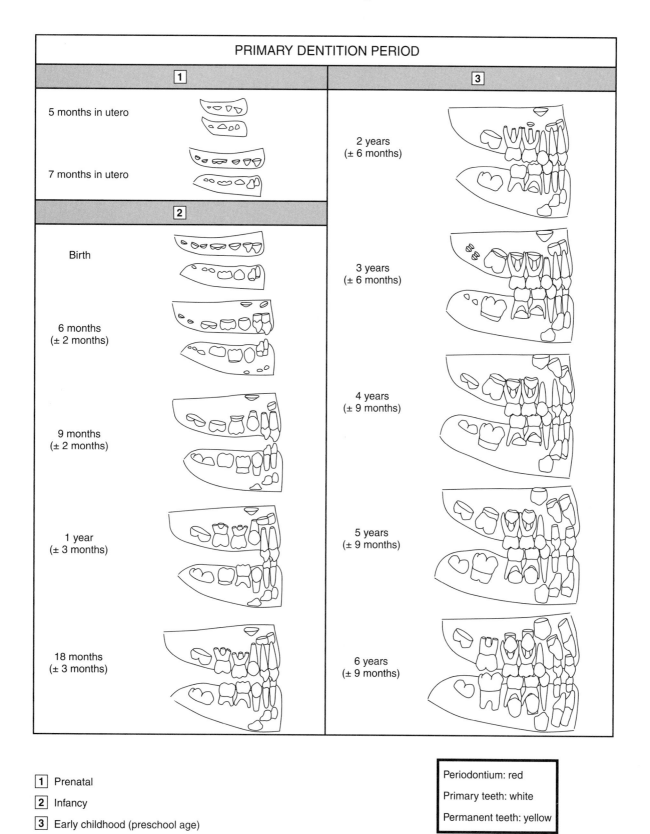

1 Prenatal

2 Infancy

3 Early childhood (preschool age)

Periodontium: red

Primary teeth: white

Permanent teeth: yellow

REVIEW QUESTIONS

Fill in the blanks by choosing the appropriate terms from the list below.

1. Although there are only two dentitions, there are three _____ throughout a person's lifetime because of the overlap of time between the dentitions.

2. Each oral cavity should be assigned a dentition period to allow for the most effective dental treatment for that period; this is especially important with the consideration of orthodontic therapy, because growth during certain dentition periods is maximized to allow expansion of both of the _____ and movement of the teeth within.

3. The first dentition period is the _____.

4. The primary dentition period begins with the eruption of the primary _____, which occurs between approximately 6 months and 6 years of age.

5. Only _____ are present in the dentition during the primary dentition period.

6. The primary dentition has its full _____ completed at 30 months.

7. The eruption of the primary teeth is usually completed when the primary _____ are in occlusion.

8. The jaws are beginning to grow during the primary dentition period to accommodate the larger _____.

9. The primary dentition period is a period that usually ends when the first permanent tooth erupts, the permanent _____.

10. The primary dentition period is followed by the _____.

jaws	mixed dentition period	permanent teeth
dentition periods	eruption	mandibular central incisor
primary teeth	primary dentition period	second molars
mandibular first molar		

References

Chapter 6, Tooth development and eruption and Chapter 15, Overview of the dentitions. In Bath-Balogh M, Fehrenbach MJ: *Illustrated dental embryology, histology, and anatomy,* ed 3, St. Louis, 2011, Saunders.

FIGURE 3-4   Permanent dentition eruption timeline

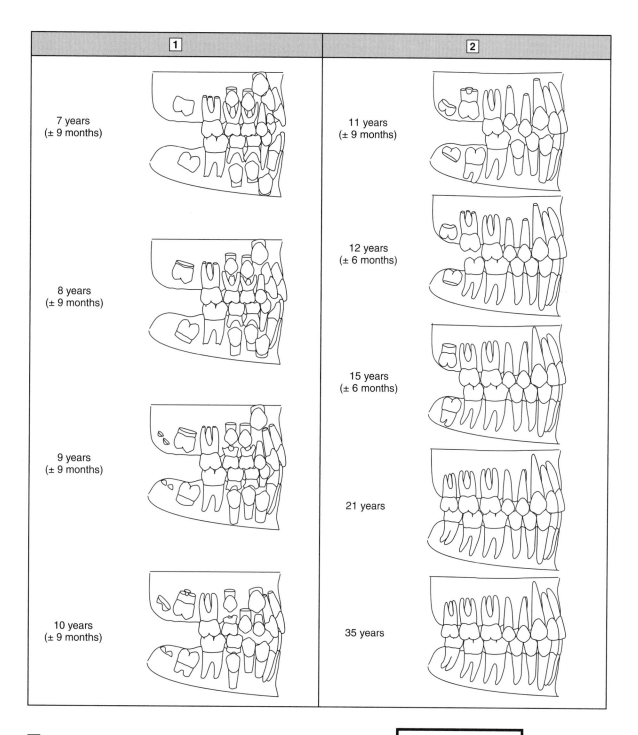

1	
7 years (± 9 months)	
8 years (± 9 months)	
9 years (± 9 months)	
10 years (± 9 months)	

2	
11 years (± 9 months)	
12 years (± 6 months)	
15 years (± 6 months)	
21 years	
35 years	

1 MIXED DENTITION PERIOD–Late childhood (school age)

2 PERMANENT DENTITION PERIOD–Adolescence and adulthood

Periodontium: red

Primary teeth: white

Permanent teeth: yellow

REVIEW QUESTIONS

Fill in the blanks by choosing the appropriate terms from the list below.

1. The _____ is a period that occurs between approximately 6 and 12 years of age with both primary and permanent teeth present, giving a possible "ugly duckling" appearance.

2. During the mixed dentition period, there is _____, or *exfoliation,* of the primary dentition, allowing for the tooth fairy to visit.

3. The mixed dentition period begins with the eruption of the first permanent tooth, the permanent _____, which is guided by the distal surface of the primary second molar.

4. During the mixed dentition period, there is _____ of the permanent teeth into the oral cavity after their crowns are completed.

5. Both _____ and permanent teeth are present during the transitional stage of the mixed dentition period.

6. The _____ differences between the primary and permanent teeth become apparent clinically during the mixed dentition period because of the fact that the permanent teeth have less overlying opaque enamel; thus the underlying yellow dentin is more visible.

7. The _____ is a period that begins with the shedding of the last primary tooth, which is approximately after 12 years of age, cutting off most of the tooth fairy visits.

8. During the permanent dentition period, there is little growth of the _____, given that puberty has passed, which contrasts with the mixed dentition period that has the fastest and most noticeable growth of the bone tissue, consistent with the onset of puberty.

9. When an oral cavity is unusually early or late regarding the usual sequential eruption of teeth, the _____ of the biological family should be reviewed for hereditary considerations.

10. The _____ are usually the only teeth present in the dentition during the permanent dentition period.

shedding	permanent dentition period	permanent teeth
primary teeth	mixed dentition period	mandibular first molar
color	eruption	jaws
dental history		

Reference

Chapter 6, Tooth development and eruption and Chapter 15, Overview of the dentitions. In Bath-Balogh M, Fehrenbach MJ: *Illustrated dental embryology, histology, and anatomy,* ed 3, St. Louis, 2011, Saunders.

FIGURE 3-5 Dental tissue and crown designations (anterior tooth: labiolingual section; posterior tooth: mesiodistal section)

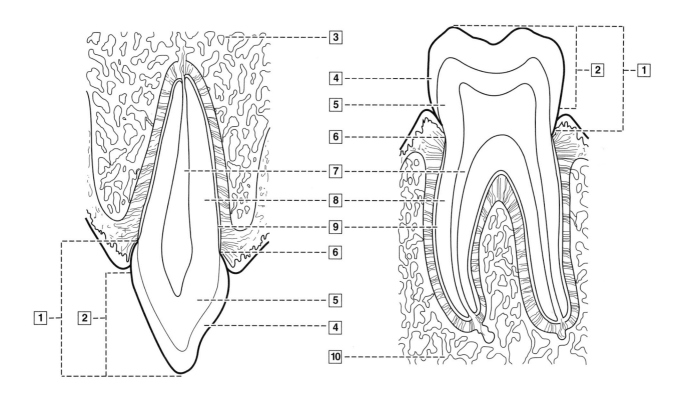

1	Anatomic crown	**6**	Cementoenamel junction (CEJ)
2	Clinical crown	**7**	Pulp cavity
3	Maxillary alveolar process	**8**	Dentin
4	Enamel	**9**	Cementum
5	Dentin	**10**	Mandibular alveolar process

REVIEW QUESTIONS

Fill in the blanks by choosing the appropriate terms from the list below.

1. Each root of a tooth consists of a(n) _____ with dentin covered by enamel, a constant throughout the life of the tooth, except for attrition and other physical wear.

2. Each root of a tooth within the jaw has dentin covered by _____.

3. The inner part of the _____ of both the crown and root of the tooth covers the innermost pulp cavity.

4. The _____ has a chamber and canal(s) with an apical foramen.

5. The _____ of the crown and cementum of the root usually meet close to the cementoenamel junction with three interfaces possibly present.

6. The _____ is an external line at the neck or cervix of the tooth and usually feels smooth or evenly grainy or possibly has a slight groove when explored.

7. The _____ of the upper jaw contains the roots of the maxillary teeth.

8. The _____ of the lower jaw contains the roots of the mandibular teeth.

9. The _____ is that part of the anatomic crown that is visible to the clinician when dental charting an oral cavity and thus not covered by gingiva.

10. The height of the clinical crown is determined by the location of the _____, or *free gingiva*, which can change over time due to gingival recession.

anatomic crown	maxillary alveolar process	cementum
pulp cavity	clinical crown	mandibular alveolar process
enamel	dentin	marginal gingiva
cementoenamel junction		

Reference

Chapter 15, Overview of the dentitions. In Fehrenbach MJ, Herring SW: *Illustrated anatomy of the head and neck,* ed 4, St. Louis, 2012, Saunders.

FIGURE 3-6 Enamel with enamel rods (cross section and longitudinal section with microanatomic views)

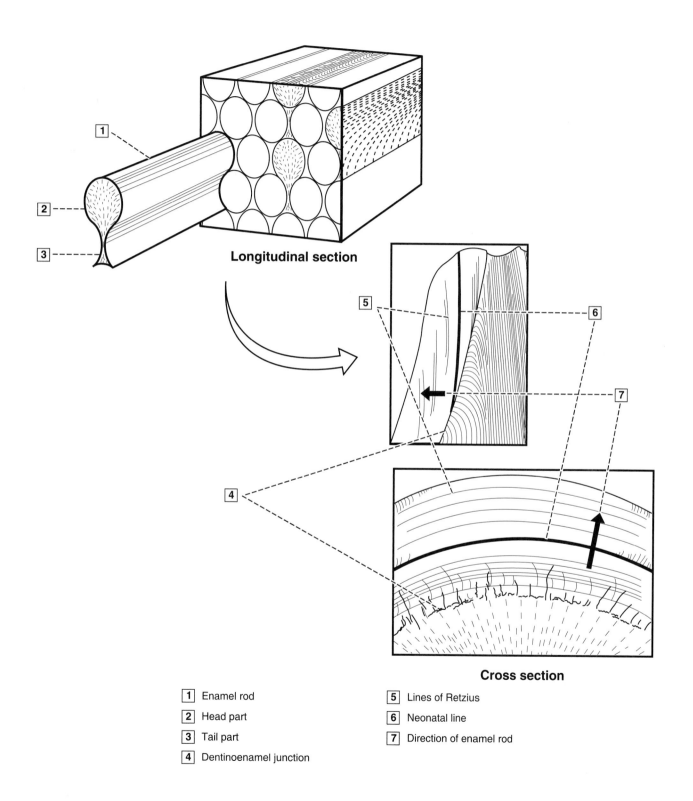

Longitudinal section

Cross section

1	Enamel rod	**5**	Lines of Retzius
2	Head part	**6**	Neonatal line
3	Tail part	**7**	Direction of enamel rod
4	Dentinoenamel junction		

REVIEW QUESTIONS

Fill in the blanks by choosing the appropriate terms from the list below.

1. Mature enamel is a highly mineralized or inorganic material, consisting of mainly

   _____.

2. The _____ is the crystalline structural unit of enamel; enamel is composed of millions of these unit structures.

3. Surrounding the outer part of each enamel rod is the _____, which appears different from the rod core on cross sections because of its different crystalline orientation.

4. The _____ appear as brown incremental lines in a stained section of mature enamel with different orientation depending on the sectioning of the tissue.

5. Associated with the lines of Retzius are the raised imbrication lines and grooves of the _____, which are noted clinically on the nonmasticatory surfaces of some teeth in the oral cavity, and which can be lost through tooth wear.

6. The _____ is a pronounced incremental line of Retzius, which marks the stress or trauma experienced by the ameloblasts during birth, illustrating the sensitivity of the ameloblasts as they form enamel matrix.

7. The _____ is a junction between mature enamel and dentin that appears scalloped on a cross section of a tooth, with the convex side toward the dentin, and the concave side toward the enamel.

8. The _____ are a microscopic feature of mature enamel and represent short dentinal tubules near the dentinoenamel junction that result from odontoblasts that crossed the basement membrane before it mineralized into the dentinoenamel junction.

9. The _____ are a microscopic feature that are noted as small, dark brushes with their bases near the dentinoenamel junction in the inner one third of enamel, representing areas of less mineralization.

10. The _____ are a microscopic feature that represent partially mineralized vertical sheets of enamel matrix that extend from the dentinoenamel junction near the tooth's cervix to the outer occlusal surface.

enamel rod	perikymata	enamel spindles
interprismatic region	neonatal line	dentinoenamel junction
enamel tufts	enamel lamellae	calcium hydroxyapatite
lines of Retzius		

Reference

Chapter 12, Enamel. In Bath-Balogh M, Fehrenbach MJ: *Illustrated dental embryology, histology, and anatomy,* ed 3, St. Louis, 2011, Saunders.

FIGURE 3-7 Development of enamel and dentin at the dentinoenamel junction

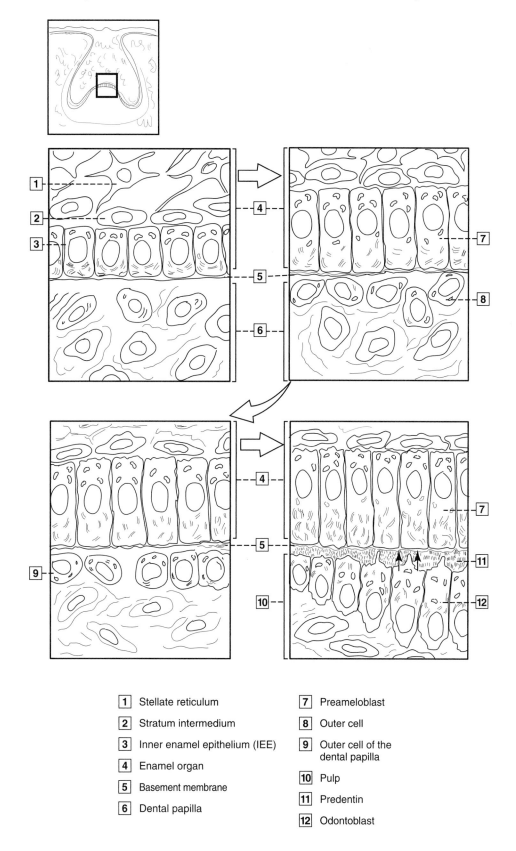

1 Stellate reticulum	**7** Preameloblast
2 Stratum intermedium	**8** Outer cell
3 Inner enamel epithelium (IEE)	**9** Outer cell of the dental papilla
4 Enamel organ	**10** Pulp
5 Basement membrane	**11** Predentin
6 Dental papilla	**12** Odontoblast

REVIEW QUESTIONS

Fill in the blanks by choosing the appropriate terms from the list below.

1. The outer cuboidal cells of the enamel organ are the _____, which will serve as a protective barrier for the rest of the enamel organ during enamel production during the bell stage.

2. Between the outer and inner enamel epithelium are the two innermost layers, the _____ and stratum intermedium.

3. One of the innermost layers of the enamel organ is the _____, which is made up of a compressed layer of flat to cuboidal cells.

4. After the formation of the _____ in the bell-shaped enamel organ, these innermost cells grow even more columnar, or elongate, as they differentiate into preameloblasts, which then will undergo repolarization.

5. In the future, the _____ will first induce dental papilla cells to differentiate into dentin-forming cells (odontoblasts) that then will differentiate into cells that secrete enamel (ameloblasts).

6. The dental papilla within the concavity of the enamel organ undergoes extensive differentiation so that it now consists of two types of tissue in layers, the _____ and central cells of the dental papilla.

7. The outer cells of the dental papilla are induced by the preameloblasts to differentiate into _____.

8. After the differentiation and repolarization, the odontoblasts now begin dentinogenesis, which is the apposition of _____ on their side of the basement membrane.

9. After the differentiation of odontoblasts from the outer cells of the dental papilla and their formation of predentin, the _____ between the preameloblasts and the odontoblasts disintegrates; this is the future dentinoenamel junction.

10. The _____ become, with further tooth development, the primordium of the pulp.

stellate reticulum	predentin	odontoblasts
preameloblasts	central cells of the dental papilla	stratum intermedium
outer cells of the dental papilla	inner enamel epithelium	basement membrane
outer enamel epithelium		

Reference

Chapter 6, Tooth development and eruption. In Bath-Balogh M, Fehrenbach MJ: *Illustrated dental embryology, histology, and anatomy,* ed 3, St. Louis, 2011, Saunders.

ANSWER KEY 1. outer enamel epithelium, 2. stellate reticulum, 3. stratum intermedium, 4. inner enamel epithelium, 5. preameloblasts, 6. outer cells of the dental papilla, 7. odontoblasts, 8. predentin, 9. basement membrane, 10. central cells of the dental papilla.

FIGURE 3-8 Apposition of enamel and dentin at the dentinoenamel junction

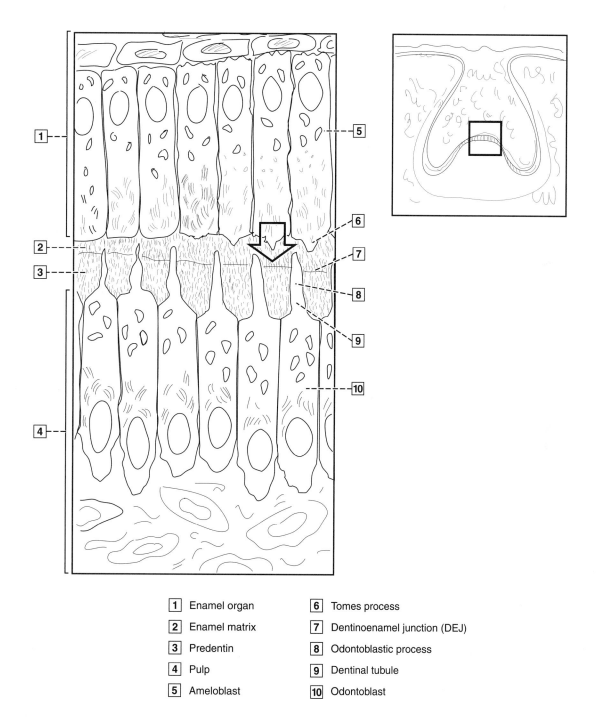

1 Enamel organ	**6** Tomes process
2 Enamel matrix	**7** Dentinoenamel junction (DEJ)
3 Predentin	**8** Odontoblastic process
4 Pulp	**9** Dentinal tubule
5 Ameloblast	**10** Odontoblast

REVIEW QUESTIONS

Fill in the blanks by choosing the appropriate terms from the list below.

1. The final stages of odontogenesis include the stage of _____, or *secretory stage*, during which the enamel, dentin, and cementum are secreted in successive layers.

2. The _____ is reached when the matrices of the hard dental tissue types subsequently fully mineralize.

3. The disintegration of the basement membrane allows the preameloblasts to contact the newly formed predentin, which induces the preameloblasts to differentiate into _____.

4. After differentiation, the ameloblasts begin amelogenesis, or the apposition of _____, laying it down on their side of the now-disintegrating basement membrane.

5. The enamel matrix is secreted from _____, an angled part of each ameloblast that faces the disintegrating basement membrane created as the ameloblasts move away from the dentin interface.

6. Continued apposition of both types of dental matrix becomes regular and rhythmic, as the cellular bodies of both the odontoblasts and ameloblasts retreat away from the _____, forming their perspective tissue types.

7. The odontoblasts, unlike the ameloblasts, will leave attached cellular extensions in the length of the predentin, the _____, as they move away from the newly formed dentinoenamel junction.

8. Each odontoblastic process is contained in a mineralized cylinder, the _____.

9. The cell bodies of _____ will remain within pulp attached by the odontoblastic processes after the apposition stage.

10. The cell bodies of the ameloblasts will be involved in the mineralization process but will be lost after _____ of the tooth into the oral cavity.

Tomes process	**dentinoenamel junction**	**odontoblasts**
apposition	**ameloblasts**	**eruption**
enamel matrix	**maturation stage**	**dentinal tubule**
odontoblastic processes		

Reference

Chapter 6, Tooth development and eruption. In Bath-Balogh M, Fehrenbach MJ: *Illustrated dental embryology, histology, and anatomy,* ed 3, St. Louis, 2011, Saunders.

FIGURE 3-9   Dentin (mesiodistal section with microanatomic view)

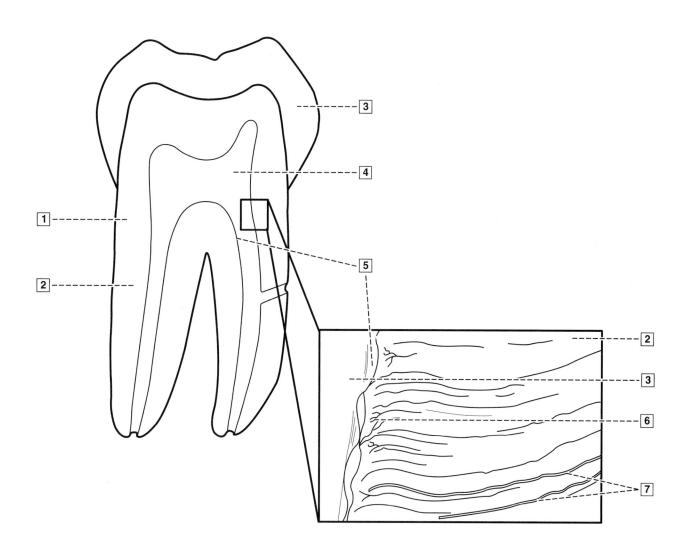

1	Mantle dentin	**5**	Dentinoenamel junction
2	Circumpulpal dentin	**6**	Odontoblastic processes
3	Enamel	**7**	Dentinal tubules
4	Pulp		

REVIEW QUESTIONS

Fill in the blanks by choosing the appropriate terms from the list below.

1. The _____ are long tubes in the dentin that extend from the dentinoenamel junction in the crown area, or dentinocemental junction in the root area, to the outer wall of the pulp and are filled with dentinal fluid.

2. The _____ is a long cellular extension located within the dentinal tubule that is still attached to the cell body of the odontoblast within the pulp.

3. Dentin that creates the wall of the dentinal tubule is the _____, which is highly mineralized after dentin maturation.

4. The dentin that is found between the tubules is the _____.

5. The _____ is the first predentin that forms and matures within the tooth.

6. Deep to the mantle dentin is the layer of dentin around the outer wall of pulp, the _____, which makes up the bulk of the dentin in a tooth.

7. The _____ is formed in a tooth before the completion of the apical foramen(s) of the root, which is the opening in the root's pulp canal and is characterized by its regular pattern of dentinal tubules.

8. The _____ is formed after the completion of the apical foramen(s), continues to form throughout the life of the tooth, and is formed more slowly than primary dentin.

9. The _____ are a microscopic feature that appear as incremental lines or bands that stain darkly in a section of dentin.

10. The _____ is a microscopic feature most often found in the peripheral part of dentin beneath the root's cementum, adjacent to the dentinocemental junction.

Tomes granular layer	circumpulpal dentin	secondary dentin
mantle dentin	odontoblastic process	peritubular dentin
dentinal tubules	imbrication lines of von Ebner	primary dentin
intertubular dentin		

Reference

Chapter 13, Dentin and pulp. In Bath-Balogh M, Fehrenbach MJ: *Illustrated dental embryology, histology, and anatomy,* ed 3, St. Louis, 2011, Saunders.

FIGURE 3-10 Pulp in primary and permanent teeth (mesiodistal section)

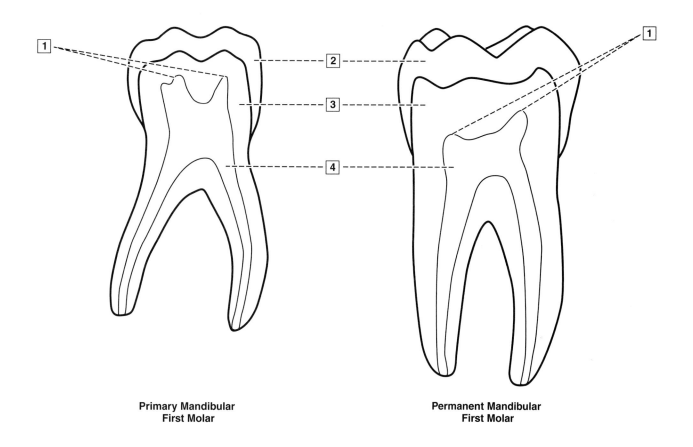

**Primary Mandibular
First Molar**

**Permanent Mandibular
First Molar**

1 Pulp horns

2 Enamel

3 Dentin

4 Pulp cavity

REVIEW QUESTIONS

Fill in the blanks by choosing the appropriate terms from the list below.

1. The _____ is the innermost tissue of the tooth and appears radiolucent (darker) because it is less dense than the radiopaque (or lighter) hard tissues of the tooth.

2. The pulp of a tooth is a(n) _____ with all the components of such a tissue such as fibroblasts, fibers, and intercellular substance.

3. The pulp forms from the _____ during tooth development for both dentitions.

4. The _____ on primary teeth shows that pulp chambers and pulp horns are relatively large in proportion to those of the permanent teeth.

5. The large mass of pulp is contained within the _____ of the tooth.

6. The pulp horns are especially prominent in the _____ dentition, under the buccal cusp of premolars and the mesiobuccal cusp of molars.

7. Smaller extensions of coronal pulp into the cusps of posterior teeth form the _____, which are at risk for exposure during restorative procedures.

8. Overall, the _____ of the primary dentition is thinner than that of the permanent counterparts; however, its thickness between the pulp chambers and the enamel is increased, especially in the primary mandibular second molar.

9. The _____ is relatively thin in comparison to permanent counterparts, but it has consistent thickness overlying the dentin of the crown.

10. The _____ teeth have whiter enamel on their crowns than the permanent teeth because of the increased opacity of the enamel, which covers the underlying yellow dentin.

pulp horns	pulp cavity	pulp chamber
enamel	central cells of the dental papilla	pulp
primary	permanent	connective tissue
dentin		

Reference

Chapter 13, Dentin and pulp, and Chapter 18, Primary dentition. In Bath-Balogh M, Fehrenbach MJ: *Illustrated dental embryology, histology, and anatomy,* ed 3, St. Louis, 2011, Saunders.

FIGURE 3-11   Pulp (mesiodistal section with microanatomic view)

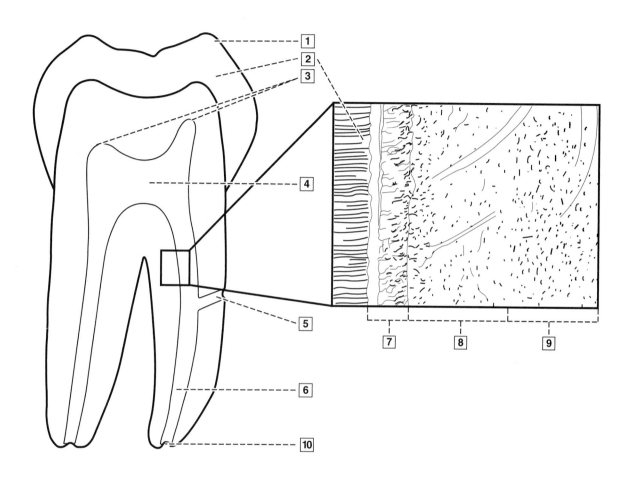

1 Enamel	**6** Radicular pulp
2 Dentin	**7** Odontoblastic layer
3 Pulp horns	**8** Cell-free zone
4 Coronal pulp	**9** Cell-rich zone
5 Accessory canal	**10** Apical foramen

REVIEW QUESTIONS

Fill in the blanks by choosing the appropriate terms from the list below.

1. An inner layer of the cell bodies of the _____ still remain in the mature tooth along the outer pulpal wall.

2. The _____ are not found on anterior teeth, but instead these smaller extensions of coronal pulp are found in the cusps of posterior teeth.

3. The _____ is the part of the pulp located in the crown of the tooth.

4. The _____, or *pulp canal,* is that part of the pulp located in the root of the tooth.

5. The _____ is the opening from the pulp into the surrounding periodontal ligament near each apex of the tooth.

6. The _____, or *lateral canals,* may be associated with the pulp and are extra openings from the pulp to the periodontal ligament; they are usually located on the lateral surface of the roots of the teeth.

7. The first zone of pulp closest to the dentin is the _____, which consists of a layer of the cell bodies of odontoblasts, whose odontoblastic processes are located in the dentinal tubules of the adjacent dentin.

8. The next zone, nearest to the odontoblastic layer and inward from the dentin, is considered the _____.

9. The next zone after the cell-free zone is the _____, inward from dentin.

10. The zone of pulp that is in the center of the pulp chamber is the _____.

pulp horns	apical foramen	coronal pulp
radicular pulp	pulpal core	cell-free zone
cell-rich zone	accessory canals	odontoblastic layer
odontoblasts		

Reference

Chapter 13, Dentin and pulp. In Bath-Balogh M, Fehrenbach MJ: *Illustrated dental embryology, histology, and anatomy,* ed 3, St. Louis, 2011, Saunders.

FIGURE 3-12 Periodontium and dentin (mesiodistal section with microanatomic view)

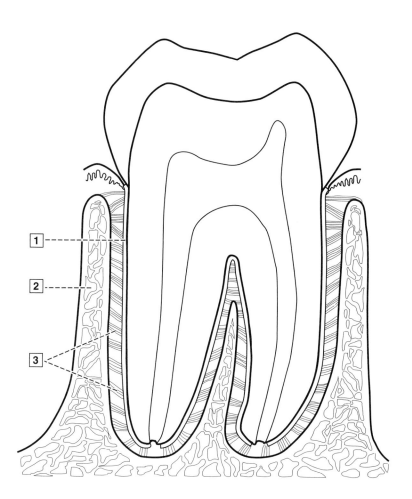

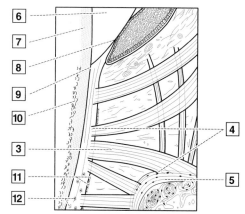

1. Cementum
2. Alveolar bone
3. Periodontal ligament
4. Sharpey fibers
5. Alveolar crest of alveolar bone proper
6. Enamel
7. Mantle dentin
8. Cementoenamel junction
9. Dentinocemental junction
10. Tomes granular layer in dentin
11. Cementoblasts in pulp
12. Cementocytes in cementum

REVIEW QUESTIONS

Fill in the blanks by choosing the appropriate terms from the list below.

1. The periodontium includes the cementum, alveolar bone, and _____.

2. The _____ is the part of the periodontium that attaches the teeth to the alveolar bone by anchoring the periodontal ligament.

3. In a healthy situation, the cementum is usually not clinically visible because it usually covers the entire root, overlying _____ in dentin.

4. Cementum is a hard tissue that is thickest at the tooth's apex or apices and in the interradicular areas of multirooted teeth and thinnest at the _____.

5. The _____ are a part of the collagen fibers from the periodontal ligament that are each partially inserted into the outer part of the cementum at 90°, or at a right angle, to the cemental surface (as well as those in alveolar bone).

6. After the apposition of cementum in layers, the _____ that do not become entrapped in cementum line up along the cemental surface along the length of the outer covering of the periodontal ligament so that they can form subsequent layers of cementum if the tooth is injured.

7. The _____ cementum consists of the first layers of cementum deposited at the dentinocemental junction, and thus is also termed *primary cementum* and contains no embedded cementocytes.

8. The _____ cementum is sometimes termed *secondary cementum* because it is deposited later than primary type and contains embedded cementocytes.

9. Each _____ lies in its lacuna (plural, lacunae), similar to the pattern noted in bone, with these lacunae having canaliculi or canals.

10. The width of cellular cementum can change during the life of the tooth, especially at the _____ of the individual teeth.

cementum	acellular	cementoenamel junction
Sharpey fibers	Tomes granular layer	apices
cementoblasts	periodontal ligament	cellular
cementocyte		

Reference

Chapter 14, Periodontium. In Bath-Balogh M, Fehrenbach MJ: *Illustrated dental embryology, histology, and anatomy,* ed 3, St. Louis, 2011, Saunders.

FIGURE 3-13 Dentin and cementum root development

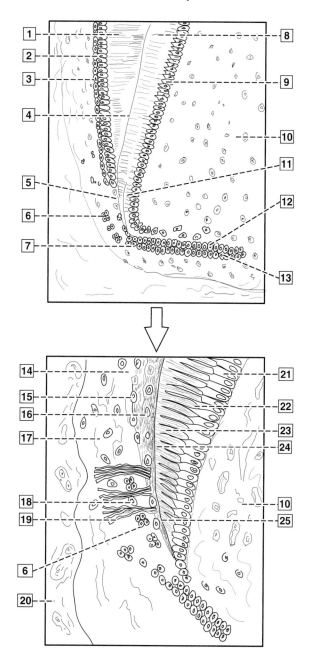

1 Enamel	**7** Disintegration of Hertwig epithelial root sheath	**13** Outer enamel epithelium (OEE)	**19** Formation of periodontal ligament
2 Ameloblasts		**14** Cementum	**20** Developing alveolar bone
3 Stratum intermedium	**8** Coronal dentin	**15** Cementoblast	**21** Odontoblast
4 Dentinoenamel junction (DEJ)	**9** Odontoblasts	**16** Cementocyte	**22** Predentin
5 Future cementoenamel junction	**10** Pulp	**17** Dental sac	**23** Root dentin
	11 Root dentin	**18** Dental sac cell becoming a cementoblast	**24** Dentinocemental junction
6 Epithelial rests of Malassez	**12** Inner enamel epithelium (IEE)		**25** Cementoid

REVIEW QUESTIONS

Fill in the blanks by choosing the appropriate terms from the list below.

1. The process of the development of the _____ takes place long after the crown is completely shaped and the tooth is starting to erupt into the oral cavity.

2. The structure responsible for root development is the _____, which is the most cervical part of the enamel organ, a bilayer rim that consists of only inner and outer enamel epithelium.

3. To form the root region, the cervical loop begins to grow deeper into the surrounding ectomesenchyme of the dental sac, elongating and moving away from the newly completed crown area to enclose more of the dental papilla, forming the _____.

4. The function of the Hertwig epithelial root sheath is to shape the root(s) by inducing _____ formation so that it is continuous with coronal dentin.

5. After this disintegration of the Hertwig epithelial root sheath, its cells may become the

   _____.

6. The _____ differentiates into cementum, as well as alveolar bone and periodontal ligament.

7. This disintegration of the root sheath allows the undifferentiated cells of the dental sac to contact the newly formed surface of root dentin, which induces these cells to become immature

   _____.

8. The cementoblasts move to cover the root dentin area and undergo cementogenesis, laying down

   _____.

9. Unlike ameloblasts and odontoblasts, which leave no cellular bodies in their secreted products, many cementoblasts become entrapped by the cementum they produce and become mature _____ in the later stages of apposition.

10. As a result of the apposition of cementum over the dentin, the _____ is formed in the area where the disintegrating basement membrane between the two tissue types was located.

cementoblasts	dentinocemental junction	Hertwig epithelial root sheath
dental sac	root	root dentin
cementoid	cervical loop	cementocytes
epithelial rests of Malassez		

Reference

Chapter 6, Tooth development and eruption. In Bath-Balogh M, Fehrenbach MJ: *Illustrated dental embryology, histology, and anatomy,* ed 3, St. Louis, 2011, Saunders.

FIGURE 3-14 Production of reduced enamel epithelium over new enamel surface

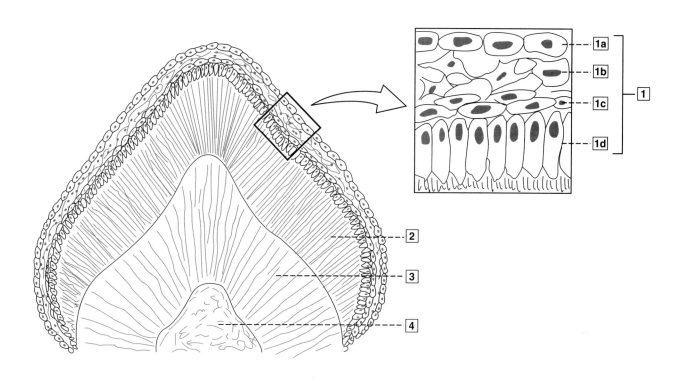

1 Compressed to form reduced enamel epithelium (REE)	**1d** Ameloblasts
1a Outer enamel epithelium	**2** Enamel
1b Stellate reticulum	**3** Dentin
1c Stratum intermedium	**4** Pulp

REVIEW QUESTIONS

Fill in the blanks by choosing the appropriate terms from the list below.

1. The _____ eruption of a primary tooth has many stages as the tooth moves into place in the alveolar process of each arch; this is not the passive eruption, which occurs with aging, when the gingival tissue recedes but no actual tooth movement takes place.

2. After enamel apposition ceases in the crown area of each primary or permanent tooth, the _____ place an acellular dental cuticle on the newly formed outer enamel surface.

3. During tooth development, the enamel organ consists of stellate reticulum, stratum intermedium, and _____, along with the ameloblasts from the inner enamel epithelium.

4. The layers of the enamel organ become compressed, forming the _____, which appears as a few layers of flattened cells overlying the enamel surface.

5. The external cells of the reduced enamel epithelium are mostly from the stratum intermedium cells, but possibly cellular remnants of the stellate reticulum and outer enamel; thus these undifferentiated epithelial cells will divide and multiply and eventually give rise to the _____.

6. When this formation of the reduced enamel epithelium occurs for a primary tooth, it can then begin the _____ into the oral cavity.

7. To allow for the eruption process, the reduced enamel epithelium first has to fuse with the _____ lining the oral cavity.

8. A residue, _____, may form on newly erupted teeth of both dentitions that may leave the teeth extrinsically stained green-gray; this residue consists of the fused tissue of the reduced enamel epithelium and oral epithelium, as well as the dental cuticle placed by the ameloblasts on the newly formed outer enamel surface.

9. Nasmyth membrane easily picks up stain from food debris and is hard to remove except by selective polishing of the newly exposed outer _____ surface.

10. With the _____ forming before the root, prevention of traumatic injury to the permanent teeth before they are fully anchored into the jaws is very important.

eruption process	reduced enamel epithelium	ameloblasts
Nasmyth membrane	initial junctional epithelium	active
enamel	oral epithelium	outer enamel epithelium
crown		

Reference

Chapter 6, Tooth development and eruption. In Bath-Balogh M, Fehrenbach MJ: *Illustrated dental embryology, histology, and anatomy,* ed 3, St. Louis, 2011, Saunders.

ANSWER KEY 1. active, 2. ameloblasts, 3. outer enamel epithelium, 4. reduced enamel epithelium, 5. initial junctional epithelium, 6. eruption process, 7. oral epithelium, 8. Nasmyth membrane, 9. enamel, 10. crown.

FIGURE 3-15 Tooth eruption

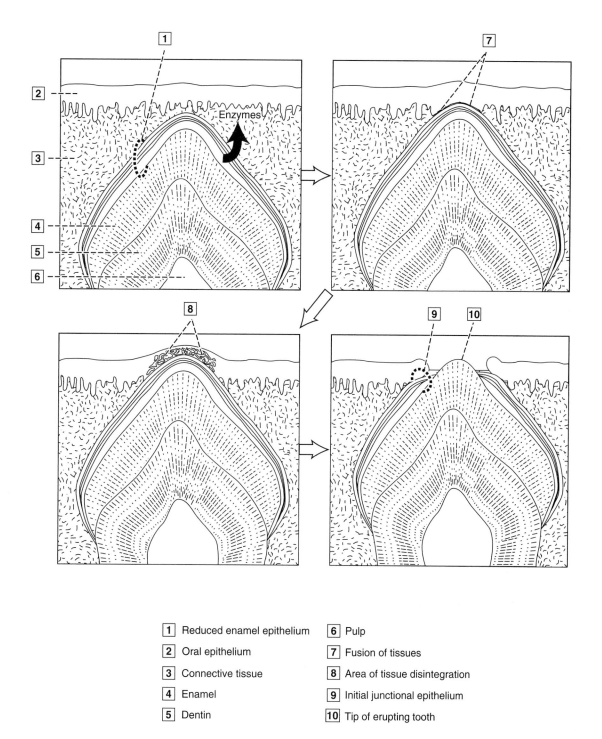

1 Reduced enamel epithelium	6 Pulp
2 Oral epithelium	7 Fusion of tissues
3 Connective tissue	8 Area of tissue disintegration
4 Enamel	9 Initial junctional epithelium
5 Dentin	10 Tip of erupting tooth

REVIEW QUESTIONS

Fill in the blanks by choosing the appropriate terms from the list below.

1. To allow for the eruption process, the reduced enamel epithelium first has to undergo _____ with the oral epithelium lining the oral cavity.

2. The _____ from the reduced enamel epithelium disintegrate the central part of the fused tissue, leaving an epithelial tunnel for the tooth to erupt through the surrounding oral epithelium into the oral cavity.

3. The tissue _____ during the eruption process can cause a localized inflammatory response known as "teething," which may be accompanied by tenderness and edema of the local tissue.

4. Proper homecare can reduce the amount of _____ and thus the discomfort associated with these oral changes in infants as their first teeth erupt, as well as in young adults when their third molars erupt.

5. A panoramic radiograph of the _____ is important in order to monitor on tooth development.

6. A permanent tooth often starts to erupt before the _____ tooth is fully shed, possibly creating problems in spacing but interceptive orthodontic therapy can prevent some of these situations.

7. As a primary tooth actively erupts, the coronal part of the fused epithelial tissue peels off the crown, leaving the cervical part still attached to the neck of the tooth, which can then serve as the _____ of the tooth, creating a seal between the tissue and the tooth surface.

8. The initial junctional epithelium of the tooth is replaced by a definitive junctional epithelium as the _____ becomes completely formed.

9. The process of eruption for a(n) _____ permanent tooth is the same as for the primary tooth.

10. The process of the _____ permanent tooth's eruption is similar to that of a succedaneous one, but no primary tooth is shed.

enzymes	inflammation	disintegration
root	succedaneous	primary
nonsuccedaneous	fusion	initial junctional epithelium
mixed dentition		

Reference

Chapter 6, Tooth development and eruption. In Bath-Balogh M, Fehrenbach MJ: *Illustrated dental embryology, histology, and anatomy*, ed 3, St. Louis, 2011, Saunders.

FIGURE 3-16 Succedaneous permanent teeth development (section of fetal mandible)

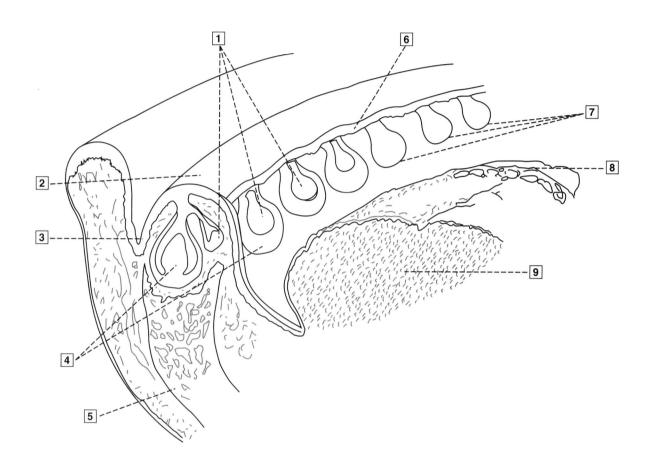

1	Successional dental lamina of permanent teeth primordia	**6**	Oral epithelium (cut to show tooth buds)
2	Developing mandibular dental arch	**7**	Tooth germs of nonsuccedaneous permanent molars
3	Vestibule	**8**	Base of tongue
4	Developing primary teeth	**9**	Body of tongue
5	Developing mandible		

REVIEW QUESTIONS

Fill in the blanks by choosing the appropriate terms from the list below.

1. To allow for the eruption process, the _____ first has to fuse with the oral epithelium lining the oral cavity.

2. When the primary tooth is then lost, exfoliated, or shed, the _____ permanent tooth develops lingual to it.

3. The process involving shedding of the primary tooth consists of differentiation of multinucleated _____ from fused macrophages, which absorb the alveolar bone between the two teeth.

4. The _____, are formed from undifferentiated mesenchyme; these cells cause resorption, or removal of parts of the primary's root of dentin and cementum, as well as small parts of the enamel crown.

5. Special _____ destroy any remaining collagen fibers during the shedding process of the primary dentition.

6. The process of shedding the primary tooth is intermittent ("on again/off again"), because at the same time that osteoclasts differentiate to resorb bone and odontoblasts differentiate to resorb dental tissue, the always-ready _____ and cementoblasts work to replace the resorbed parts of the root.

7. The succedaneous permanent tooth usually erupts into the oral cavity in a position lingual to the roots of the shedding or shed _____ tooth, just as it develops that way.

8. The only exception to the lingual eruption placement is the _____ maxillary incisors, which move to a more facially placed position as they erupt into the oral cavity.

9. It is common on a partially erupted tooth to have a(n) _____ cyst that appears as fluctuant, blue vesicle-like lesion.

10. Both succedaneous and nonsuccedaneous permanent teeth erupt in _____, or sequential, order.

reduced enamel epithelium	osteoclasts	primary
fibroclasts	odontoblasts	permanent
succedaneous	eruption	chronological
odontoclasts		

Reference

Chapter 6, Tooth development and eruption. In Bath-Balogh M, Fehrenbach MJ: *Illustrated dental embryology, histology, and anatomy,* ed 3, St. Louis, 2011, Saunders.

FIGURE 3-17 Multiroot development

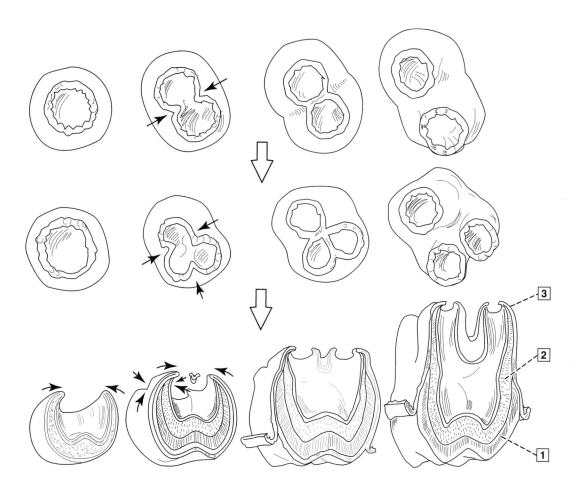

1 Enamel
2 Dentin
3 Pulp

REVIEW QUESTIONS

Fill in the blanks by choosing the appropriate terms from the list below.

1. Like anterior teeth, _____ premolars and molars originate as a single root on the base of the crown, with this part of the posterior teeth considered the root trunk.

2. The cervical cross section of the _____ initially follows the form of the crown; however, the root of a posterior tooth divides from the root trunk into the correct number of root branches for its tooth type.

3. Differential growth of _____ causes the root trunk of the multirooted teeth to divide into two or three roots.

4. During the formation of the enamel organ on a multirooted tooth, elongation of its _____ occurs, which allows the development of long, tongue-like horizontal epithelial extensions or flaps within it.

5. Two or three epithelial extensions or flaps can be present on multirooted teeth from the elongation of the cervical loop, depending on the similar number of _____ on the mature tooth.

6. The usually single cervical opening of the coronal _____ is divided into two or three openings by these horizontal extensions from the cervical loop to produce the correct number of roots.

7. On the pulpal surfaces of these holes that correspond to each root, dentin formation starts after the induction of the odontoblasts and _____ of Hertwig epithelial root sheath and the associated basement membrane.

8. The _____ are induced to form cementum on the newly formed dentin only at the periphery of each opening on the pulpal surface corresponding to each root needed.

9. The posterior molars of the _____ of the permanent dentition usually have three roots.

10. The posterior molars of the _____ of the permanent dentition usually have two roots.

disintegration	cervical loop	enamel organ
maxillary teeth	multirooted	cementoblasts
roots	root trunk	mandibular teeth
Hertwig epithelial root sheath		

Reference

Chapter 6, Tooth development and eruption. In Bath-Balogh M, Fehrenbach MJ: *Illustrated dental embryology, histology, and anatomy,* ed 3, St. Louis, 2011, Saunders.

FIGURE 3-18 Alveolar bone

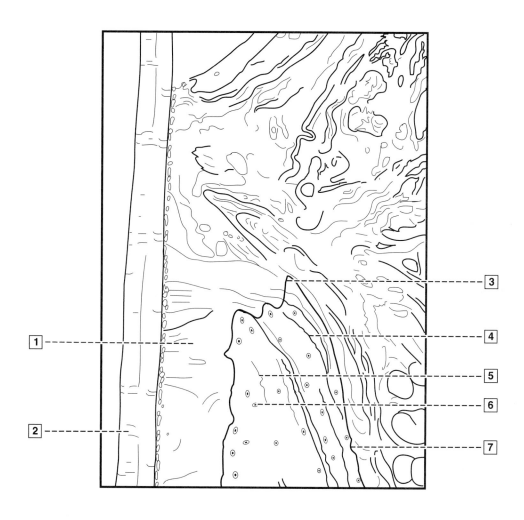

1 Periodontal ligament	**5** Reversal line
2 Cementum	**6** Osteocyte in lacuna
3 Alveolar crest	**7** Howship lacuna
4 Arrest line	

REVIEW QUESTIONS

Fill in the blanks by choosing the appropriate terms from the list below.

1. The _____ is that part of either the maxillae or mandible that supports and protects the teeth.

2. The alveolar bone is that part of the periodontium in which the cementum of the tooth is attached to it through the _____.

3. The _____ is the lining of the tooth socket or alveolus.

4. The _____ is the most cervical rim of the alveolar bone proper.

5. Within fully mineralized bone are _____, which are entrapped mature osteoblasts.

6. The cell body of the osteocyte is surrounded by bone, except for the space immediately around it, the _____.

7. The cytoplasmic processes of the osteocyte radiate outward in all directions in the bone and are located in tubular canals of matrix, or _____.

8. The _____, with layered formation of bone along its periphery, is accomplished by the osteoblasts, which later become entrapped as osteocytes.

9. The _____ appear as smooth lines between the layers of bone because of osteoblasts having rested, formed bone, and then rested again after appositional growth, showing the incremental or layered nature of appositional growth.

10. The _____ appear as scalloped lines between the layers of bone showing where bone resorption has first taken place, followed quickly by appositional growth of new bone.

arrest lines	alveolar crest	canaliculi
lacuna	alveolar bone	periodontal ligament
reversal lines	alveolar bone proper	appositional growth
osteocytes		

Reference

Chapter 14, Periodontium. In Bath-Balogh M, Fehrenbach MJ: *Illustrated dental embryology, histology, and anatomy,* ed 3, St. Louis, 2011, Saunders.

FIGURE 3-19 Periodontal ligament and alveolar bone (mesiodistal section)

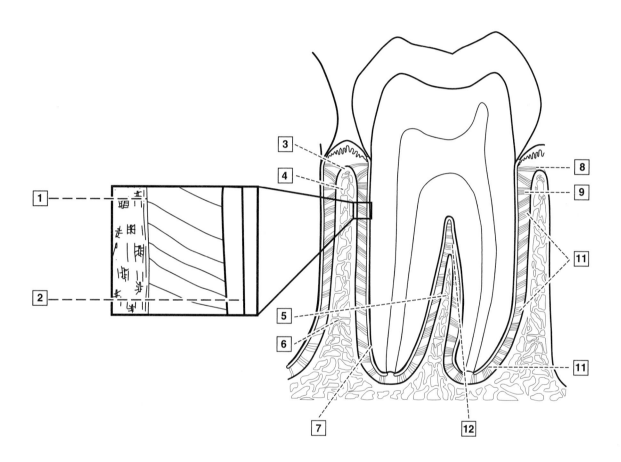

1 Sharpey fibers within alveolar bone	**7** Cementum
2 Sharpey fibers within cementum	**8** Alveolar crest group
3 Alveolar crest	**9** Horizontal group
4 Alveolar bone	**10** Oblique group
5 Interradicular septum	**11** Apical group
6 Interdental bone	**12** Interradicular group

REVIEW QUESTIONS

Fill in the blanks by choosing the appropriate terms from the list below.

1. The _____ consists of both cortical bone and trabecular bone.

2. The alveolar bone between two neighboring teeth is the _____.

3. The alveolar bone between roots is the _____.

4. A part of the alveolar bone proper is seen on radiographs as the _____, which is uniformly radiopaque (or lighter).

5. The ends of the principal fibers that are within either cementum or alveolar bone proper are considered _____.

6. The main principal fiber group is the alveolodental ligament, which consists of five fiber subgroups: alveolar crest, horizontal, oblique, apical, and _____ on multirooted teeth.

7. The _____ of the alveolodental ligament is attached to the cementum just below the cementoenamel junction and runs in an inferior and outward direction to insert into the alveolar crest of the alveolar bone proper.

8. The _____ of the alveolodental ligament is just apical to the alveolar crest subgroup and runs at right angles to the long axis of the tooth from cementum to the alveolar bone proper, just inferior to its alveolar crest.

9. The _____ of the alveolodental ligament is the most numerous of the fiber subgroups and covers the apical two thirds of the root, with this subgroup running from the cementum in an oblique direction to insert into the alveolar bone proper more coronally.

10. The _____ of the alveolodental ligament radiates from cementum around the apex of the root to the surrounding alveolar bone proper at the base of the alveolus.

lamina dura	horizontal group	Sharpey fibers
interradicular septum	interdental bone	oblique group
apical group	alveolar crest group	interradicular groups
supporting alveolar bone		

Reference

Chapter 14, Periodontium. In Bath-Balogh M, Fehrenbach MJ: *Illustrated dental embryology, histology, and anatomy,* ed 3, St. Louis, 2011, Saunders.

ANSWER KEY 1. supporting alveolar bone, 2. interdental bone, 3. interradicular septum, 4. lamina dura, 5. Sharpey fibers, 6. interradicular groups, 7. alveolar crest group, 8. horizontal group, 9. oblique group, 10. apical group.

FIGURE 3-20 Interdental ligament (anterior view and mesiodistal section)

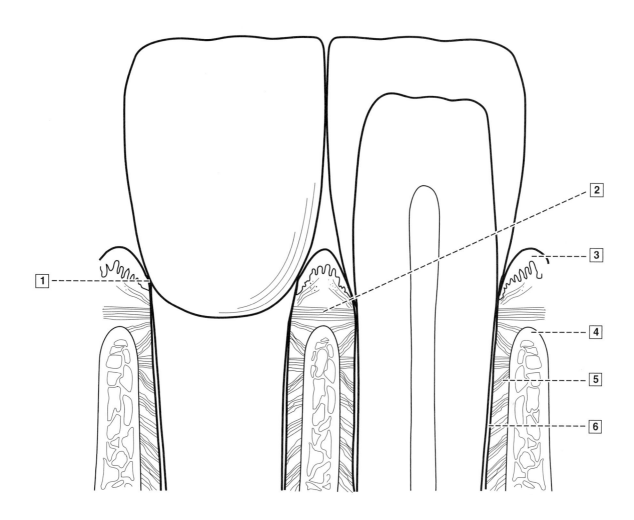

1	Cementoenamel junction
2	Interdental ligament
3	Interdental papilla
4	Alveolar crest
5	Alveolodental ligament
6	Cementum

REVIEW QUESTIONS

Fill in the blanks by choosing the appropriate terms from the list below.

1. The other fiber group of the _____ (besides the alveolodental ligament) is the interdental ligament.

2. The interdental ligament inserts mesiodistally or interdentally into the cervical _____ of neighboring teeth.

3. The interdental ligament is at a height that is superior to the _____ of the alveolar bone proper.

4. The interdental ligament is at a height that is inferior to the base of the _____.

5. The interdental ligament's fibers travel from cementum to cementum without any attachment to the _____.

6. The interdental ligament helps to hold the teeth in _____.

7. The _____ connects all the teeth of each arch, both maxillary and mandibular.

8. The interdental ligament is sometimes termed the _____ because of its direction.

9. The function of the interdental ligament is to resist _____ that can be applied to the teeth or twisting of the tooth in its alveolus.

10. The fibers that are inserted from the interdental ligament into both cementum and alveolar bone are considered _____.

periodontal ligament	junctional epithelium	interproximal contact
interdental ligament	Sharpey fibers	transseptal ligament
alveolar crest	alveolar bone	rotational forces
cementum		

Reference

Chapter 14, Periodontium. In Bath-Balogh M, Fehrenbach MJ: *Illustrated dental embryology, histology, and anatomy,* ed 3, St. Louis, 2011, Saunders.

ANSWER KEY 1. periodontal ligament, 2. cementum, 3. alveolar crest, 4. junctional epithelium, 5. alveolar bone, 6. interproximal contact, 7. interdental ligament, 8. transseptal ligament, 9. rotational forces, 10. Sharpey fibers.

FIGURE 3-21 Gingival fiber group (frontal view and labiolingual section)

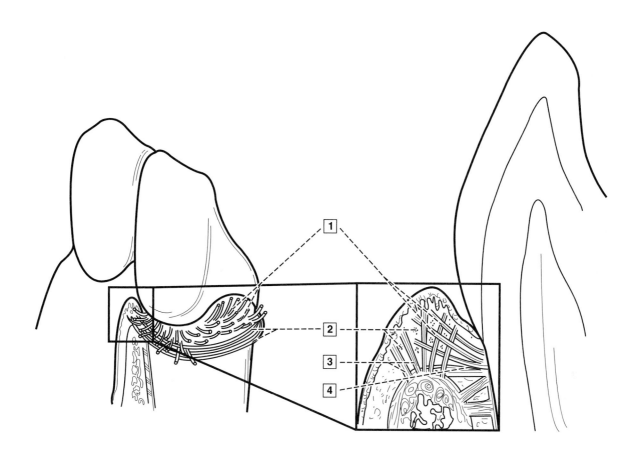

1 Dentogingival ligament
2 Circular ligament
3 Alveologingival ligament
4 Dentoperiosteal ligament

REVIEW QUESTIONS

Fill in the blanks by choosing the appropriate terms from the list below.

1. The _____ is considered by some histologists to be part of the principal fibers of the periodontal ligament.

2. The gingival fiber group is a separate but adjacent group to the _____ and interdental ligament.

3. The gingival fiber group is found within the _____ of the marginal gingiva.

4. The gingival fiber group does not support the tooth in relationship to the jaw, resisting any forces of mastication or speech; rather it supports only the _____ to maintain its relationship to the tooth.

5. The _____ of the gingival fiber group encircles the tooth, as shown on a cross section of a tooth, interlacing with the other gingival fiber subgroups.

6. The _____ is the most extensive of the gingival fiber group, as it inserts in the cementum on the root, apical to the epithelial attachment, and extends into the lamina propria of the marginal and attached gingiva.

7. The dentogingival ligament works with the circular ligament to maintain _____ integrity, mainly that of the marginal gingiva so as to maintain its relationship to the tooth.

8. The _____ radiates from the alveolar crest of the alveolar bone proper and extends coronally into the overlying lamina propria of the marginal gingiva.

9. The alveologingival ligament helps to attach the gingiva to the _____ because of its one mineralized attachment.

10. The _____ courses from the cementum, near the cementoenamel junction, across the alveolar crest to anchor the tooth to the alveolar bone and protect the deeper periodontal ligament.

circular ligament	dentogingival ligament	alveolar bone
dentoperiosteal ligament	gingival fiber group	alveolodental ligament
marginal gingiva	lamina propria	gingival
alveologingival ligament		

Reference

Chapter 14, Periodontium. In Bath-Balogh M, Fehrenbach MJ: *Illustrated dental embryology, histology, and anatomy,* ed 3, St. Louis, 2011, Saunders.

ANSWER KEY 1. gingival fiber group, 2. alveolodental ligament, 3. lamina propria, 4. marginal gingiva, 5. circular ligament, 6. dentogingival ligament, 7. gingival, 8. alveologingival ligament, 9. alveolar bone, 10. dentoperiosteal ligament.

FIGURE 3-22 Primary dentition: occlusal view with facial and lingual views in dental chart

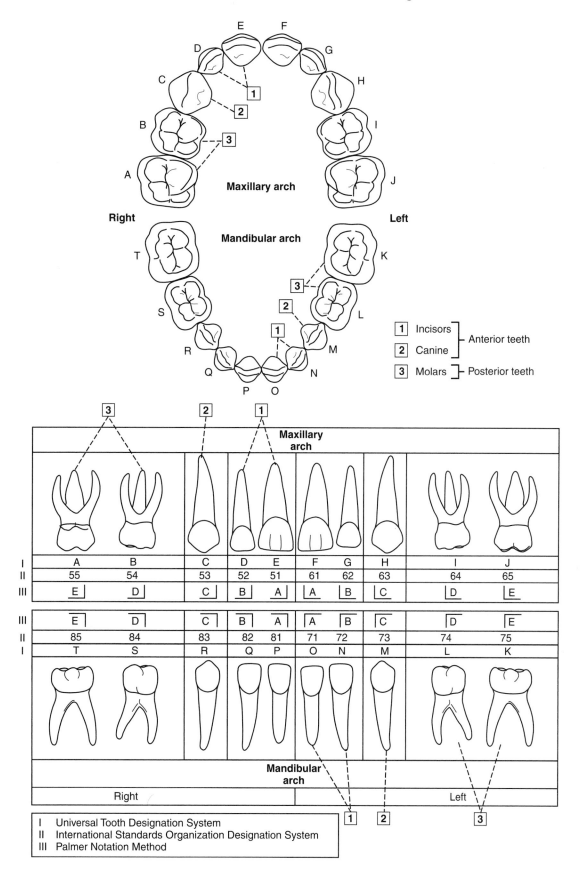

REVIEW QUESTIONS

Fill in the blanks by choosing the appropriate terms from the list below.

1. The tooth types of both arches within the primary dentition, which is also termed the _____ dentition, include eight incisors, four canines, and eight molars, for a total of 20 teeth.

2. It is important to note that only the permanent dentition has premolars; in contrast, the primary dentition does not have _____.

3. The _____ function as instruments for biting and cutting food during mastication, because of their triangular proximal form.

4. The _____, because of their tapered shape and their prominent cusp, function to pierce or tear food during mastication.

5. As the teeth with the largest and strongest crowns, the _____ function in grinding food during mastication.

6. It is the wide occlusal surfaces of the molars, with their prominent _____, that help with mastication.

7. Both the primary teeth and the permanent teeth can be designated by either letters or numbers using the _____.

8. With the Universal Tooth Designation System, the primary teeth are designated in a consecutive arrangement by using capital letters, *A* through *T*, starting with the maxillary right second molar, moving _____, and ending with the mandibular right second molar.

9. Another tooth designation system that is commonly used during orthodontic therapy is the _____, also known as the *Military Tooth Numbering System*.

10. Within the Palmer Notation Method, the teeth are designated with a right-angle symbol indicating the _____, with the tooth number inside indicating the position of the tooth in regards to the median line of the quadrant of the dental arch.

molars	Universal Tooth Designation System	canines
Palmer Notation Method	cusps	quadrants
deciduous	clockwise	premolars
incisors		

Reference

Chapter 15, Overview of the dentitions. In Bath-Balogh M, Fehrenbach MJ: *Illustrated dental embryology, histology, and anatomy,* ed 3, St. Louis, 2011, Saunders.

FIGURE 3-23 Permanent dentition: occlusal view with facial and lingual views in dental chart

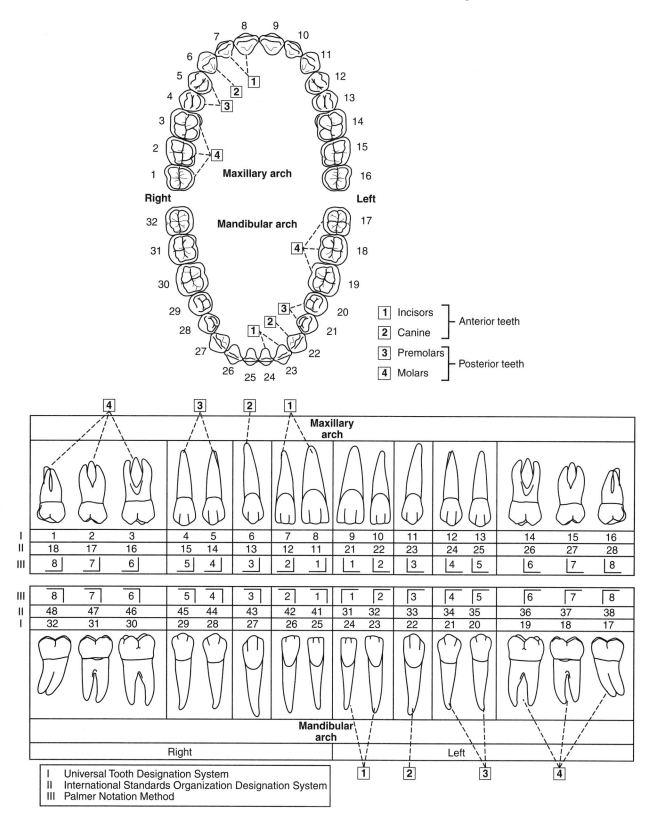

REVIEW QUESTIONS

Fill in the blanks by choosing the appropriate terms from the list below.

1. The tooth types of both dental arches within the permanent dentition, which is also called the _____ dentition, include eight incisors, four canines, eight premolars, and 12 molars, for a total of 32 teeth.

2. Note that only the permanent dentition has _____; in contrast, the primary dentition does not have this tooth type.

3. The premolars, which are found only during the permanent dentition period, function to assist the _____ in grinding food during mastication because of their broad occlusal surface and their prominent cusps.

4. The premolars assist the _____ in piercing and tearing food with their multiple cusps.

5. As the teeth with the largest and strongest crowns, the molars function in grinding food during _____, as assisted by the premolars.

6. The molars of the permanent dentition are _____, because they are without any primary predecessors.

7. Only the anterior teeth and premolars of the permanent dentition are _____, because they have primary predecessors.

8. The permanent teeth are designated by the _____, a consecutive arrangement of the oral cavity as observed from the front and using the digits *1* through *32*, starting with the maxillary right third molar, moving clockwise, and ending with the mandibular right third molar.

9. The _____ as instituted by the World Health Organization has the teeth designated by using a two-digit code with the first digit of the code indicating the quadrant, and the second digit indicating the position of the tooth in the quadrant from the median line.

10. Using the International Standards Organization Designation System, the second digit, which indicates the tooth, the digits *1* through *8* are used for the permanent teeth, with this designation using the _____ as the standard and then numbering in a distal direction.

Universal Tooth Designation System	premolars	succedaneous
molars	International Standards	median line
nonsuccedaneous	Organization Designation System	mastication
	secondary	canines

Reference

Chapter 15, Overview of the dentitions. In Bath-Balogh M, Fehrenbach MJ: *Illustrated dental embryology, histology, and anatomy,* ed 3, St. Louis, 2011, Saunders.

ANSWER KEY 1. secondary, 2. premolars, 3. molars, 4. canines, 5. mastication, 6. nonsuccedaneous, 7. succedaneous, 8. Universal Tooth Designation System, 9. International Standards Organization Designation System, 10. median line.

FIGURE 3-24 Orientational terms for tooth surfaces

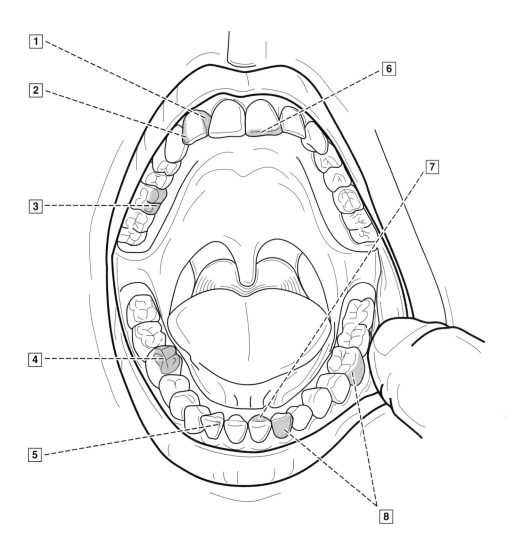

1	Mesial surface	**5**	Proximal surface with contact area
2	Distal surface	**6**	Incisal surface
3	Palatal surface	**7**	Lingual surface
4	Occlusal surface	**8**	Facial surfaces: labial and buccal surfaces

REVIEW QUESTIONS

Fill in the blanks by choosing the appropriate terms from the list below.

1. The tooth surfaces closest to the surface of the face are considered _____ surfaces.

2. Those facial tooth surfaces closest to the lips are termed the _____ surfaces.

3. Those facial tooth surfaces closest to the inner cheek are considered the _____ surfaces.

4. Those tooth surfaces closest to the tongue are termed the _____ surfaces.

5. Those lingual surfaces closest to the palate on the maxillary arch are sometimes also termed the _____ surfaces.

6. The masticatory surface is the chewing surface on the most superior surface of the crown, and this is the _____ surface for anterior teeth.

7. The masticatory surface is the chewing surface on the most superior surface of the crown, and this is the _____ surface for posterior teeth.

8. The surface closest to the midline is considered the _____ surface.

9. The surface farthest away from the midline is considered the _____ surface.

10. Together, both the mesial and the distal surfaces between adjacent teeth are considered the _____ surface.

mesial	facial	palatal
distal	labial	occlusal
incisal	buccal	proximal
lingual		

Reference

Chapter 15, Overview of the dentitions. In Bath-Balogh M, Fehrenbach MJ: *Illustrated dental embryology, histology, and anatomy,* ed 3, St. Louis, 2011, Saunders.

FIGURE 3-25 Embrasures of teeth

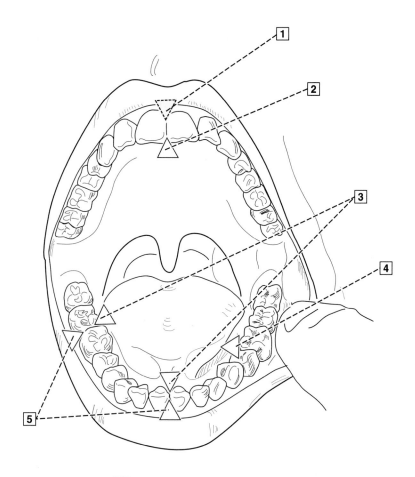

1. Apical embrasure (if diseased)
2. Incisal embrasure
3. Lingual embrasures
4. Occlusal embrasure
5. Facial embrasures

REVIEW QUESTIONS

Fill in the blanks by choosing the appropriate terms from the list below.

1. When two teeth in the same arch come into contact, their curvatures next to the contact areas form spaces considered _____.

2. The embrasures are continuous with the _____ between the teeth, and there is an increasing angle of the occlusal embrasures anteroposteriorly.

3. The embrasures in the oral cavity form _____ between teeth to direct food away from the gingiva.

4. The embrasures provide a mechanism for teeth to be more _____, so as to be healthier against dental biofilm or food product buildup.

5. The embrasures protect the _____ from undue frictional trauma but also provide the proper degree of stimulation to the soft tissue covering the alveolar process of both arches.

6. The area where the crowns of adjacent teeth in the same arch physically touch each proximal surface is the _____.

7. The _____, or *crest of curvature,* is the greatest elevation of the tooth either incisocervically or occlusocervically on a specific surface of the crown.

8. It is noted when viewing teeth overall that the proximal _____ curvature is greatest on the anterior teeth and the least on the posterior teeth.

9. The cementoenamel junction curvature is approximately similar on _____ and distal surfaces of the two teeth that face each other.

10. On any given tooth, the height of the cementoenamel junction curvature is greater on the mesial aspect of that tooth than it is on the _____.

gingiva	contact area	interproximal spaces
spillways	self-cleansing	cementoenamel junction
mesial	embrasures	distal
height of contour		

Reference

Chapter 15, Overview of the dentitions. In Bath-Balogh M, Fehrenbach MJ: *Illustrated dental embryology, histology, and anatomy,* ed 3, St. Louis, 2011, Saunders.

ANSWER KEY 1. embrasures, 2. interproximal spaces, 3. spillways, 4. self-cleansing, 5. gingiva, 6. contact area, 7. height of contour, 8. cementoenamel junction, 9. mesial, 10. distal.

FIGURE 3-26 Maxillary right central incisor (lingual and incisal views)

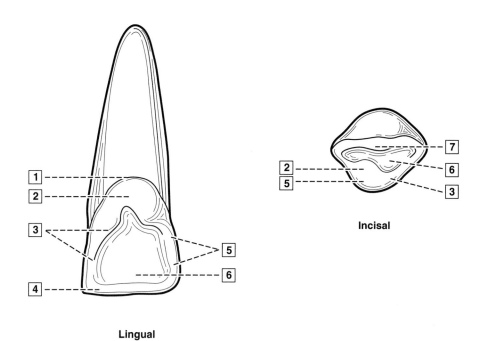

Lingual

Incisal

1	Cementoenamel junction
2	Cingulum
3	Mesial marginal ridge
4	Linguoincisal ridge
5	Distal marginal ridge
6	Lingual fossa
7	Incisal ridge

REVIEW QUESTIONS

Fill in the blanks by choosing the appropriate terms from the list below.

1. The permanent maxillary central incisors erupt between 7 to 8 years of age (root completion at age 10), usually _____ the mandibular central incisors.

2. They are the most prominent teeth in the permanent dentition because of both their large size and their _____ position.

3. They are the largest of all the incisors, and the two usually share a mesial _____ .

4. The maxillary central incisor has a single conical _____, smooth and slightly straight, usually with a rounded apex.

5. From the facial view, the _____ is nearly straight, with two labial developmental depressions that may extend the length of the crown from the cervical to the incisal, showing the division of the surface into three labial developmental lobes.

6. The overall mesial outline is slightly rounded, with a sharp mesioincisal _____ in comparison with the distoincisal one.

7. On the lingual surface, the single _____ is wide and well developed in size, as well as being located slightly off center toward the distal.

8. From the lingual view, the mesial _____ is longer than the distal one.

9. The single _____ is wide yet shallow and is located immediately incisal to the cingulum.

10. There may be a vertically placed _____, which originates in the lingual pit and extends cervically and slightly distally onto the cingulum.

angle	anterior arch	marginal ridge
linguogingival groove	contact area	lingua fossa
root	cingulum	incisal ridge
after		

Reference

Chapter 16, Permanent anterior teeth. In Bath-Balogh M, Fehrenbach MJ: *Illustrated dental embryology, histology, and anatomy,* ed 3, St. Louis, 2011, Saunders.

ANSWER KEY 1. after, 2. anterior arch, 3. contact area, 4. root, 5. incisal ridge, 6. angle, 7. cingulum, 8. marginal ridge, 9. lingual fossa, 10. linguogingival groove.

FIGURE 3-27   Maxillary right lateral incisor (lingual and incisal views)

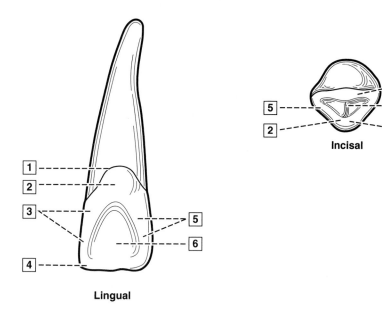

Incisal

Lingual

1 Cementoenamel junction
2 Cingulum
3 Mesial marginal ridge
4 Linguoincisal ridge
5 Distal marginal ridge
6 Lingual fossa
7 Incisal ridge

REVIEW QUESTIONS

Fill in the blanks by choosing the appropriate terms from the list below.

1. The permanent maxillary lateral incisors erupt between 8 to 9 years of age (root completion at age 11), usually _____ the maxillary central incisors.

2. The _____ of a maxillary lateral incisor has the greatest degree of variation in form of any permanent tooth except for the third molars.

3. It has a prominent, yet centered and narrower _____ than does a maxillary central incisor on the lingual surface.

4. It has a deeper _____ on the lingual surface than does the maxillary central incisor.

5. The longer mesial _____ on the lingual surface is nearly straight, and the shorter distal one is quite straight.

6. The _____ is noticeably well developed in size, as noted from the lingual view.

7. A(n) _____ is more common on a lateral than on a maxillary central incisor and is located on the incisal surface of the cingulum, along the lingual groove.

8. The _____ is more common on the tooth than on a maxillary central incisor and originates in the lingual pit, extending cervically and slightly distally onto the cingulum; it may also extend onto the root surface as seen from the lingual view.

9. Similar to a maxillary central incisor, the _____ on a lateral is more curved on the mesial surface than the distal surface of this tooth.

10. The _____ is usually labial to the long axis of the tooth as noted in its proximal view features.

linguoincisal ridge	lingual pit	crown
cementoenamel junction	marginal ridge	linguogingival groove
cingulum	incisal edge	lingual fossa
after		

Reference

Chapter 16, Permanent anterior teeth. In Bath-Balogh M, Fehrenbach MJ: *Illustrated dental embryology, histology, and anatomy,* ed 3, St. Louis, 2011, Saunders.

FIGURE 3-28   Mandibular right central incisor (lingual and incisal views)

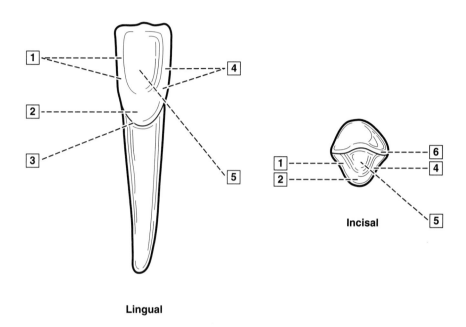

Lingual

Incisal

1	Mesial marginal ridge
2	Cingulum
3	Cementoenamel junction
4	Distal marginal ridge
5	Lingual fossa
6	Incisal ridge

REVIEW QUESTIONS

Fill in the blanks by choosing the appropriate terms from the list below.

1. The permanent mandibular central incisors erupt between 6 to 7 years of age (root completion at age 9), usually _____ the maxillary central incisors.

2. Due to its smallness, the tooth has only one antagonist in the _____.

3. The crown of a mandibular central incisor is quite _____ from the labial view, having a fan shape.

4. The _____ of a mandibular central incisor is narrower on the lingual surface than the labial surface, with its outline that is the reverse of the labial view.

5. Overall, the lingual surface is smooth and has a small, centered _____.

6. On the lingual surface, the single _____ is barely noticeable.

7. Because the cingulum is centered, the faint mesial and distal _____ have the same length.

8. The _____ curvature is higher incisally on the mesial than on the distal surface.

9. The _____ is usually at a right angle, or perpendicular, to the labiolingual axis of the crown of the tooth and overall is just lingual to the long axis of the root.

10. They are the smallest and simplest teeth of the permanent dentition; thus they are smaller than the lateral incisors of the _____.

lingual fossa	marginal ridges	crown
mandibular arch	before	maxillary arch
symmetrical	cingulum	incisal edge
cementoenamel junction		

Reference

Chapter 16, Permanent anterior teeth. In Bath-Balogh M, Fehrenbach MJ: *Illustrated dental embryology, histology, and anatomy,* ed 3, St. Louis, 2011, Saunders.

FIGURE 3-29   Mandibular right lateral incisor (lingual and incisal views)

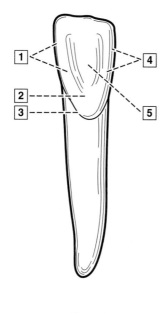

Lingual

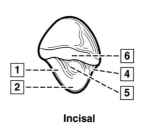

Incisal

1	Mesial marginal ridge
2	Cingulum
3	Cementoenamel junction
4	Distal marginal ridge
5	Lingual fossa
6	Incisal ridge

REVIEW QUESTIONS

Fill in the blanks by choosing the appropriate terms from the list below.

1. The permanent mandibular lateral incisors erupt between 7 to 8 years of age (root completion at age 10), usually _____ the mandibular central incisors.

2. From both the labial and lingual views, the _____ appears tilted or *twisted* distally in comparison with the long axis of the tooth.

3. The mesioincisal _____ of the incisal edge is sharper than the distoincisal one.

4. The small single _____ lies just distal to the long axis of the root on its lingual surface.

5. On the lingual surface, both the mesial _____ and distal one are more developed than on a mandibular central incisor, although the mesial one is longer than the distal one.

6. A single _____ is present on the lingual surface of the tooth.

7. A(n) _____ is rarely present on a mandibular lateral incisor, although it is more often present than on a mandibular central incisor.

8. The height of the _____ curvature is greater on the mesial surface than the distal surface.

9. The crown of a mandibular lateral incisor lacks bilateral _____, unlike the central incisor of the same arch.

10. The tooth has a single root, and like the mandibular central incisor, has pronounced _____, especially on the distal surface.

symmetry	lingual fossa	crown
cementoenamel junction	root concavities	lingual pit
angle	marginal ridge	after
cingulum		

Reference

Chapter 16, Permanent anterior teeth. In Bath-Balogh M, Fehrenbach MJ: *Illustrated dental embryology, histology, and anatomy,* ed 3, St. Louis, 2011, Saunders.

ANSWER KEY   1. after, 2. crown, 3. angle, 4. cingulum, 5. marginal ridge, 6. lingual fossa, 7. lingual pit, 8. cementoenamel junction, 9. symmetry, 10. root concavities.

FIGURE 3-30 Maxillary right canine (lingual and incisal views)

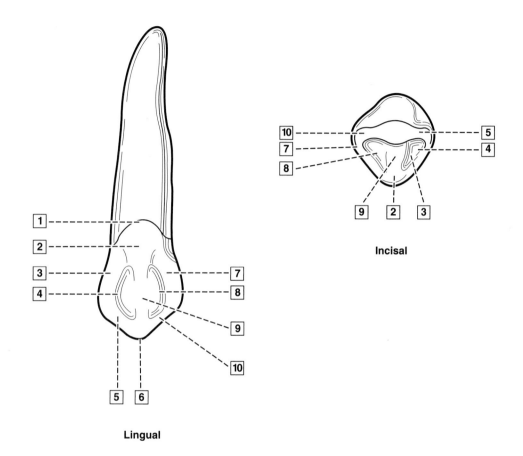

Incisal

Lingual

1	Cementoenamel junction		6	Cusp tip
2	Cingulum		7	Distal marginal ridge
3	Mesial marginal ridge		8	Distolingual fossa
4	Mesiolingual fossa		9	Lingual ridge
5	Mesial cusp slopes		10	Distal cusp slopes

REVIEW QUESTIONS

Fill in the blanks by choosing the appropriate terms from the list below.

1. The permanent maxillary canines erupt between 11 to 12 years of age (root completion between ages 13 to 15), usually _____ the mandibular canines, the maxillary incisors, and possibly the maxillary premolars.

2. The long _____ is single and has a blunt apex; it is the longest one in the maxillary arch.

3. The _____ on the lingual surface is more developed and larger than that of a central incisor of the same arch, making the tooth stronger during mastication.

4. A maxillary canine does somewhat resemble a mandibular canine; however, the cusp is more developed and larger, and the _____ is sharper on a maxillary tooth.

5. All lingual surface features of the maxillary canine are more prominent than on the mandibular canine, including the _____ and marginal ridges.

6. The lingual surface has prominent mesial and distal _____, with one on each side of the cingulum.

7. The tooth has a shallow but visible _____ and distolingual fossa on the lingual surface.

8. The cingulum and the incisal half of the lingual surface are sometimes separated by a shallow lingual groove, and this groove may contain a _____ near its center, or it may be present without the lingual groove.

9. The _____ curves higher incisally on the mesial surface than on the distal surface.

10. The _____ seem to form a nearly straight line, and the mesial marginal ridge is longer than the distal marginal ridge.

lingual ridge	root	cingulum
mesiolingual fossa	cusp slopes	after
lingual pit	cusp tip	marginal ridges
cementoenamel junction		

Reference

Chapter 16, Permanent anterior teeth. In Bath-Balogh M, Fehrenbach MJ: *Illustrated dental embryology, histology, and anatomy,* ed 3, St. Louis, 2011, Saunders.

ANSWER KEY 1. after, 2. root, 3. cingulum, 4. cusp tip, 5. lingual ridge, 6. marginal ridges, 7. mesiolingual fossa, 8. lingual pit, 9. cementoenamel junction, 10. cusp slopes.

FIGURE 3-31 Mandibular right canine (lingual and incisal views)

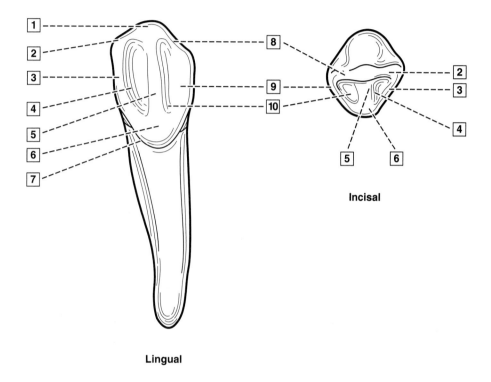

Lingual

Incisal

1	Cusp tip	6	Cingulum
2	Mesial cusp slopes	7	Cementoenamel junction
3	Mesial marginal ridge	8	Distal cusp slopes
4	Mesiolingual fossa	9	Distal marginal ridge
5	Lingual ridge	10	Distolingual fossa

REVIEW QUESTIONS

Fill in the blanks by choosing the appropriate terms from the list below.

1. The permanent mandibular canines erupt between 9 to 10 years of age (root completion between ages 12 to 14), usually _____ the maxillary canines and after most of the incisors have erupted.

2. The lingual surface of the crown of a mandibular canine is smoother than that of a maxillary canine and has a less developed _____, as well as the two marginal ridges.

3. The single _____ of a mandibular canine may be as long as that of a maxillary canine, but it is usually somewhat shorter, although it is still the longest of the mandibular arch.

4. The _____ outline is shorter and rounder than the mesial outline, similar to that of a maxillary canine.

5. The mesial _____ of a mandibular canine is shorter than the one on the distal cusp when first erupted, as noted from the labial view.

6. The lingual surface is relatively smooth, except for the faintly demarcated features of a _____, mesial marginal ridge, distal marginal ridge, and two lingual fossae, the distolingual fossa and mesiolingual fossa.

7. Rarely are there _____ or even lingual grooves on the lingual surface.

8. The _____ is more lingually inclined without incisal wear, unlike the labially placed one on a cusp of the maxillary canine.

9. The _____ curvature on the mesial surface is more toward the incisal when compared to the same surface of a maxillary canine.

10. From the incisive view, the mesial _____ is longer than the distal marginal one.

lingual pits	cementoenamel junction	distal
cusp tip	lingual ridge	cingulum
root	cusp slope	before
marginal ridge		

Reference

Chapter 16, Permanent anterior teeth. In Bath-Balogh M, Fehrenbach MJ: *Illustrated dental embryology, histology, and anatomy,* ed 3, St. Louis, 2011, Saunders.

FIGURE 3-32 Maxillary right first premolar (mesial and occlusal views)

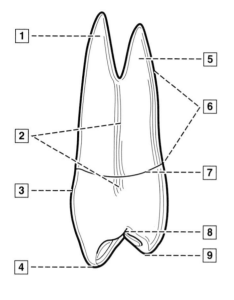

Mesial

Occlusal

1 Buccal root	**9** Lingual cusp	**17** Buccal cusp ridge of the buccal cusp
2 Mesial developmental depression	**10** Distal cusp ridge of buccal cusp	**18** Mesial cusp ridge of the buccal cusp
3 Buccal cervical ridge	**11** Lingual cusp ridge of buccal cusp (buccal triangular ridge)	**19** Mesiobuccal triangular groove
4 Buccal cusp	**12** Distobuccal triangular groove	**20** Mesial triangular fossa (with mesial pit)
5 Lingual root	**13** Distal triangular fossa (with distal pit)	**21** Mesial marginal ridge
6 Root trunk	**14** Distal marginal ridge	**22** Mesiolingual triangular groove
7 Cementoenamel junction	**15** Distolingual triangular groove	**23** Lingual triangular ridge
8 Mesial marginal groove	**16** Central groove	**24** Transverse ridge

REVIEW QUESTIONS

Fill in the blanks by choosing the appropriate terms from the list below.

1. The permanent maxillary first premolars erupt between 10 and 11 years of age (root completion between ages 12 to 13), _____ to the primary maxillary canines or their arch space, and thus are the succedaneous replacements for the primary maxillary first molars.

2. Most maxillary first premolars are _____, having two root branches in the apical third, with a buccal root and a lingual root, or *palatal root.*

3. A distinct mesial _____ is present on the root trunk of the maxillary first premolar, extending from the contact area to the bifurcation.

4. The _____ for a two-rooted tooth usually shows two pulp horns (one for each cusp) and two pulp canals (one for each root).

5. From the buccal view, the _____ of a maxillary first premolar is the widest mesiodistally of all the premolars.

6. This tooth is the only tooth in the permanent dentition that has a buccal cusp with the mesial _____ longer than the distal one.

7. The shorter _____ is sharp but not as sharp as the buccal cusp and is offset toward the mesial.

8. The _____ curvature is more occlusally located on the mesial surface than on the distal surface.

9. Extending mesiodistally, across the occlusal table of the maxillary first premolar, there is a long _____, evenly dividing the tooth buccolingually.

10. The _____ triangular fossa, which surrounds the mesiobuccal triangular groove, is deeper than the shallower distal triangular fossa, which surrounds the distobuccal triangular groove, with the deepest parts of these fossae being the occlusal developmental pits, mesial and distal.

bifurcated	cusp slope	pulp cavity
mesial	crown	root concavity
central groove	cementoenamel junction	distal
lingual cusp		

Reference

Chapter 17, Permanent posterior teeth. In Bath-Balogh M, Fehrenbach MJ: *Illustrated dental embryology, histology, and anatomy,* ed 3, St. Louis, 2011, Saunders.

ANSWER KEY 1. distal, 2. bifurcated, 3. root concavity, 4. pulp cavity, 5. crown, 6. cusp slope, 7. lingual cusp, 8. cementoenamel junction, 9. central groove, 10. mesial.

FIGURE 3-33 Maxillary right second premolar (mesial and occlusal views)

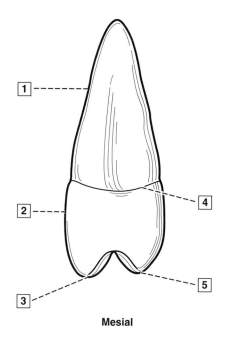

Mesial

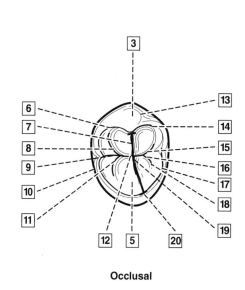

Occlusal

1 Root	**8** Distobuccal triangular groove	**15** Mesiobuccal triangular groove
2 Buccal cervical ridge	**9** Distal triangular fossa (with distal pit)	**16** Mesial triangular fossa (with mesial pit)
3 Buccal cusp	**10** Distal marginal ridge	**17** Mesial marginal ridge
4 Cementoenamel junction	**11** Distolingual triangular groove	**18** Mesiolingual triangular groove
5 Lingual cusp	**12** Central groove	**19** Lingual triangular ridge
6 Distal cusp ridge of buccal cusp	**13** Buccal cusp ridge of the buccal cusp	**20** Transverse ridge
7 Lingual cusp ridge of buccal cusp (buccal triangular ridge)	**14** Mesial cusp ridge of the buccal cusp	

REVIEW QUESTIONS

Fill in the blanks by choosing the appropriate terms from the list below.

1. The permanent maxillary second premolars erupt between 10 to 12 years of age (root completion between ages 12 to 14), _____ to the permanent maxillary first premolars, and thus are the succedaneous replacements for the primary maxillary second molars.

2. A maxillary second premolar resembles a first premolar, except that its _____ is less angular and more rounded.

3. Unlike a maxillary first premolar, a maxillary second premolar usually has only a single _____.

4. The _____ of this tooth has two pulp horns and one single pulp canal.

5. The _____ of a maxillary second premolar is neither as long nor as sharp as that same cusp on a maxillary first premolar.

6. All lingual surface features of a maxillary second premolar are similar to those of a maxillary first premolar; one noteworthy exception is that the _____ is larger, almost the same height as the buccal cusp on a maxillary second premolar, and slightly displaced to the mesial.

7. The mesial surface of a maxillary second premolar is similar to that of a maxillary first premolar, except that the cusps are closer to being the same size, and no mesial _____ is present on the crown and root surfaces. Instead this area is rounder.

8. Both the contact areas and _____ marginal ridge are more cervically located than those on a maxillary first premolar.

9. The _____ is shorter on a maxillary second premolar than on a maxillary first premolar and ends in a mesial pit and distal pit, which are closer together and thus more to the middle of the occlusal table.

10. A maxillary second premolar has numerous _____ radiating from the central groove, giving the tooth a more wrinkled appearance compared with a maxillary first premolar.

root concavity	supplemental grooves	mesial
central groove	root	crown
pulp cavity	lingual cusp	distal
buccal cusp		

Reference

Chapter 17, Permanent posterior teeth. In Bath-Balogh M, Fehrenbach MJ: *Illustrated dental embryology, histology, and anatomy,* ed 3, St. Louis, 2011, Saunders.

FIGURE 3-34 Mandibular right first premolar (mesial and occlusal views)

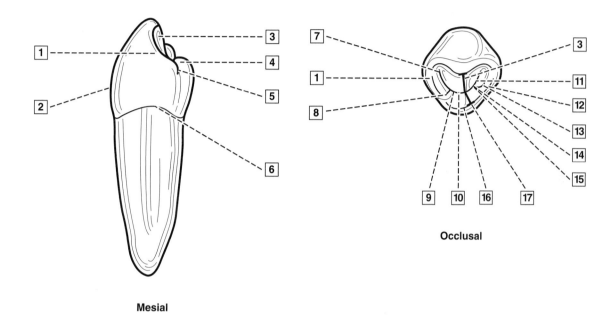

Mesial

Occlusal

1	Mesial marginal ridge	10	Central groove
2	Buccal cervical ridge	11	Distobuccal triangular groove
3	Buccal triangular ridge	12	Distal marginal ridge
4	Lingual cusp	13	Distal marginal groove
5	Mesiolingual groove	14	Distolingual triangular groove
6	Cementoenamel junction	15	Distal fossa (with distal pit)
7	Mesiobuccal triangular groove	16	Lingual triangular ridge
8	Mesiolingual groove	17	Transverse ridge
9	Mesial fossa (with mesial pit)		

REVIEW QUESTIONS

Fill in the blanks by choosing the appropriate terms from the list below.

1. The permanent mandibular first premolars erupt between 10 to 12 years of age (root completion between ages 12 to 13), _____ to the permanent mandibular canines, and thus are the succedaneous replacements for the primary mandibular first molars.

2. A mandibular first premolar resembles a mandibular _____ in many more ways than it does a mandibular second premolar.

3. A mandibular first premolar has a(n) _____ that is long and sharp and is the only functional cusp during occlusion, similar to a mandibular canine.

4. The _____ of a mandibular first premolar is usually small and nonfunctioning and is similar in appearance to the cingulum found on some maxillary canines.

5. The outline of the _____ of a mandibular first premolar from the buccal view is nearly symmetrical.

6. The mesial _____ of the buccal cusp is shorter than the distal one.

7. Because the lingual cusp is small, most of the _____ can be seen from the lingual view.

8. From the proximal view, the mesial _____ is nearly parallel to the angulation of the transverse ridge at a more cervical level.

9. The _____ curvature is more occlusal on the mesial surface.

10. The crown outline of the mandibular first premolar is diamond shaped from the occlusal, with a notch in the mesial outline at the _____.

mesiolingual groove	canine	lingual cusp
crown	cusp slope	occlusal surface
marginal ridge	distal	cementoenamel junction
buccal cusp		

Reference

Chapter 17, Permanent posterior teeth. In Bath-Balogh M, Fehrenbach MJ: *Illustrated dental embryology, histology, and anatomy,* ed 3, St. Louis, 2011, Saunders.

FIGURE 3-35 Mandibular right second premolar (mesial and occlusal views of the three-cusp type)

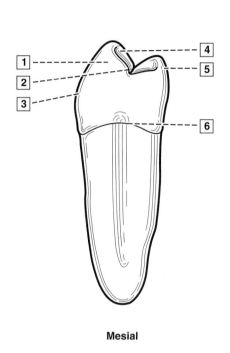

Mesial

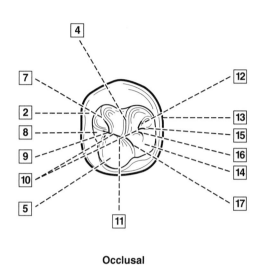

Occlusal

1	Buccal cusp	10	Central groove
2	Mesial marginal ridge	11	Central pit
3	Buccal cervical ridge	12	Distobuccal triangular groove
4	Buccal triangular ridge	13	Distal marginal ridge
5	Mesiolingual cusp	14	Distolingual cusp
6	Cementoenamel junction	15	Distal marginal groove
7	Mesiobuccal triangular groove	16	Distal fossa (with distal pit)
8	Mesial marginal groove	17	Lingual groove
9	Mesial fossa (with mesial pit)		

REVIEW QUESTIONS

Fill in the blanks by choosing the appropriate terms from the list below.

1. The permanent mandibular second premolars erupt between 11 to 12 years of age (root completion between ages 13 to 14), _____ to the mandibular first premolars, and thus are the succedaneous replacements for the primary mandibular second molars.

2. Unlike mandibular first premolars, the more common three-cusp type has three cusps: one large _____ composed of the three buccal lobes and two smaller lingual cusps composed of the two lingual lobes.

3. Similar to mandibular first premolars, the less common two-cusp type has a larger buccal cusp and a single smaller _____.

4. The _____ of the three-cusp type shows three pointed pulp horns.

5. The lingual cusp or cusps, depending on the type, are longer, causing less of the _____ to be seen from the lingual view.

6. From the proximal view, the mesial _____ is at almost a right angle, or 90°, to the long axis of the tooth and there is no mesiolingual groove present.

7. On the three-cusp type, the cusps are separated by two developmental grooves, a V-shaped _____, and a linear lingual groove.

8. The central groove on the two-cusp type is most often crescent shaped, forming a U-shaped groove pattern on the _____; less often, the central groove may be straight, forming an H-shaped groove pattern on the same tooth surface.

9. On the three-cusp type, a deep _____ is located at the junction of the central groove and the lingual groove, toward the lingual.

10. The central groove of the two-cusp type has its terminal ends centered in the mesial fossa and distal fossa, which are circular depressions having _____ radiating from them and none of the two-cusp types have a lingual groove or central pit.

marginal ridge	pulp cavity	distal
supplemental grooves	buccal cusp	central pit
central groove	lingual cusp	occlusal table
occlusal surface		

Reference

Chapter 17, Permanent posterior teeth. In Bath-Balogh M, Fehrenbach MJ: *Illustrated dental embryology, histology, and anatomy,* ed 3, St. Louis, 2011, Saunders.

FIGURE 3-36 Maxillary right first molar (lingual, mesial, and occlusal views)

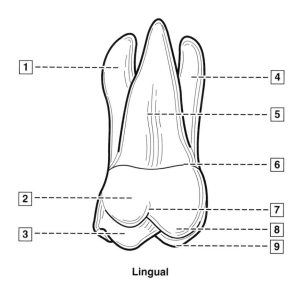

Lingual

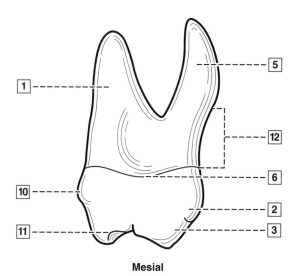

Mesial

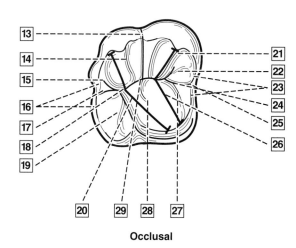

Occlusal

1	Mesiobuccal root
2	Cusp of Carabelli
3	Mesiolingual cusp
4	Distobuccal root
5	Lingual root
6	Cementoenamel junction
7	Distolingual groove
8	Distolingual cusp
9	Distobuccal cusp
10	Cervical ridge
11	Mesiobuccal cusp
12	Root trunk
13	Buccal groove
14	Distal marginal ridge
15	Distal marginal ridge groove
16	Distal fossa with distal pit
17	Distolingual cusp ridge
18	Distal fossa (with distal pit)
19	Distolingual cusp ridge
20	Oblique ridge
21	Mesiobuccal cusp ridge
22	Mesiobuccal triangular groove
23	Mesial marginal ridge
24	Mesial fossa (with mesial pit)
25	Mesial marginal ridge groove
26	Transverse ridge
27	Mesiolingual triangular groove
28	Mesiolingual cusp ridge
29	Central groove with central pit

REVIEW QUESTIONS

Fill in the blanks by choosing the appropriate terms from the list below.

1. The permanent maxillary first molars erupt between 6 to 7 years of age (root completion between ages 9 to 10), _____ to the primary maxillary second molars and thus nonsuccedaneous because there are no primary predecessors.

2. These teeth are the first permanent teeth to erupt into the _____.

3. The maxillary first molar is the largest tooth in the maxillary arch, as well as having the largest _____ in the permanent dentition.

4. The three _____ of maxillary first molars are larger and more divergent than those of the second molars and are also more complex in form than those of the maxillary premolars.

5. The _____, or lingual root is the largest and longest, inclines lingually, and extends beyond the crown outline with a banana-like curvature toward the buccal.

6. The _____ of a maxillary first molar usually has one pulp horn for each major cusp.

7. From the buccal view, the occlusal outline of a maxillary first molar is divided symmetrically by the _____.

8. A developmental groove extends between the two buccal cusps, runs apically about halfway to the cementoenamel junction, and is parallel with the long axis of the tooth, where it can fade out but it may end in a _____.

9. The _____ is initially with a primary maxillary second molar, until that tooth is shed; later it is with the permanent second premolar after that tooth erupts.

10. From the lingual view, since it is the largest cusp on the occlusal surface, the _____ outline is much longer and larger, but the cusp is not as sharp as the distolingual cusp; commonly arising from the lingual surface of this cusp is a fifth nonfunctioning cusp, the cusp of Carabelli.

buccal groove	buccal pit	crown
mesiolingual cusp	palatal	distal
mesial contact	roots	maxillary arch
pulp cavity		

Reference

Chapter 17, Permanent posterior teeth. In Bath-Balogh M, Fehrenbach MJ: *Illustrated dental embryology, histology, and anatomy,* ed 3, St. Louis, 2011, Saunders.

ANSWER KEY 1. distal, 2. maxillary arch, 3. crown, 4. roots, 5. palatal, 6. pulp cavity, 7. buccal groove, 8. buccal pit, 9. mesial contact, 10. mesiolingual cusp.

FIGURE 3-37 Maxillary second first molar: rhomboidal crown outline (lingual, mesial, and occlusal views)

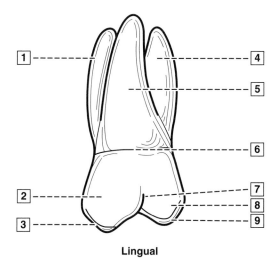

Lingual

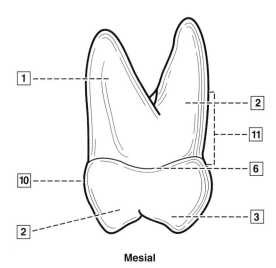

Mesial

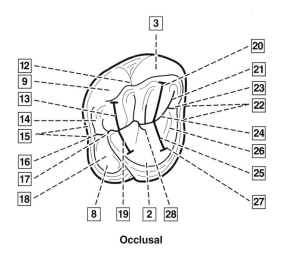

Occlusal

1	Mesiobuccal root
2	Mesiolingual cusp
3	Mesiobuccal cusp
4	Distobuccal root
5	Lingual root
6	Cementoenamel junction
7	Distolingual groove
8	Distolingual cusp
9	Distobuccal cusp
10	Cervical ridge
11	Root trunk
12	Buccal groove
13	Distobuccal cusp ridge
14	Distobuccal triangular groove
15	Distal marginal ridge
16	Distal marginal ridge groove
17	Distal fossa (with distal pit)
18	Distolingual cusp ridge
19	Oblique ridge
20	Mesiobuccal cusp ridge
21	Mesiobuccal triangular groove
22	Mesial marginal ridge
23	Mesial marginal ridge groove
24	Mesial fossa (with mesial pit)
25	Mesiolingual cusp ridge
26	Mesiolingual triangular groove
27	Transverse ridge
28	Central groove with central pit

REVIEW QUESTIONS

Fill in the blanks by choosing the appropriate terms from the list below.

1. The permanent maxillary second molars erupt between 12 to 13 years of age (root completion between ages 14 to 16), _____ to the permanent maxillary first molars and thus nonsuccedaneous because there are no primary predecessors.

2. The _____ usually has four cusps similar to the four major cusps of the maxillary first molar, but it can have three cusps.

3. The three _____ within the alveolar process on maxillary second molars are smaller than the maxillary first molars, less divergent, and placed at a more parallel position than on the maxillary first molars.

4. The _____ of a maxillary second molar consists of a pulp chamber and three main pulp canals, one for each of the three roots.

5. The more common rhomboidal type has four sides with opposite sides parallel; this type is similar to that of the maxillary _____ but with an even more accentuated outline.

6. The heart-shaped type is the less common and is similar to the typical maxillary

   _____.

7. However, the _____ is less prominent on the second than on the first molar as seen on the occlusal table of the tooth.

8. An increased number of _____ are usually present on the occlusal table of the second, making it seem wrinkled.

9. With the heart-shaped type, the _____ is quite small, with the other three cusps completely overshadowing it.

10. It is important to note that no _____ is present until the maxillary third molar possibly erupts and moves into occlusion.

oblique ridge	supplemental grooves	distal
distal contact area	pulp cavity	crown
first molar	roots	third molar
distolingual cusp		

Reference

Chapter 17, Permanent posterior teeth. In Bath-Balogh M, Fehrenbach MJ: *Illustrated dental embryology, histology, and anatomy,* ed 3, St. Louis, 2011, Saunders.

ANSWER KEY 1. distal, 2. crown, 3. roots, 4. pulp cavity, 5. first molar, 6. third molar, 7. oblique ridge, 8. supplemental grooves, 9. distolingual cusp, 10. distal contact area.

FIGURE 3-38 Mandibular right first molar (lingual, mesial, and occlusal views)

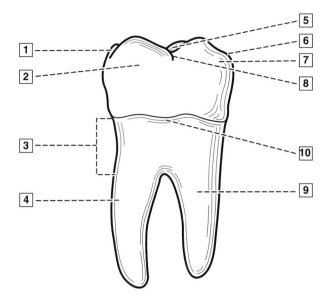

Lingual

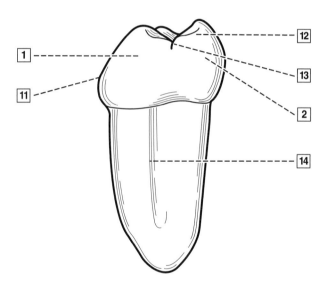

Mesial

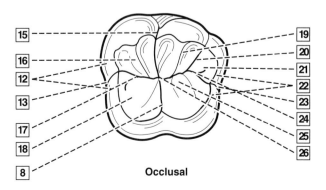

Occlusal

1	Mesiobuccal cusp
2	Mesiolingual cusp
3	Root trunk
4	Mesial root
5	Distobuccal cusp
6	Distal cusp
7	Distolingual cusp
8	Lingual groove
9	Distal root
10	Cementoenamel junction
11	Cervical ridge
12	Mesial marginal ridge
13	Mesial marginal ridge groove
14	Mesial fluting
15	Mesiobuccal groove
16	Mesiobuccal cusp ridge
17	Mesial triangular fossa (with mesial pit)
18	Mesiolingual cusp ridge
19	Distobuccal cusp ridge
20	Distobuccal groove
21	Distal cusp ridge
22	Distal marginal ridge
23	Distal marginal ridge groove
24	Distal triangular fossa (with distal pit)
25	Distolingual cusp ridge
26	Central groove with central pit

REVIEW QUESTIONS

Fill in the blanks by choosing the appropriate terms from the list below.

1.   The permanent mandibular first molars erupt between 6 to 7 years of age (root completion between ages 9 to 10), _____ to the primary mandibular second molars and thus are nonsuccedaneous because they have no primary predecessors.

2.   These teeth are usually the first _____ to erupt in the oral cavity.

3.   The _____ of a mandibular first molar usually has five cusps: three buccal and two lingual.

4.   The two _____ , mesial and distal, of a mandibular first molar are larger and more divergent than on the mandibular second molar, leaving them widely separated buccally.

5.   There is the presence of _____, an elongated developmental depression, noted on many surfaces of the root branches, especially on the mesial surface of the mesial root, but none is observed on the distal surface of the distal root.

6.   The _____ of a mandibular first molar is more likely to have three root canals: distal, mesiobuccal, and mesiolingual, and five pulp horns.

7.   The mesiobuccal groove extends straight cervically to a point about midway occlusocervically, but slightly mesial to the center mesiodistally, and usually ends in the _____.

8.   A(n) _____, which has a mesiodistally-oriented roundness in the cervical third of the buccal surface, is apparent; it is usually more prominent in its mesial part.

9.   The _____ is the smallest cusp and has a sharp tip.

10.   The Y-shaped groove pattern is formed on the _____ around the cusps by the mesiobuccal groove, distobuccal groove, and lingual groove; it also has three fossae: large central fossa, smaller mesial triangular fossa, and distal triangular fossa, with associated pits.

crown	fluting	permanent teeth
occlusal table	roots	distal
distal cusp	buccal cervical ridge	buccal pit
pulp cavity		

Reference

Chapter 17, Permanent posterior teeth. In Bath-Balogh M, Fehrenbach MJ: *Illustrated dental embryology, histology, and anatomy,* ed 3, St. Louis, 2011, Saunders.

FIGURE 3-39 Mandibular right second molar (lingual, mesial, and occlusal views)

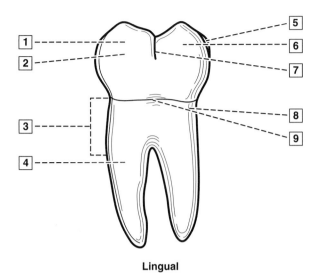

Lingual

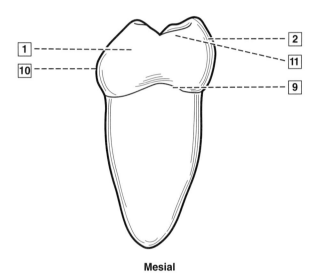

Mesial

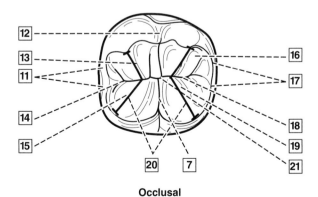

Occlusal

1	Mesiobuccal cusp
2	Mesiolingual cusp
3	Root trunk
4	Mesial root
5	Distobuccal cusp
6	Distolingual cusp

7	Lingual groove
8	Distal root
9	Cementoenamel junction
10	Cervical ridge
11	Mesial marginal ridge
12	Buccal groove

13	Mesiobuccal cusp ridge
14	Mesial triangular fossa (with mesial pit)
15	Mesiolingual cusp ridge
16	Distobuccal cusp ridge
17	Distal marginal ridge
18	Distal triangular fossa (with distal pit)

19	Distolingual cusp ridge
20	Transverse ridges
21	Central groove with central pit

REVIEW QUESTIONS

Fill in the blanks by choosing the appropriate terms from the list below.

1. The permanent mandibular second molars erupt between 11 to 12 years of age (root completion between ages 14 to 15), _____ to the permanent mandibular first molars and thus nonsuccedaneous because there are no primary predecessors.

2. The _____ measurements of a mandibular second molar are generally smaller when compared to a first molar, and the four cusps of a second molar are nearly equal in size compared with the five cusps of differing sizes of a mandibular first molar.

3. The two _____ of a second molar are smaller, shorter, and less divergent in placement than those of a mandibular first molar.

4. Although the _____ of a mandibular second molar can have two pulp canals (one for each root), it is more likely to have three pulp canals, similar to a mandibular first molar: distal, mesiobuccal, and mesiolingual canals (the latter two being together in the mesial root).

5. From the buccal view, the _____ divides the same-sized mesiobuccal cusp and distobuccal cusp of a mandibular second molar.

6. The occlusal surface of a mandibular second molar is considerably different from that of a mandibular first molar because there is no _____, and all cusps present are of equal size.

7. A cross-shaped groove pattern is formed where the well-defined central groove is crossed by the buccal groove and lingual groove, dividing the _____ into four parts that are nearly equal.

8. On the occlusal table there are three _____ present: central, mesial, and distal.

9. The cusp slopes on a mandibular second molar are less smooth than on a mandibular first molar because second molars have an increased number of _____.

10. Unlike a mandibular first molar, this tooth has two _____; the triangular ridges of the mesiobuccal and mesiolingual cusps meet to form this, as do the distobuccal and distolingual cusps.

crown	distal cusp	occlusal pits
supplemental grooves	distal	transverse ridges
occlusal table	roots	pulp cavity
buccal groove		

Reference

Chapter 17, Permanent posterior teeth. In Bath-Balogh M, Fehrenbach MJ: *Illustrated dental embryology, histology, and anatomy,* ed 3, St. Louis, 2011, Saunders.

FIGURE 4-1 Skull bones (frontal view)

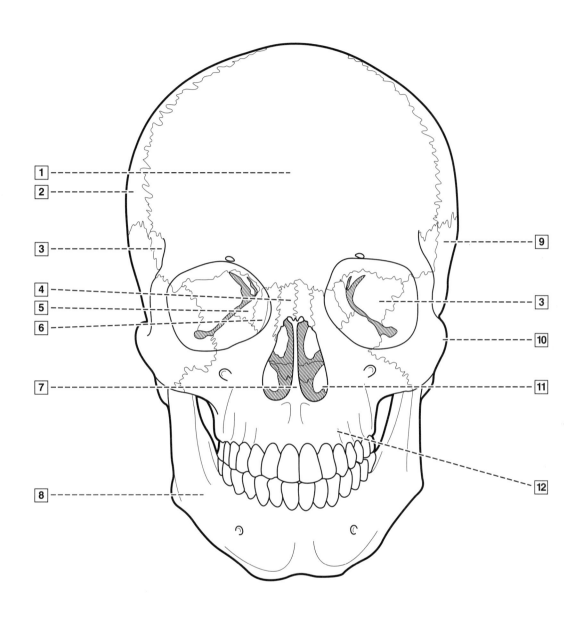

1	Frontal bone	**7**	Vomer
2	Parietal bone	**8**	Mandible
3	Sphenoid bone	**9**	Temporal bone
4	Nasal bone	**10**	Zygomatic bone
5	Ethmoid bone	**11**	Inferior nasal concha
6	Lacrimal bone	**12**	Maxilla

REVIEW QUESTIONS

Fill in the blanks by choosing the appropriate terms from the list below.

1. The _____ is a single cranial bone of the skull that forms the posterior part of the skull and the base of the cranium with four sides that articulate with the first cervical vertebra, the atlas.

2. The _____ is a single fused cranial bone of the skull that forms the anterior part of the skull, superior to the eyes, and includes the forehead and the roof of the orbits.

3. Each _____ is one of a pair of cranial bones of the skull that articulate with each other at the sagittal suture and that together form the greater part of the right and left lateral walls and roof of the skull.

4. Each _____ is one of a pair of cranial bones of the skull that together form the lateral walls of the skull and part of the base of the skull; each is composed of three parts: the squamous, tympanic, and petrous parts.

5. The _____ is a single cranial bone of the skull in the shape of a bat or butterfly and located in the midline, assisting in the formation of the base of the cranium, the sides of the skull, and the floors and walls of each orbit.

6. The _____ is a single midline cranial bone of the skull that helps connect the cranial skeleton to the facial skeleton and includes two unpaired plates: the perpendicular plate and cribriform plate, which cross each other.

7. Each _____ is one of a pair of small, oblong facial bones of the skull that together lie side by side, fused to each other to form the bridge of the nose in the midline; each is located superior to the piriform aperture, the anterior opening of the nasal cavity.

8. Each _____ is one of a pair of facial bones of the skull in the shape of a diamond, which together form the cheekbones and also help form the walls and floor of the orbits; it is composed of three processes: the frontal, temporal, and maxillary processes.

9. The _____ is one of a pair of facial bones of the skull that fuse developmentally and together form the upper jaw; each has a body and four processes: the frontal, zygomatic, palatine, and alveolar processes.

10. The _____ is a single fused facial bone of the skull that forms the lower jaw and is the only freely movable bone of the skull, having an articulation with each of the paired temporal bones at each temporomandibular joint.

frontal bone	ethmoid bone	zygomatic bone
parietal bone	mandible	maxilla
sphenoid bone	temporal bone	occipital bone
nasal bone		

Reference

Chapter 3, Skeletal system. In Fehrenbach MJ, Herring SW: *Illustrated anatomy of the head and neck,* ed 4, St. Louis, 2012, Saunders.

FIGURE 4-2   Skull bones and landmarks (lateral view)

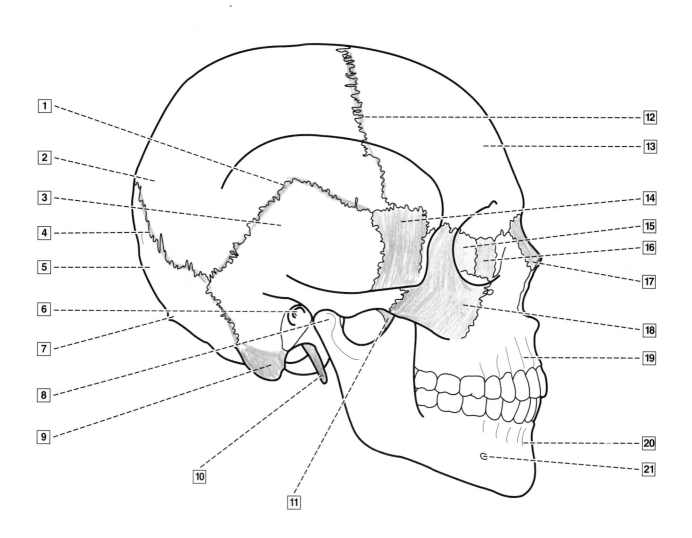

1 Squamosal suture	8 Condyloid process	15 Ethmoid bone
2 Parietal bone	9 Mastoid process of temporal bone	16 Lacrimal bone
3 Temporal bone	10 Styloid process	17 Nasal bone
4 Lambdoidal suture	11 Pterygoid process	18 Zygomatic bone
5 Occipital bone	12 Coronal suture	19 Maxilla
6 External acoustic meatus	13 Frontal bone	20 Mandible
7 External occipital protuberance	14 Sphenoid bone	21 Mental foramen

REVIEW QUESTIONS

Fill in the blanks by choosing the appropriate terms from the list below.

1. The paired _____ extends across the skull, between the frontal bone and the parietal bone on each side; it is also the location of the diamond-shaped *anterior fontanelle* or "soft spot" in a newborn that remains open until 2 years of age.

2. The single _____ extends from the front to the back of the skull at the midline between the parietal bones, is parallel with the sagittal plane, and also at a right angle to the coronal suture of the skull.

3. The single _____ is located between the occipital bone and the parietal bone and is more serrated-looking than the others, resembling an upside down V-shape.

4. The paired _____ is arched and located between the temporal bone and the parietal bone.

5. The tympanic part of the temporal bone forms most of the _____, a short canal leading to the tympanic cavity that is located posterior to the articular fossa.

6. On the inferior aspect of the petrous part of the temporal bone and posterior to the external acoustic meatus is the _____, a large roughened projection that is composed of air spaces that communicate with the middle ear cavity and that serves as a site for the attachment of the sternocleidomastoid muscle.

7. Inferior and medial to the external acoustic meatus and on the petrous part of the temporal bone is a long, pointed projection, the _____, a structure that serves for attachment of tongue and pharyngeal muscles and ligaments.

8. Inferior to the greater wing of the sphenoid bone is the _____, an area of attachment for some of the muscles of mastication; it consists of two plates that project inferiorly, the lateral and medial pterygoid plates.

9. Each paired _____ is an irregular, thin plate of bone that forms a small part of the anterior medial wall of the orbit and is considered the most fragile and smallest of all of the facial bones.

10. The _____ consists of two parts: the mandibular condyle and the constricted part that supports it, the neck of the mandible.

mastoid process	sagittal suture	condyloid process
lambdoidal suture	external acoustic meatus	coronal suture
lacrimal bone	squamosal suture	pterygoid process
styloid process		

Reference

Chapter 3, Skeletal system. In Fehrenbach MJ, Herring SW: *Illustrated anatomy of the head and neck,* ed 4, St. Louis, 2012, Saunders.

FIGURE 4-3   Skull bones and landmarks (inferior view)

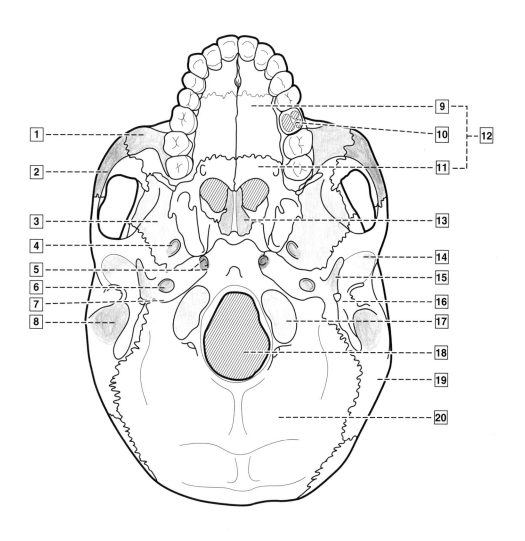

1 Zygomatic process of maxilla	8 Mastoid process	15 Styloid process
2 Zygomatic bone	9 Palatine process of maxilla	16 Stylomastoid foramen
3 Sphenoid bone	10 Alveolar process	17 Occipital condyle
4 Foramen ovale	11 Horizontal plate of palatine bone	18 Foramen magnum
5 Foramen lacerum	12 Hard palate	19 Temporal bone
6 Carotid canal	13 Vomer	20 Occipital bone
7 Jugular foramen	14 Mandibular fossa	

REVIEW QUESTIONS

Fill in the blanks by choosing the appropriate terms from the list below.

1. The hard palate of the skull is formed by the two palatine processes of the maxilla anteriorly and the two horizontal plates of the _____(s) posteriorly, which is(are) noted by the median palatine suture.

2. The larger anterior opening on the sphenoid bone is the _____, which is the passageway for the mandibular nerve of the fifth cranial or trigeminal nerve.

3. The large, irregularly shaped _____ is filled with cartilage during life.

4. A round opening, the _____, is located in the petrous part of the temporal bone and carries both the internal carotid artery and sympathetic carotid plexus.

5. Immediately posterior to the styloid process is the _____, an opening through which the seventh cranial or facial nerve exits from the skull to the face.

6. The _____ is located just medial to the styloid process and through which passes the internal jugular vein and three cranial nerves: the ninth cranial nerve or glossopharyngeal nerve, the tenth cranial nerve or vagus nerve, and the eleventh cranial nerve or accessory nerve.

7. The largest opening on the inferior view of the skull is the _____ of the occipital bone, through which the spinal cord, vertebral arteries, and eleventh cranial nerve, or accessory nerve pass.

8. Lateral and anterior to each side of the foramen magnum is the _____, which is a curved and smooth projection that has an articulation with the atlas, the first cervical vertebra.

9. On the inferior surface of the zygomatic process of the temporal bone is the _____, located posterior to the articular eminence; together they comprise the parts of the bony surface that articulate with the mandible on each side at the temporomandibular joint.

10. The _____ is a thin, flat, single midline facial bone of the skull that forms the posterior part of the nasal septum.

occipital condyle	**carotid canal**	**foramen lacerum**
foramen ovale	**jugular foramen**	**articular fossa**
stylomastoid foramen	**palatine bone**	**foramen magnum**
vomer		

Reference

Chapter 3, Skeletal system. In Fehrenbach MJ, Herring SW: *Illustrated Anatomy of the Head and Neck*, ed 4, St. Louis, 2012, Saunders.

FIGURE 4-4 Skull bones and landmarks (internal view)

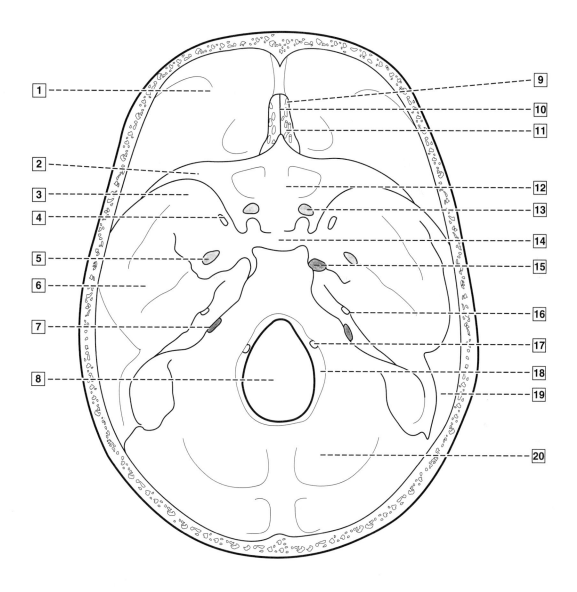

1 Frontal bone	8 Foramen magnum	15 Foramen lacerum
2 Lesser wing of sphenoid bone	9 Ethmoid bone	16 Internal acoustic meatus
3 Greater wing of sphenoid bone	10 Crista galli	17 Hypoglossal canal
4 Foramen rotundum	11 Cribriform plate	18 Hypoglossal foramen
5 Foramen ovale	12 Sphenoid bone	19 Parietal bone
6 Temporal bone	13 Optic foramen	20 Occipital bone
7 Jugular foramen	14 Sella turcica	

REVIEW QUESTIONS

Fill in the blanks by choosing the appropriate terms from the list below.

1.   The perforated _____ has foramina for the first cranial nerve or olfactory nerve.

2.   The _____ carries the maxillary nerve of the fifth cranial nerve or trigeminal nerve.

3.   As with an external skull surface view, the _____ is also present on the superior view of the internal skull, along with other nearby foramina, and carries the spinal cord, vertebral arteries, and the eleventh cranial nerve or accessory nerve.

4.   The _____ is the passageway for the seventh cranial nerve or facial nerve and the eighth cranial or vestibulocochlear nerve.

5.   The anterior process of the midline cranial bone of the skull, the _____, helps form the base of the orbital apex.

6.   The large posterolateral process of the midline cranial bone of the skull is the

     _____.

7.   The _____ is a bony canal that is located in the occipital bone of the skull, and that transmits the twelfth cranial nerve or the hypoglossal nerve from its point of entry near the medulla oblongata to its exit from the base of the skull near the jugular foramen.

8.   The _____ is the opening to the optic canal.

9.   The _____ is a saddle-shaped depression in the sphenoid bone, with its hypophyseal fossa holding the pituitary gland.

10. The _____ is a wedge-shaped vertical midline continuation of the perpendicular plate of the ethmoid bone superiorly into the cranial cavity; it serves as an attachment for layers covering the brain.

internal acoustic meatus	crista galli	sella turcica
hypoglossal canal	cribriform plate	lesser wing of the sphenoid bone
greater wing of the sphenoid bone	optic foramen	foramen rotundum
foramen magnum		

References

Chapter 3, Skeletal system. In Fehrenbach MJ, Herring SW: *Illustrated anatomy of the head and neck,* ed 4, St. Louis, 2012, Saunders; and Chapter 8, Head and neck. In Drake R, Vogl AW, Mitchell AWM: *Gray's anatomy for students,* ed 2, Philadelphia, 2010, Churchill Livingstone.

FIGURE 4-5   Skull bones and landmarks (midsagittal section)

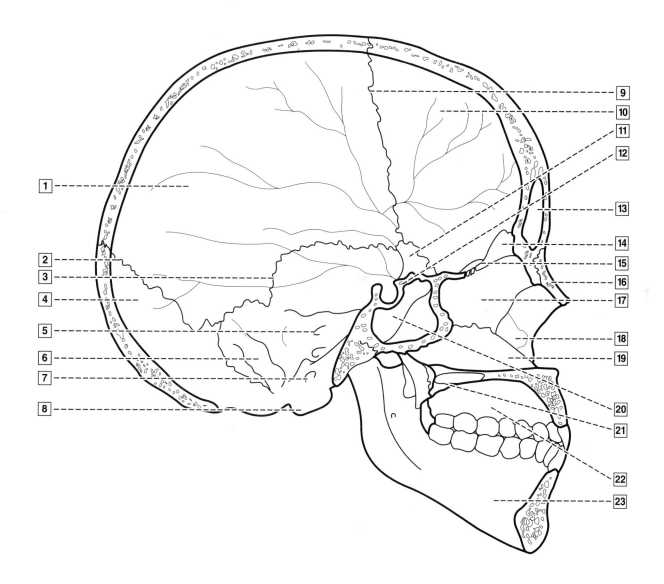

1 Parietal bone	**9** Coronal suture	**17** Perpendicular plate of ethmoid bone
2 Lambdoidal suture	**10** Frontal bone	**18** Inferior nasal concha
3 Squamosal suture	**11** Sphenoid bone	**19** Vomer
4 Occipital bone	**12** Sella turcica	**20** Sphenoidal sinus
5 Internal acoustic meatus	**13** Frontal sinus	**21** Palatine bone
6 Temporal bone	**14** Crista galli of ethmoid bone	**22** Maxilla
7 Hypoglossal canal	**15** Cribriform plate	**23** Mandible
8 Occipital condyle	**16** Nasal bone	

REVIEW QUESTIONS

Fill in the blanks by choosing the appropriate terms from the list below.

1. The body of each _____ has orbital, nasal, infratemporal, and facial surfaces; each body contains the maxillary sinuses, which are air-filled spaces, or paranasal sinuses.

2. The _____ articulates with each maxilla by way of their contained respective mandibular and maxillary arches of the dentition.

3. The _____ are paired facial bones that project from the maxillae to form a part of the lateral walls of the nasal cavity.

4. The _____ has four borders and is shaped like a curved plate.

5. Lateral and anterior to the foramen magnum are the paired condyles, curved and smooth projections of the _____.

6. The _____ articulates with one zygomatic and one parietal bone, the occipital and sphenoid bones, and the mandible.

7. The _____ fit between the frontal processes of the maxillae.

8. The paired _____ are located in the frontal bone just superior to the nasal cavity and are asymmetric, with the left and right structures always separated by a septum.

9. The paired _____ are located in the body of the sphenoid bone and are often asymmetric because of the lateral displacement of the intervening septum.

10. The _____ form the posterior part of the hard palate and the floor of the nasal cavity; anteriorly they join with the maxillae.

maxilla	mandible	palatine bones
parietal bone	sphenoidal sinuses	temporal bone
occipital bone	inferior nasal conchae	nasal bones
frontal sinuses		

Reference

Chapter 3, Skeletal system. In Fehrenbach MJ, Herring SW: *Illustrated anatomy of the head and neck,* ed 4, St. Louis, 2012, Saunders.

FIGURE 4-6 Orbit (anterior view)

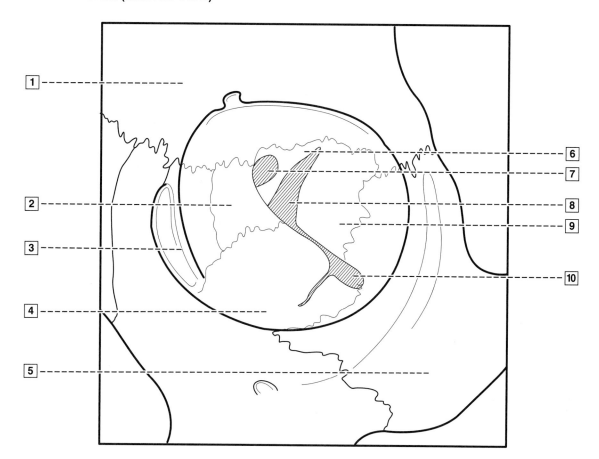

1 Frontal bone	6 Lesser wing of sphenoid bone
2 Ethmoid bone	7 Optic canal
3 Lacrimal bone	8 Superior orbital fissure
4 Maxilla	9 Greater wing of sphenoid bone
5 Zygomatic bone	10 Inferior orbital fissure

REVIEW QUESTIONS

Fill in the blanks by choosing the appropriate terms from the list below.

1. The _____ contains and protects the eyeball and is a prominent feature of the anterior part of the skull.

2. The round opening in the orbital apex is the _____.

3. The optic canal lies between the two roots of the _____.

4. Lateral to the optic canal is the curved and slitlike _____, which is located between the greater and lesser wings of the sphenoid bone.

5. The inferior orbital fissure can also be seen between the _____ and the maxilla.

6. The _____ connects the orbit with the infratemporal and pterygopalatine fossae; the infraorbital and zygomatic nerves, branches of the maxillary nerve, and infraorbital artery all enter the orbit through this structure.

7. The _____ forms the anterior part of the lateral wall of the orbit.

8. The orbital plates of the _____ create the roof or superior wall of the orbit.

9. The _____ forms the greatest part of the medial wall of the orbit.

10. The _____ is located at the anterior medial corner of the orbit, with the orbital surfaces of the maxilla forming the floor or inferior wall.

optic canal	orbit	lacrimal bone
superior orbital fissure	frontal bone	zygomatic bone
greater wing of the sphenoid bone	ethmoid bone	lesser wing of the sphenoid bone
inferior orbital fissure		

Reference

Chapter 3, Skeletal system. In Fehrenbach MJ, Herring SW: *Illustrated anatomy of the head and neck,* ed 4, St. Louis, 2012, Saunders.

FIGURE 4-7 Nasal region (anterior view)

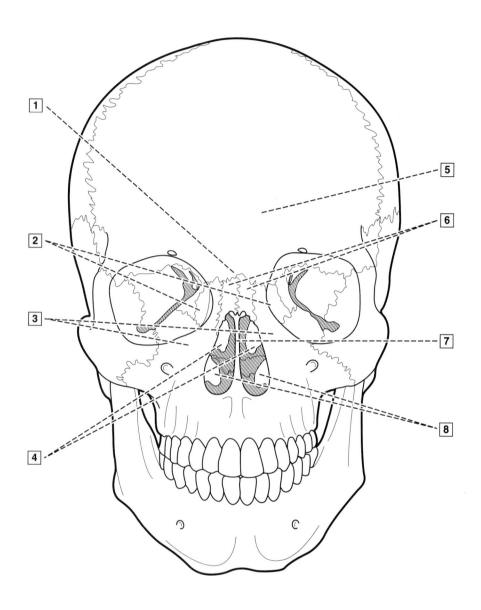

1	Nasion	**5**	Frontal bone
2	Lacrimal bones	**6**	Nasal bones
3	Maxillae	**7**	Nasal septum
4	Middle nasal conchae	**8**	Inferior nasal conchae

REVIEW QUESTIONS

Fill in the blanks by choosing the appropriate terms from the list below.

1. The _____ is the upper part of the respiratory tract and is located between the orbits, having both lateral walls and a floor, with anterior and posterior openings; it is lined by a respiratory mucosa like the rest of the respiratory system.

2. The bridge of the nose is formed from the paired _____.

3. Each lateral wall of the nasal cavity has three projecting structures or turbinates that extend inward from each maxilla: the superior nasal concha, the _____, and the inferior nasal concha, with each extending like a scroll into the nasal cavity.

4. The vertical partition, the _____, divides the nasal cavity into two parts.

5. The posterior part of the nasal septum is formed by the _____.

6. The _____ is a separate facial bone of the skull that forms off the lateral wall of the nasal cavity.

7. The _____, a midpoint landmark, is located at the junction of the frontal and nasal bones.

8. The anterior opening of the nasal cavity, the _____, is large and triangular.

9. The floor of the nasal cavity is formed from the bones of the hard palate: the palatine processes of the _____ anteriorly and the horizontal plates of the palatine bones posteriorly.

10. Anteriorly, the nasal septum is formed by both the perpendicular plate of the _____ superiorly and the nasal septal cartilage inferiorly.

nasal cavity	**nasal septum**	**nasion**
ethmoid bone	**vomer**	**piriform aperture**
nasal bones	**inferior nasal concha**	**maxillae**
middle nasal concha		

References

Chapter 3, Skeletal system. In Fehrenbach MJ, Herring SW: *Illustrated anatomy of the head and neck,* ed 4, St. Louis, 2012, Saunders; and Chapter 1, Face and neck regions. In Bath-Balogh M, Fehrenbach MJ: *Illustrated dental embryology, histology, and anatomy,* ed 3, St. Louis, 2011, Saunders.

FIGURE 4-8 Nasal cavity (sagittal section of the lateral wall)

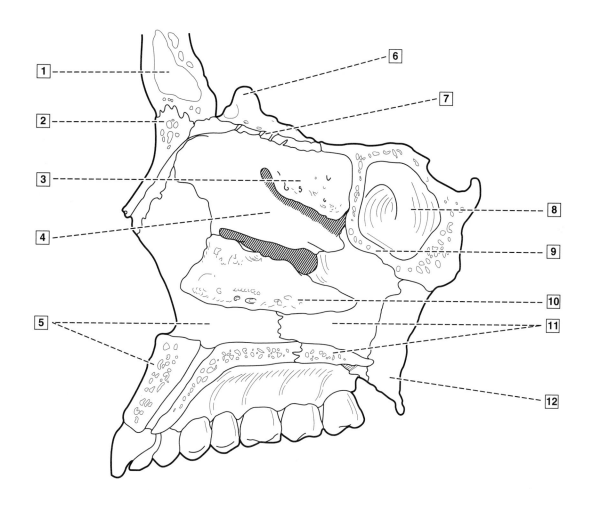

1	Frontal bone	8	Sphenoidal sinus
2	Nasal bone	9	Sphenoid bone
3	Superior nasal concha	10	Inferior nasal concha
4	Middle nasal concha	11	Palatine bone
5	Maxilla	12	Medial pterygoid plate
6	Crista galli		
7	Cribriform plate		

REVIEW QUESTIONS

Fill in the blanks by choosing the appropriate terms from the list below.

1. Each _____ communicates with and drains into the nasal cavity by the frontonasal duct, a constricted canal to the middle nasal meatus.

2. Each lateral wall of the nasal cavity has three projecting structures or turbinates that extend inward from the maxilla: the _____, the middle nasal concha, and the inferior nasal concha.

3. The lateral boundaries of the nasal cavity are formed by the _____ along with the palatine bones.

4. Protected by each nasal concha is a channel, the _____, with each having openings through which the paranasal sinuses or nasolacrimal duct communicates with the nasal cavity.

5. The anterior openings to the nasal cavities are the _____, and the posterior openings are choanae, or *posterior nasal apertures.*

6. A vertical midline continuation of the perpendicular plate superiorly into the cranial cavity is the wedge-shaped _____.

7. The _____, visible from viewing the inside of the cranial cavity and present on the superior aspect of the bone and surrounding the crista galli, is perforated by foramina to allow the passage of olfactory nerves for the sense of smell.

8. The vertical plates of the _____ form a part of the lateral walls of the nasal cavity.

9. The _____ are paired facial bones of the skull that project from the maxillae to form a part of the lateral walls of the nasal cavity.

10. The _____ communicate with and drain into the nasal cavity through an opening superior to each superior nasal concha.

palatine bones	superior nasal concha	inferior nasal conchae
frontal sinus	maxillae	cribriform plate
nares	crista galli	sphenoidal sinuses
nasal meatus		

References

Chapter 3, Skeletal system. In Fehrenbach MJ, Herring SW: *Illustrated anatomy of the head and neck,* ed 4, St. Louis, 2012, Saunders; and Chapter 11, Head and neck structures. In Bath-Balogh M, Fehrenbach MJ: *Illustrated dental embryology, histology, and anatomy,* ed 3, St. Louis, 2011, Saunders.

ANSWER KEY 1. frontal sinus, 2. superior nasal concha, 3. maxillae, 4. nasal meatus, 5. nares, 6. crista galli, 7. cribriform plate, 8. palatine bones, 9. inferior nasal conchae, 10. sphenoidal sinuses.

FIGURE 4-9   Occipital bone (inferior, lateral, and posterior views)

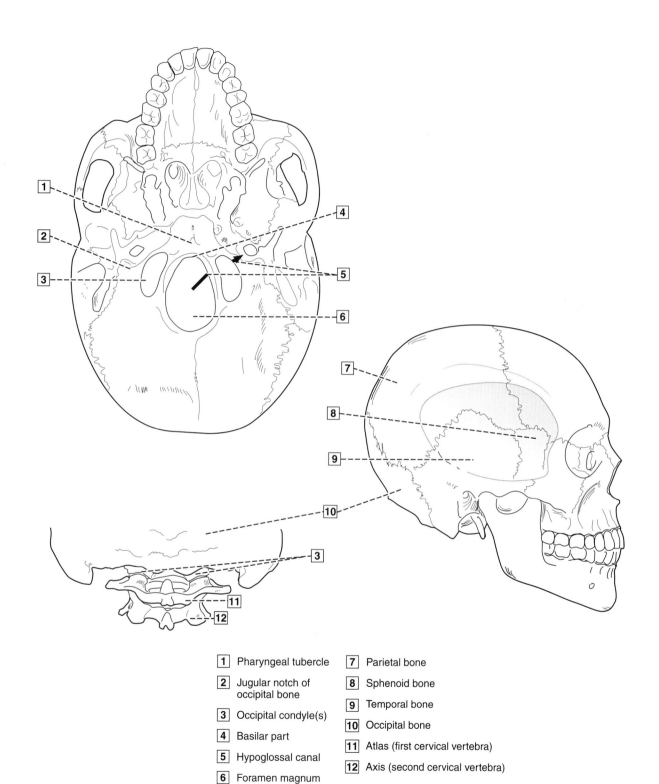

1	Pharyngeal tubercle	**7**	Parietal bone
2	Jugular notch of occipital bone	**8**	Sphenoid bone
3	Occipital condyle(s)	**9**	Temporal bone
4	Basilar part	**10**	Occipital bone
5	Hypoglossal canal	**11**	Atlas (first cervical vertebra)
6	Foramen magnum	**12**	Axis (second cervical vertebra)

REVIEW QUESTIONS

Fill in the blanks by choosing the appropriate terms from the list below.

1. The _____ is a single cranial bone of the skull.

2. The occipital bone articulates with the _____, temporal bone, and sphenoid bone of the skull.

3. The occipital bone articulates with the first cervical vertebra or, _____ of the neck.

4. On the external surface of the occipital bone from an inferior view, it can be seen that the large_____ is completely formed by this bone.

5. Lateral and anterior to the foramen magnum are the _____, a pair of curved and smooth projections on the occipital bone.

6. On the stout _____, a four-sided plate anterior to the foramen magnum has a midline projection on the occipital bone, the pharyngeal tubercle.

7. When tilting the skull model, the openings anterior and lateral to the foramen magnum are visible on the inferior view of the occipital bone, the paired _____.

8. The _____ of the occipital bone, the medial part that forms the jugular foramen (the lateral part is from the temporal bone), is noted on the inferior view.

9. The occipital bone is an irregular bone with _____ sides that is somewhat curved upon itself.

10. The occipital bone forms the posterior part of the skull and the base of the _____ of the brain.

jugular notch	foramen magnum	parietal bone
cranium	hypoglossal canals	four
atlas	occipital bone	basilar part
occipital condyles		

Reference

Chapter 3, Skeletal system. In Fehrenbach MJ, Herring SW: *Illustrated anatomy of the head and neck,* ed 4, St. Louis, 2012, Saunders.

FIGURE 4-10   Frontal bone (lateral, anterior, and inferior views)

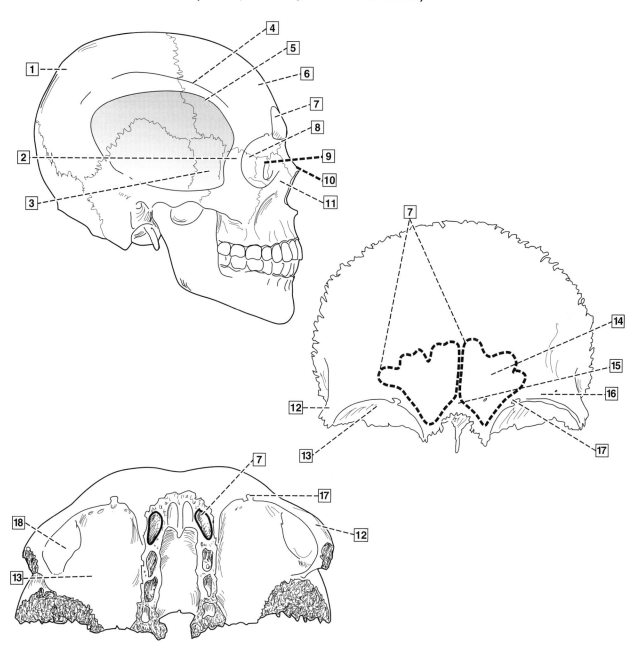

1 Parietal bone	**7** Location of frontal sinus(es)	**13** Orbital roof
2 Zygomatic bone	**8** Ethmoid bone	**14** Frontal eminence
3 Sphenoid bone	**9** Lacrimal bone	**15** Glabella
4 Superior temporal line	**10** Nasal bone	**16** Supraorbital ridge
5 Inferior temporal line	**11** Maxilla	**17** Supraorbital notch
6 Frontal bone	**12** Zygomatic process of frontal bone	**18** Lacrimal fossa

REVIEW QUESTIONS

Fill in the blanks by choosing the appropriate terms from the list below.

1. The _____ is a single cranial bone of the skull that forms the anterior part of the skull superior to the eyes in the frontal region and includes the forehead, the roof of the orbits, and part of the nasal cavity.

2. The frontal bone articulates with the _____, sphenoid bone, lacrimal bones, nasal bones, ethmoid bone, zygomatic bones, and maxillae.

3. The frontal bone's part of the superior temporal line and _____ is visible when the bone is viewed from the lateral aspect.

4. Internally, the frontal bone contains the paired paranasal sinuses, the _____.

5. The _____ is located on the medial part of the supraorbital ridge of the frontal bone and is where the supraorbital artery and nerve travel from the orbit to the forehead.

6. Between the supraorbital ridges of the frontal bone is the _____, the smooth elevated area between the eyebrows.

7. Lateral to the orbit is a projection, the orbital surface of the _____ of the frontal bone.

8. From the inferior view of the frontal bone, each _____ is visible and is located just inside the lateral part of the supraorbital ridge.

9. Each lacrimal fossa of the frontal bone contains the _____, which produces lacrimal fluid, or *tears.*

10. The curved elevations over the superior part of the orbit are the _____ of the frontal bone, subjacent to the eyebrows.

lacrimal gland	lacrimal fossa	zygomatic process
frontal sinuses	parietal bones	supraorbital ridges
inferior temporal line	supraorbital notch	glabella
frontal bone		

Reference

Chapter 3, Skeletal system. In Fehrenbach MJ, Herring SW: *Illustrated anatomy of the head and neck,* ed 4, St. Louis, 2012, Saunders.

ANSWER KEY 1. frontal bone, 2. parietal bones, 3. inferior temporal line, 4. frontal sinuses, 5. supraorbital notch, 6. glabella, 7. zygomatic process, 8. lacrimal fossa, 9. lacrimal gland, 10. supraorbital ridges.

FIGURE 4-11   Parietal bones (posterior view)

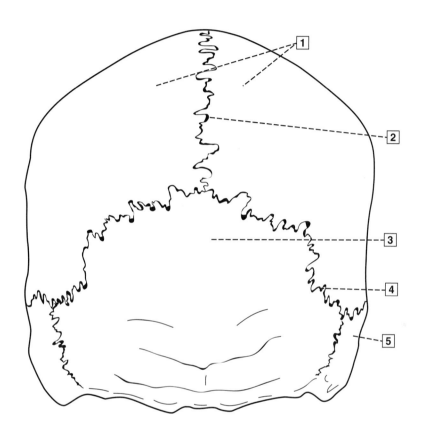

1 Parietal bones

2 Sagittal suture

3 Occipital bone

4 Lambdoidal suture

5 Temporal bone

REVIEW QUESTIONS

Fill in the blanks by choosing the appropriate terms from the list below.

1. The _____ are paired cranial bones of the skull.

2. The two parietal bones articulate with each other at the single _____, which extends from the front to the back of the skull at the midline between the bones and is parallel with the sagittal plane of the skull.

3. The parietal bones are located posterior to the _____.

4. The two parietal bones together form the greater part of the right and left lateral walls and the roof of the _____.

5. The parietal bones articulate with other bones of the skull: the occipital, frontal, temporal, and _____ bones.

6. The paired parietal bones articulate with the occipital bone at the single _____, which is by far more serrated-looking than the other sutures, resembling an upside down V.

7. Each parietal bone has _____ borders and is shaped like a curved plate.

8. The external surface of the parietal bone is convex, smooth, and marked near the center by, the _____, which indicates the point where ossification commenced.

9. The _____, the longest and thickest part of each parietal bone articulates with the bone of the opposite side at the sagittal suture.

10. Occasionally the parietal bone can be divided into two parts, upper and lower, by a(n) _____.

parietal eminence	sagittal suture	skull
sagittal border	anteroposterior suture	frontal bone
four	parietal bones	lambdoidal suture
sphenoid		

Reference

Chapter 3, Skeletal system. In Fehrenbach MJ, Herring SW: *Illustrated anatomy of the head and neck,* ed 4, St. Louis, 2012, Saunders.

FIGURE 4-12 Temporal bone(s) (lateral and inferior views)

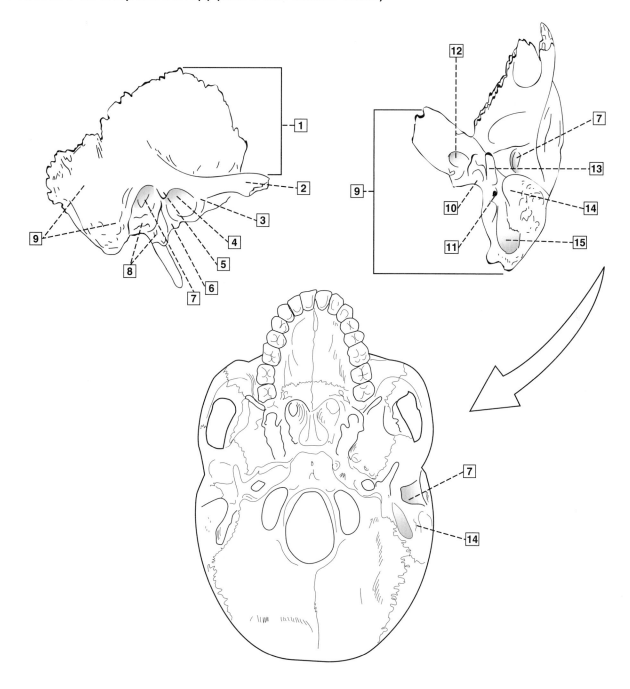

1	Squamous part	**6**	Petrotympanic fissure	**11**	Stylomastoid foramen
2	Zygomatic process	**7**	External acoustic meatus	**12**	Carotid canal
3	Articular eminence	**8**	Tympanic part	**13**	Styloid process
4	Articular fossa	**9**	Petrous part	**14**	Mastoid process
5	Postglenoid process	**10**	Jugular notch	**15**	Mastoid notch

REVIEW QUESTIONS

Fill in the blanks by choosing the appropriate terms from the list below.

1. The _____ are paired cranial bones that form the lateral walls of the skull in the temporal region.

2. The temporal bones are part of the base of the _____ in the auricular region.

3. Each temporal bone is deep to the _____, as well as overlying the sphenoid bone, forming one side of the head posterior to the eyes.

4. Each temporal bone articulates with one zygomatic and one parietal bone, the occipital and sphenoid bones, and the _____.

5. Each temporal bone is composed of _____ parts: the squamous, tympanic, and petrous parts.

6. The small, irregularly shaped _____ of the temporal bone is associated with the ear canal and forms most of the external acoustic meatus.

7. The large, fan-shaped part on each of the temporal bones is the _____ of the temporal bone.

8. The _____ of the temporal bone is inferiorly located and helps form the cranial floor.

9. Anterior to the articular fossa of the temporal bone is the _____, and posterior is the postglenoid process, with the tympanic part separated from the petrous part by the petrotympanic fissure.

10. On the inferior aspect of the petrous part of the temporal bone and posterior to the external acoustic meatus is a large roughened projection, the _____.

three	temple	skull
mandible	petrous part	squamous part
tympanic part	temporal bones	articular eminence
mastoid process		

Reference

Chapter 3, Skeletal system. In Fehrenbach MJ, Herring SW: *Illustrated anatomy of the head and neck,* ed 4, St. Louis, 2012, Saunders.

FIGURE 4-13 Sphenoid bone (inferior view, superior view of internal skull surface, and lateral aspect)

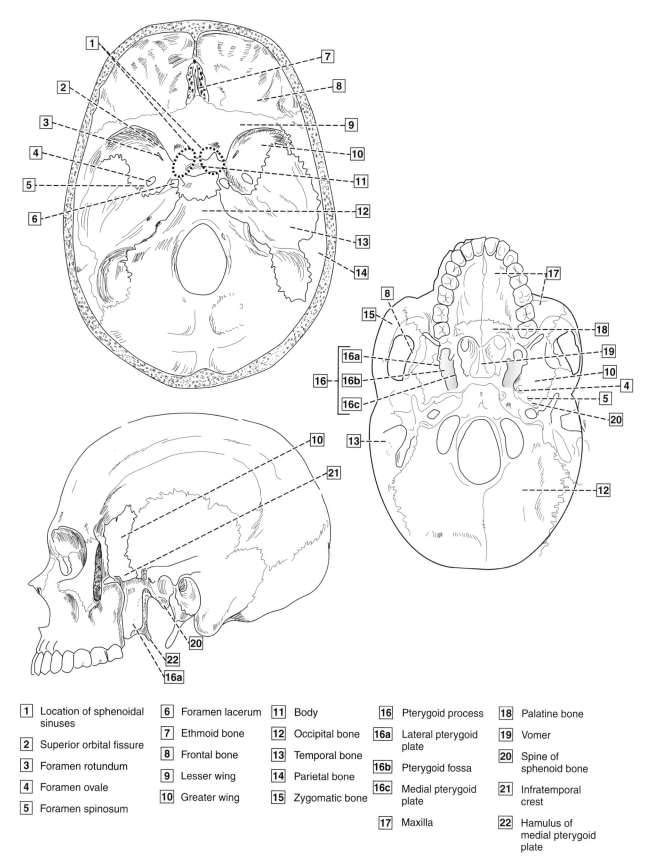

1 Location of sphenoidal sinuses	**6** Foramen lacerum	**11** Body	**16** Pterygoid process	**18** Palatine bone
2 Superior orbital fissure	**7** Ethmoid bone	**12** Occipital bone	**16a** Lateral pterygoid plate	**19** Vomer
3 Foramen rotundum	**8** Frontal bone	**13** Temporal bone	**16b** Pterygoid fossa	**20** Spine of sphenoid bone
4 Foramen ovale	**9** Lesser wing	**14** Parietal bone	**16c** Medial pterygoid plate	**21** Infratemporal crest
5 Foramen spinosum	**10** Greater wing	**15** Zygomatic bone	**17** Maxilla	**22** Hamulus of medial pterygoid plate

REVIEW QUESTIONS

Fill in the blanks by choosing the appropriate terms from the list below.

1. The _____ is a midline cranial bone of the skull, because it runs through the midsagittal section and thus is internally wedged between several other bones in the anterior part of the cranium, looking like a bat or butterfly taking flight.

2. The sphenoid bone articulates with the frontal, parietal, ethmoid, temporal, zygomatic, maxillae, palatine, vomer, and _____ bones, helping to connect the cranial skeleton to the facial skeleton.

3. The sphenoid bone consists of a(n) _____ and its processes and has a number of features, projections, and important foramina.

4. The body of the sphenoid bone articulates on its anterior surface with the _____ and posteriorly with the basilar part of the occipital bone.

5. The projections of the sphenoid bone include an anterior process, the lesser wing of the sphenoid bone that forms the base of the orbital apex, and a posterolateral process, the _____ of the sphenoid bone.

6. A sharp, pointed area, the _____ of the sphenoid bone, is located at the posterior corner of each greater wing of the sphenoid bone.

7. Each greater wing of the sphenoid bone is divided into two smaller surfaces by the _____: the temporal and infratemporal surfaces.

8. The depression of the _____ is located lateral to the lateral pterygoid plate of the sphenoid bone.

9. The _____, a thin curved process, is the inferior termination of the medial pterygoid plate of the sphenoid bone.

10. The vertical pterygomaxillary fissure is between the lateral pterygoid plate of the _____ of the sphenoid bone and the maxillary tuberosity on the maxilla; it descends at right angles to the medial end of the inferior orbital fissure and gives passage to part of the maxillary artery and vein.

hamulus	pterygoid process	occipital
infratemporal fossa	ethmoid bone	greater wing
spine	sphenoid bone	infratemporal crest
body		

Reference

Chapter 3, Skeletal system. In Fehrenbach MJ, Herring SW: *Illustrated anatomy of the head and neck,* ed 4, St. Louis, 2012, Saunders.

FIGURE 4-14 Ethmoid bone (anterior view, superior view of internal skull surface, and oblique anterior view)

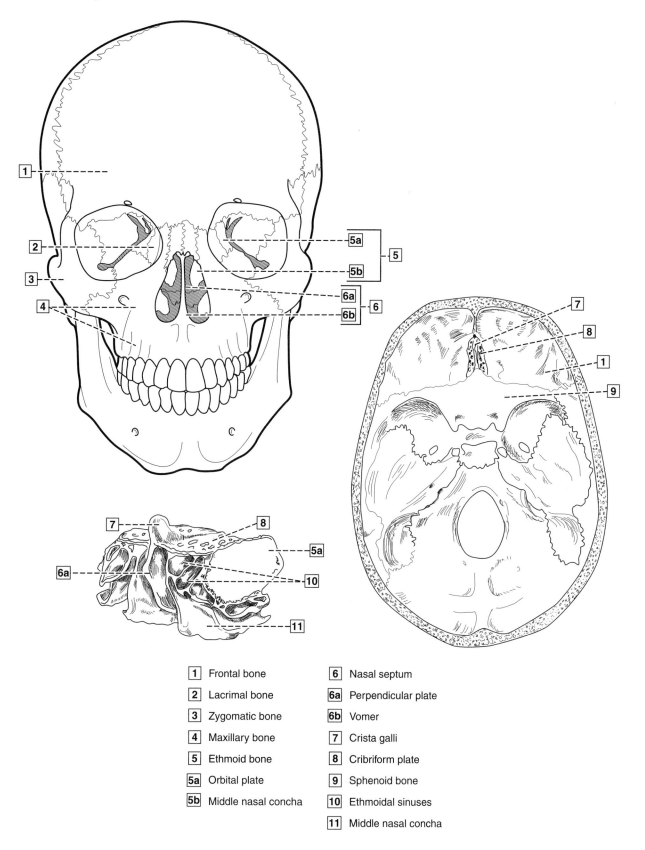

1	Frontal bone	6	Nasal septum
2	Lacrimal bone	6a	Perpendicular plate
3	Zygomatic bone	6b	Vomer
4	Maxillary bone	7	Crista galli
5	Ethmoid bone	8	Cribriform plate
5a	Orbital plate	9	Sphenoid bone
5b	Middle nasal concha	10	Ethmoidal sinuses
		11	Middle nasal concha

REVIEW QUESTIONS

Fill in the blanks by choosing the appropriate terms from the list below.

1. The _____ is a single midline cranial bone of the skull that runs through the midsagittal plane and helps connect the cranial skeleton to the facial skeleton similarly to the sphenoid bone.

2. The ethmoid bone is located anterior to the sphenoid bone in the anterior part of the _____.

3. The ethmoid bone articulates with the frontal, sphenoid, and lacrimal bones as well as the maxilla as it adjoins the _____ at its inferior and posterior borders.

4. The ethmoid bone has two unpaired plates that form it: the midline vertical perpendicular plate and the horizontal _____, which it crosses.

5. The cribriform plate, visible from the inside of the cranial cavity and present on the superior aspect of the ethmoid bone and surrounding the _____, is perforated by foramina to allow the passage of olfactory nerves for the sense of smell.

6. The lateral parts of the ethmoid bone form the superior nasal and middle nasal _____ in the nasal cavity and the paired orbital plates.

7. The _____ of the ethmoid bone forms the medial orbital wall.

8. Between the orbital plate and the conchae are the _____, or *ethmoid air cells*, which are a variable number of small cavities in the lateral mass of the ethmoid bone.

9. The _____ of the ethmoid bone is easily seen in the nasal cavity when viewing the skull and aids the nasal septal cartilage and vomer in forming the nasal septum.

10. A vertical midline continuation of the perpendicular plate superiorly into the _____ is the wedge-shaped crista galli on the ethmoid bone, which serves as an attachment for layers covering the brain.

perpendicular plate	ethmoidal sinuses	ethmoid bone
cranial cavity	cribriform plate	cranium
conchae	vomer	crista galli
orbital plate		

Reference

Chapter 3, Skeletal system. In Fehrenbach MJ, Herring SW: *Illustrated anatomy of the head and neck,* ed 4, St. Louis, 2012, Saunders.

ANSWER KEY 1. ethmoid bone, 2. cranium, 3. vomer, 4. cribriform plate, 5. crista galli, 6. conchae, 7. orbital plate, 8. ethmoidal sinuses, 9. perpendicular plate, 10. cranial cavity.

FIGURE 4-15   Vomer (medial wall of the nasal cavity)

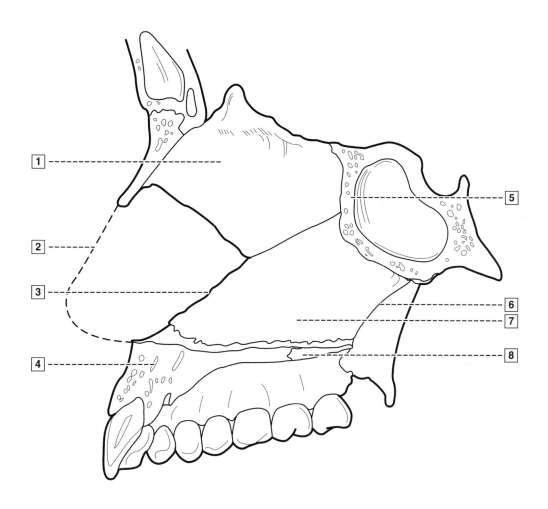

1	Ethmoid bone	**5**	Sphenoid bone
2	Outline of nasal septal cartilage	**6**	Free border
3	Articulation with nasal cartilage	**7**	Vomer
4	Maxilla	**8**	Palatine bone

REVIEW QUESTIONS

Fill in the blanks by choosing the appropriate terms from the list below.

1. The _____ is a thin, flat, single midline facial bone of the skull.

2. The vomer is almost _____ in shape.

3. The vomer forms the posterior part of the _____, with the anterior part formed by the ethmoid bone and nasal septal cartilage.

4. The perpendicular plate of the _____ is easily seen in the nasal cavity and aids the nasal septal cartilage and vomer in forming the nasal septum.

5. The floor of the nasal cavity is formed from the bones of the hard palate: palatine processes of the maxillae anteriorly and the horizontal plates of the _____ posteriorly.

6. The vomer articulates with the ethmoid bone on its anterosuperior border, the nasal cartilage anteriorly, the palatine bones and maxillae inferiorly, and the _____ on its posterosuperior border.

7. The posteroinferior border of the vomer is considered a(n) _____, because it is free of bony articulation.

8. The vomer is in noted within the _____ and thus located inside the midline placed nasal cavity, and its articulations are easily seen on a lateral view of the bone.

9. Unlike other skull bones, the vomer has no _____ attachments.

10. The vomer is not a cranial bone but is considered a(n) _____.

palatine bones	vomer	free border
facial bone	nasal septum	midsagittal plane
muscle	sphenoid bone	trapezoid
ethmoid bone		

Reference

Chapter 3, Skeletal system. In Fehrenbach MJ, Herring SW: *Illustrated anatomy of the head and neck,* ed 4, St. Louis, 2012, Saunders.

ANSWER KEY   1. vomer, 2. trapezoid, 3. nasal septum, 4. ethmoid bone, 5. palatine bones, 6. sphenoid bone, 7. free border, 8. midsagittal plane, 9. muscle, 10. facial bone.

FIGURE 4-16 Nasal bones, lacrimal bones, and inferior nasal conchae (anterior view)

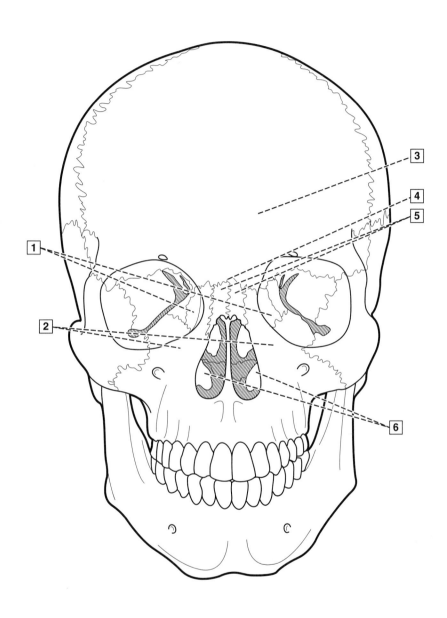

1	Lacrimal bones	4	Frontonasal suture
2	Maxillae	5	Nasal bones
3	Frontal bone	6	Inferior nasal conchae

REVIEW QUESTIONS

Fill in the blanks by choosing the appropriate terms from the list below.

1. Each paired _____ is an irregular, thin plate of bone that forms a small part of the anterior medial wall of the orbit of the skull.

2. Each lacrimal bone as a facial bone of the skull articulates with the ethmoid bone and the _____, as well as the maxilla.

3. The nasolacrimal duct is formed at the junction of the lacrimal and _____ bones.

4. Lacrimal fluid, or *tears,* from the lacrimal gland are drained through this duct into the _____.

5. The _____, paired, small, oblong facial bones of the skull, lie side by side, fused to each other to form the bridge of the nose in the midline that is superior to the piriform aperture; the fusion line between the two bones is called the *internasal suture.*

6. The nasal bones fit between the frontal processes of the maxillae and thus articulate with the frontal bone superiorly at the _____ and the maxillae laterally.

7. The _____ are paired facial bones of the skull that project from the maxillae to form a part of the lateral walls of the nasal cavity.

8. Unlike the superior and middle nasal conchae that also project from the maxillae, the inferior nasal conchae are separate _____.

9. The inferior nasal conchae articulate with the ethmoid, lacrimal, and _____, as well as the maxillae.

10. Each inferior nasal concha is composed of fragile, thin, spongy bone curved onto itself like a(n) _____.

scroll	palatine bones	inferior nasal meatus
maxillary	frontal bone	inferior nasal conchae
facial bones	lacrimal bone	nasal bones
frontonasal suture		

Reference

Chapter 3, Skeletal system. In Fehrenbach MJ, Herring SW: *Illustrated anatomy of the head and neck,* ed 4, St. Louis, 2012, Saunders.

ANSWER KEY 1. lacrimal bone, 2. frontal bone, 3. maxillary, 4. inferior nasal meatus, 5. nasal bones, 6. frontonasal suture, 7. inferior nasal conchae, 8. facial bones, 9. palatine bones, 10. scroll.

FIGURE 4-17 **Zygomatic bone(s) (lateral and anterior views)**

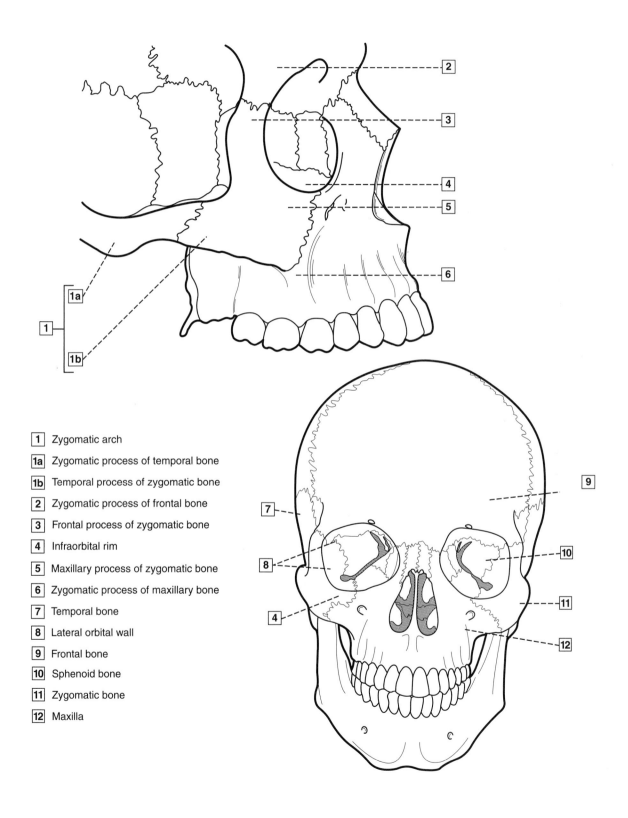

1 Zygomatic arch
1a Zygomatic process of temporal bone
1b Temporal process of zygomatic bone
2 Zygomatic process of frontal bone
3 Frontal process of zygomatic bone
4 Infraorbital rim
5 Maxillary process of zygomatic bone
6 Zygomatic process of maxillary bone
7 Temporal bone
8 Lateral orbital wall
9 Frontal bone
10 Sphenoid bone
11 Zygomatic bone
12 Maxilla

REVIEW QUESTIONS

Fill in the blanks by choosing the appropriate terms from the list below.

1. Each _____, or *zygoma,* is a paired facial bone of the skull that forms the malar surfaces, or *cheekbones.*

2. The zygomatic bones articulate with the frontal, temporal, sphenoid bones, as well as the

   _____.

3. Each zygomatic bone is diamond-shaped and composed of _____ processes with similarly named associated bony articulations: the frontal, temporal, and maxillary processes.

4. The orbital surface of the _____ of the zygomatic bone forms the anterior lateral orbital wall, with usually a paired small foramen, the zygomaticofacial foramen, as an opening on its lateral surface.

5. The _____ of the zygomatic bone forms the zygomatic arch along with the zygomatic process of the temporal bone, with a paired zygomaticotemporal foramen present on the surface of the bone.

6. The orbital surface of the _____ of the zygomatic bone forms a part of the infraorbital rim and a small part of the anterior part of the lateral orbital wall.

7. The zygomatic bone helps to form the walls and floor of the _____.

8. The lower border and medial surface of the zygomatic bone give origin to the

   _____.

9. Near the center of the temporal surface of the zygomatic bone is the _____ for the transmission of the zygomaticotemporal nerve.

10. The malar surface of the zygomatic bone is convex and perforated near its center by a small aperture, the _____, for the passage of the zygomaticofacial nerve and vessels.

zygomaticotemporal foramen	**three**	**zygomatic bone**
orbit	**zygomaticofacial foramen**	**maxillae**
masseter muscle	**maxillary process**	**frontal process**
temporal process		

Reference

Chapter 3, Skeletal system. In Fehrenbach MJ, Herring SW: *Illustrated anatomy of the head and neck,* ed 4, St. Louis, 2012, Saunders.

FIGURE 4-18 Palatine bone(s) (inferior and lateral views) with the maxillae

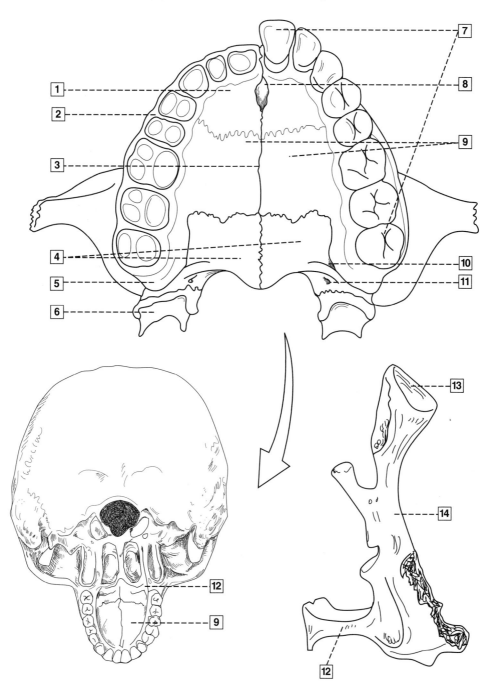

1 Palatine process of maxilla	**6** Sphenoid bone	**11** Lesser palatine foramen
2 Alveolar process of maxilla	**7** Maxillary teeth	**12** Horizontal plate of palatine bone
3 Median palatine suture	**8** Incisive foramen	**13** Orbital process at apex of orbit
4 Palatine bones	**9** Maxillae	**14** Vertical plate of palatine bone
5 Maxillary tuberosity	**10** Greater palatine foramen	

REVIEW QUESTIONS

Fill in the blanks by choosing the appropriate terms from the list below.

1. The _____ are paired bones of the skull that form the posterior part of the hard palate and the floor of the nasal cavity; anteriorly they join with the maxillae.

2. Each palatine bone is somewhat L-shaped and consists of two plates: the _____ and vertical plate.

3. The horizontal plates of each palatine bone form the lesser or posterior part of the _____.

4. The _____ of each palatine bone forms a part of the lateral walls of the nasal cavity, and each plate contributes a small lip of bone to the orbital apex.

5. The palatine bones serve as a link between the _____ and the sphenoid bone with which they articulate.

6. The two horizontal plates of each palatine bone articulate with each other at the posterior part of the _____.

7. The two horizontal plates of each palatine bone articulate anteriorly with the maxillae at the _____.

8. The large _____ is located in the posterolateral region of each palatine bone, usually at the apex of the maxillary third molar, and transmits the greater palatine nerve and blood vessels, providing an important landmark for the administration of the greater palatine nerve block.

9. A smaller opening nearby the greater palatine foramen, the _____, transmits the lesser palatine nerve and blood vessels to the soft palate and tonsils.

10. The _____ is the opening between the sphenoid bone and orbital processes of each palatine bone; it opens into the nasal cavity and gives passage to branches from the pterygopalatine ganglion and the sphenopalatine artery from the maxillary artery.

vertical plate	greater palatine foramen	maxillae
sphenopalatine foramen	palatine bones	horizontal plate
median palatine suture	lesser palatine foramen	hard palate
transverse palatine suture		

Reference

Chapter 3, Skeletal system. In Fehrenbach MJ, Herring SW: *Illustrated anatomy of the head and neck,* ed 4, St. Louis, 2012, Saunders.

FIGURE 4-19   Maxillae and landmarks (anterior view)

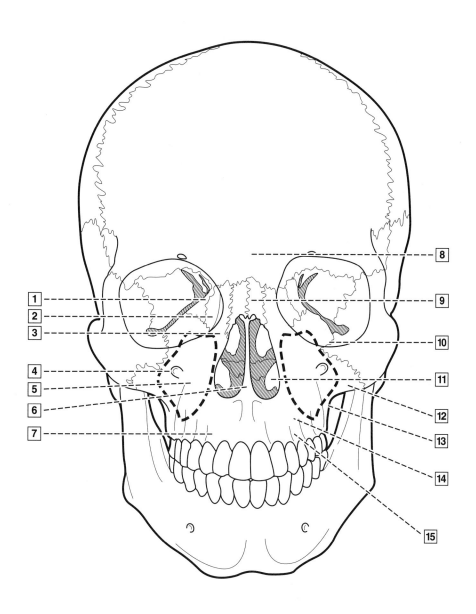

1 Ethmoid bone	**6** Vomer	**11** Inferior nasal concha
2 Lacrimal bone	**7** Alveolar process of maxilla	**12** Zygomatic process of maxilla
3 Frontal process of maxilla	**8** Frontal bone	**13** Location of maxillary sinus
4 Infraorbital foramen	**9** Nasal bone	**14** Canine fossa
5 Body of maxilla	**10** Infraorbital sulcus	**15** Canine eminence

REVIEW QUESTIONS

Fill in the blanks by choosing the appropriate terms from the list below.

1. The _____ consist of paired maxillary bones or maxilla.

2. The two parts of the maxillae are fused together at the _____.

3. Each maxilla articulates with the _____, lacrimal, nasal, inferior nasal conchal, vomer, sphenoid, ethmoid, palatine, and zygomatic bones.

4. Each maxilla includes a body and _____ processes: frontal, zygomatic, palatine, and alveolar processes.

5. The _____ of the maxilla has orbital, nasal, infratemporal, and facial surfaces.

6. Each of the bodies of the maxillae contain the _____, which are air-filled spaces, or paranasal sinuses.

7. The paired maxillary bones together form the upper _____ as the facial bones of the skull that contain the maxillary teeth.

8. From the anterior view, each _____ of the maxilla articulates with the frontal bone and forms the medial orbital rim with the lacrimal bone on its anterior surface.

9. The inferior orbital fissure carries the infraorbital and zygomatic nerves, infraorbital artery, and inferior ophthalmic vein, and then it becomes the groove in the floor of the orbital surface or infraorbital sulcus; even later the infraorbital sulcus becomes the infraorbital canal, and finally terminates on the facial surface of each maxilla as the _____.

10. An elongated depression, the _____, is just posterosuperior to the roots of each of the maxillary canine teeth.

maxillary sinuses	canine fossa	four
body	jaw	intermaxillary suture
frontal process	infraorbital foramen	maxillae
frontal bone		

Reference

Chapter 3, Skeletal system. In Fehrenbach MJ, Herring SW: *Illustrated anatomy of the head and neck,* ed 4, St. Louis, 2012, Saunders.

FIGURE 4-20 Maxilla and landmarks (cutaway lateral aspect)

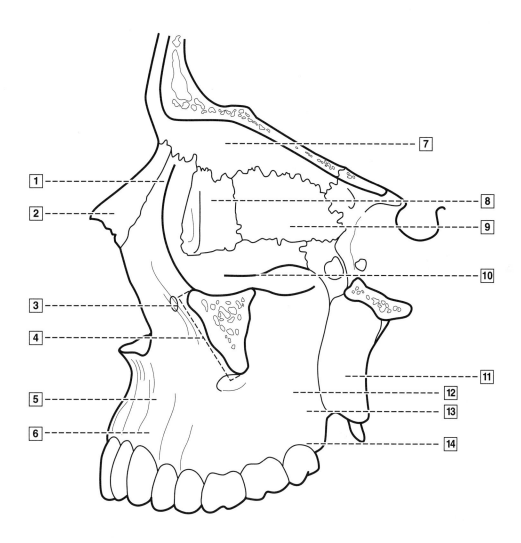

1	Frontal process of maxilla	**8**	Lacrimal bone
2	Nasal bone	**9**	Ethmoid bone
3	Infraorbital foramen	**10**	Infraorbital sulcus
4	Zygomatic process of maxilla	**11**	Sphenoid bone
5	Canine fossa	**12**	Body of maxilla
6	Canine eminence	**13**	Posterior superior alveolar foramina
7	Frontal bone	**14**	Maxillary tuberosity

REVIEW QUESTIONS

Fill in the blanks by choosing the appropriate terms from the list below.

1. The facial ridge over each of the maxillary canines, the _____, is especially prominent, providing an important landmark for the administration of the anterior superior alveolar nerve block.

2. The maxillary bone over the facial surface of the maxillary teeth is _____ than the mandibular bone over similar teeth as can be viewed on a panoramic radiograph, which allows a greater incidence of clinically adequate local anesthesia for the maxillary teeth when the agent is administered as a local infiltration than would occur with similar teeth on the mandibular arch.

3. From the lateral view, each _____ of the maxilla articulates with the zygomatic bone laterally, completing the infraorbital rim.

4. On the posterior part of the body of the maxilla is a rounded, roughened elevation, the _____, just posterior to the most distal molar of the maxillary arch of the dentition, which is an important landmark for mounting radiographs and serving as the one of the boundaries of the fossae of the skull, as well as providing an important landmark for the administration of the posterior superior alveolar nerve block.

5. The superolateral part of the maxillary tuberosity is perforated by the _____, where the posterior superior alveolar nerve and blood vessel branches enter the bone from the posterior, providing an important landmark for the administration of the posterior superior alveolar nerve block.

6. Each maxilla articulates with the frontal, lacrimal, nasal, inferior nasal conchal, vomer, sphenoid, ethmoid, palatine, and _____.

7. An elongated depression, the canine fossa, is just posterosuperior to the roots of each of the _____ canine teeth in the alveolar process of the maxilla.

8. The body of the maxilla has orbital, nasal, infratemporal, and _____ surfaces.

9. The groove in the floor of the orbital surface of each maxilla is the _____.

10. The infraorbital sulcus becomes the infraorbital canal and then terminates on the facial surface of each maxilla as the _____.

maxillary tuberosity	infraorbital foramen	zygomatic bone
zygomatic process	infraorbital sulcus	maxillary
posterior superior alveolar foramina	canine eminence	facial
less dense		

Reference

Chapter 3, Skeletal system. In Fehrenbach MJ, Herring SW: *Illustrated anatomy of the head and neck,* ed 4, St. Louis, 2012, Saunders.

FIGURE 4-21 Mandible and landmarks (lateral and internal views)

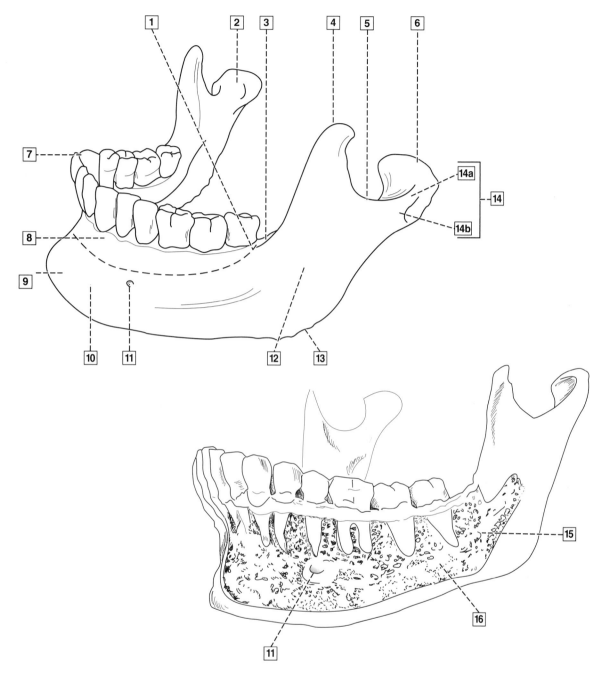

1 External oblique line	**6** Articulating surface of mandibular condyle	**11** Mental foramen	**14b** Mandibular condyle
2 Pterygoid fovea	**7** Mandibular teeth	**12** Ramus	**15** Mandibular foramen
3 Coronoid notch	**8** Alveolar process	**13** Angle	**16** Mandibular canal
4 Coronoid process	**9** Mental protuberance	**14** Condyloid process	
5 Mandibular notch	**10** Body	**14a** Neck of mandibular condyle	

REVIEW QUESTIONS

Fill in the blanks by choosing the appropriate terms from the list below.

1. The _____ is a single facial bone that forms the lower jaw and is the only freely movable bone of the skull.

2. The heavy horizontal part of the lower jaw inferior to the mental foramen is the _____ of the mandible, or *base.*

3. The _____ is the midline bony prominence of the chin, located inferior to the roots of the mandibular incisors.

4. Farther posteriorly on the lateral surface of the mandible, usually inferior to the apices of the mandibular first and second premolars, is an opening, the _____, which allows the entrance of the mental nerve and blood vessels into the mandibular canal.

5. Superior to the body of the mandible, the part of the lower jaw that contains the roots of the mandibular teeth is the _____ of the mandible.

6. On the lateral aspect of the mandible, the stout flat plate of the _____, extends superiorly and posteriorly from the body of the mandible on each side.

7. The posterior border of the ramus is thicker and extends from the angle of the mandible, which is the juncture between the ramus and the body of the mandible, to a large more posterior projection, the _____.

8. The condyloid process consists of two parts: the mandibular condyle, and the constricted part that supports it, the _____.

9. The anterior border of the ramus is a thin, sharp margin that terminates in the

   _____.

10. The main part of the anterior border of the ramus forms a concave forward curve, the _____, which is the greatest depression on the anterior border of the ramus, providing an important landmark for the administration of the inferior alveolar nerve block.

mental protuberance	alveolar process	ramus
mental foramen	body	condyloid process
mandible	coronoid notch	neck
coronoid process		

Reference

Chapter 3, Skeletal system. In Fehrenbach MJ, Herring SW: *Illustrated anatomy of the head and neck,* ed 4, St. Louis, 2012, Saunders.

FIGURE 4-22 Mandible and landmarks (medial and internal views)

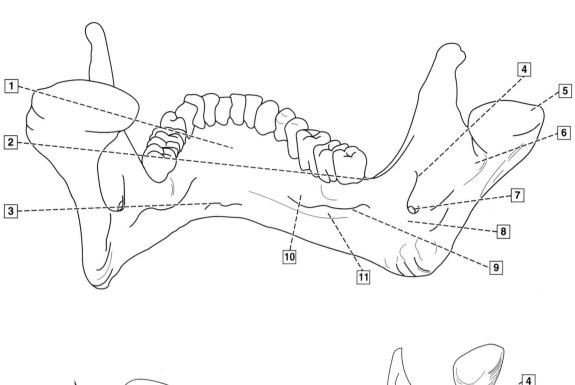

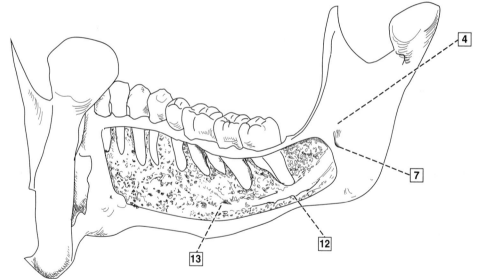

1 Alveolar process	**6** Ramus	**11** Submandibular fossa
2 Retromolar triangle	**7** Mandibular foramen	**12** Mandibular canal
3 Genial tubercles	**8** Mylohyoid groove	**13** Mental foramen
4 Lingula	**9** Mylohyoid line	
5 Articulating surface of condyle	**10** Sublingual fossa	

REVIEW QUESTIONS

Fill in the blanks by choosing the appropriate terms from the list below.

1. Near the midline of the mandible on its medial surface are the _____, or *mental spines*, a cluster of small projections that serve as a muscle attachment area.

2. At the lateral edge of each mandibular alveolar process is a rounded, roughened area, the _____, just posterior to the most distal molar of the mandibular arch of the dentition, which is a bony landmark that when covered with soft tissue is the retromolar pad.

3. Along each medial surface of the body of the mandible is the *internal oblique ridge,* or _____, that extends posteriorly and superiorly, becoming more prominent as it ascends each body; this line is the point of attachment of the mylohyoid muscle that forms the floor of the mouth.

4. A shallow depression, the _____, which contains the sublingual salivary gland, is located superior to the anterior part of the mylohyoid line.

5. Inferior to the posterior part of the mylohyoid line and inferior to the mandibular posterior teeth is a deep depression, the _____, which contains the submandibular salivary gland.

6. On the medial surface of the ramus is the _____, which is the opening of the mandibular canal, with the inferior alveolar nerve and blood vessels exiting the mandible through it.

7. Overhanging the mandibular foramen is a bony spine, the _____, which serves as an attachment for the sphenomandibular ligament associated with the temporomandibular joint.

8. A small groove, the _____, passes anteriorly to and inferiorly from the mandibular foramen, with the mylohyoid nerve and blood vessels traveling in it.

9. The _____ of the condyle is where the mandible articulates with the temporal bone at the temporomandibular joint.

10. Inferior to the articular surface of the condyle on the anterior surface of the neck is a triangular depression, the _____, which serves for the attachment of the lateral pterygoid muscle.

mylohyoid line	mylohyoid groove	sublingual fossa
pterygoid fovea	retromolar triangle	submandibular fossa
articulating surface	genial tubercles	mandibular foramen
lingula		

Reference

Chapter 3, Skeletal system. In Fehrenbach MJ, Herring SW: *Illustrated anatomy of the head and neck,* ed 4, St. Louis, 2012, Saunders.

FIGURE 4-23 Temporomandibular joint with associated bones: temporal and mandible (lateral views)

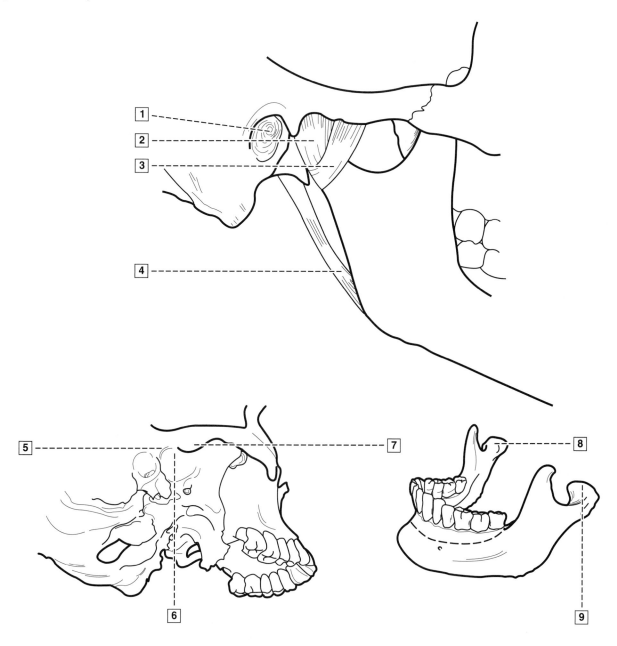

1	External acoustic meatus	6	Articular fossa
2	Joint capsule	7	Articular eminence
3	Temporomandibular ligament	8	Articulating surface of condyle
4	Stylomandibular ligament	9	Mandibular condyle
5	Postglenoid process		

REVIEW QUESTIONS

Fill in the blanks by choosing the appropriate terms from the list below.

1. The _____ is a joint on each side of the head that allows for movement of the mandible for speech and mastication.

2. The _____ is a cranial bone of the skull that articulates with the facial skull bone of the mandible at the temporomandibular joint by way of the disc of the joint.

3. The _____, or *glenoid fossa,* is posterior to the articular eminence and consists of an oval-shaped depression on the temporal bone, which is posterior and medial to the zygomatic process of the temporal bone.

4. Posterior to the articular fossa is a sharper ridge, the _____.

5. The _____ of the condyle is strongly convex in the anteroposterior direction and only slightly convex mediolaterally and is where the mandible articulates with the temporal bone.

6. A fibrous _____ completely encloses the temporomandibular joint, with it superiorly wrapping around the margin of the temporal bone's articular eminence and articular fossa and inferiorly wrapping around the circumference of the mandibular condyle including the neck.

7. The _____, or *meniscus,* is located between the temporal bone and mandibular condyle on each side, allowing articulation between the two bones at the temporomandibular joint.

8. The _____ is a variable ligament formed from thickened cervical fascia in the area that runs from the styloid process of the temporal bone to the angle of the mandible and separates the parotid and submandibular salivary glands.

9. The _____ is located on the lateral side of each joint forming a reinforcement of the lateral part of the joint capsule of the temporomandibular joint.

10. The disc of the joint completely divides the temporomandibular joint into two compartments, or _____, consisting of an upper and a lower one.

synovial cavities	postglenoid process	articulating surface
temporomandibular ligament	stylomandibular ligament	temporal bone
disc of the joint	articular fossa	temporomandibular joint
joint capsule		

References

Chapter 5, Temporomandibular joint. In Fehrenbach MJ, Herring SW: *Illustrated anatomy of the head and neck,* ed 4, St. Louis, 2012, Saunders; and Chapter 19, Temporomandibular joint. In Bath-Balogh M, Fehrenbach MJ: *Illustrated dental embryology, histology, and anatomy,* ed 3, St. Louis, 2011, Saunders.

FIGURE 4-24   Temporomandibular joint (internal view)

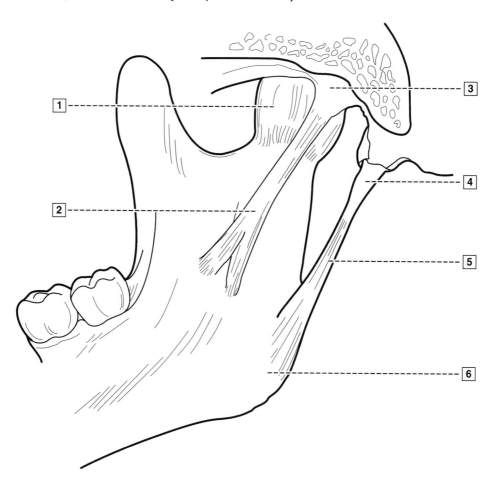

1   Joint capsule
2   Sphenomandibular ligament
3   Spine of sphenoid bone
4   Styloid process of temporal bone
5   Stylomandibular ligament
6   Angle of mandible

REVIEW QUESTIONS

Fill in the blanks by choosing the appropriate terms from the list below.

1. The mandible is joined to the cranium by ligaments of the _____, which include temporomandibular, stylomandibular, and sphenomandibular ligaments.

2. The _____ is located on the lateral side of each joint, forming a reinforcement of the lateral part of the joint capsule, and is considered the major ligament for the joint.

3. The triangle-shaped temporomandibular joint ligament has a base that is attached to the zygomatic process of the _____ and the articular tubercle; its apex is fixed to the lateral side of the neck of the mandible.

4. The temporomandibular joint ligament prevents excessive _____, or moving backward of the mandible.

5. The _____ runs from the styloid process of the temporal bone to the angle of the mandible, separates the parotid and submandibular salivary glands, and becomes taut when the mandible is protruded.

6. The _____ runs from the angular spine of the sphenoid bone to the lingula of the mandibular foramen on the medial aspect of the mandible.

7. The inferior alveolar nerve descends between the sphenomandibular ligament and the ramus of the mandible to gain access to the _____, and because of its attachment to the lingula, overlaps the opening.

8. The sphenomandibular ligament provides an important landmark for the administration of inferior alveolar nerve block; however, it may actually act as an outer barrier to the agent during the administration of the block if the medial surface of the _____ is not contacted with the needle at the deeper mandibular foramen.

9. The sphenomandibular ligament is not strictly considered part of the temporomandibular joint, because it is located on the _____ side of the mandible, some distance from the joint.

10. The stylomandibular ligament is a variable ligament formed from thickened cervical _____ in the area.

medial	**temporomandibular ligament**	**mandibular foramen**
temporal bone	**fascia**	**mandible**
stylomandibular ligament	**retraction**	**sphenomandibular ligament**
temporomandibular joint		

References

Chapter 5, Temporomandibular joint. In Fehrenbach MJ, Herring SW: *Illustrated anatomy of the head and neck,* ed 4, St. Louis, 2012, Saunders; and Chapter 19, Temporomandibular joint. In Bath-Balogh M, Fehrenbach MJ: *Illustrated dental embryology, histology, and anatomy,* ed 3, St. Louis, 2011, Saunders.

ANSWER KEY 1. temporomandibular joint, 2. temporomandibular ligament, 3. temporal bone, 4. retraction, 5. stylomandibular ligament, 6. sphenomandibular ligament, 7. mandibular foramen, 8. mandible, 9. medial, 10. fascia.

FIGURE 4-25 Temporomandibular joint (sagittal section with joint capsule removed)

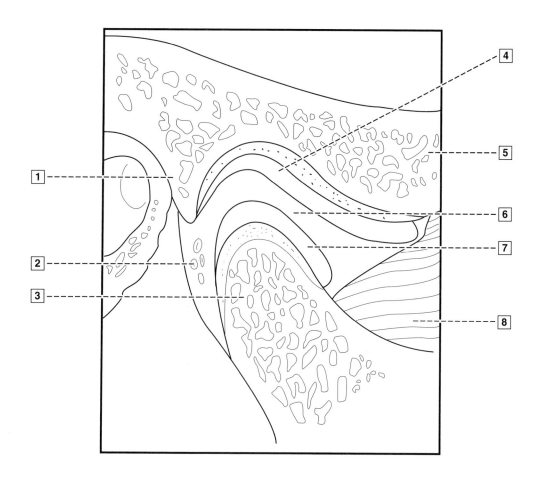

1 Postglenoid process		**5** Articular eminence
2 Blood vessels		**6** Disc of the joint
3 Mandibular condyle		**7** Lower synovial cavity
4 Upper synovial cavity		**8** Lateral pterygoid muscle

REVIEW QUESTIONS

Fill in the blanks by choosing the appropriate terms from the list below.

1. The shape of the _____ that divides the temporomandibular joint conforms to the shape of the adjacent articulating bones of the joint and is related to normal joint movements.

2. The disc of the joint is considered an extension of the _____.

3. On parasagittal section, the disc of the joint appears caplike on the _____, with its superior aspect concavoconvex from anterior to posterior and its inferior aspect concave.

4. The disc of the joint completely divides the temporomandibular joint into two compartments: the _____ and the lower synovial cavity.

5. The membranes lining the inside of the joint capsule secrete _____, which is a clear, viscous liquid that helps lubricate the joint and fills the synovial cavities.

6. The disc of the joint is not attached to the _____ anteriorly, except indirectly through the joint capsule.

7. Posteriorly, the disc of the joint is divided into two areas or divisions: upper and lower, with the upper division of the posterior part of the disc attached to the _____ of the temporal bone, and the lower division attached to the neck of the condyle.

8. The _____ area of attachment of the disc of the joint to the joint capsule is one of the locations where nerves and blood vessels enter the joint.

9. The medial and lateral ends of the articulating surface of the condyle are considered _____; the medial one extends farther beyond the neck than the lateral one does and is positioned more posteriorly; thus the long axis of each condyle deviates posteriorly and meets a similarly drawn axis from the contralateral condyle at the anterior border of the foramen magnum.

10. The disc of the joint is attached to the _____ and medial poles of the mandibular condyle.

posterior	lateral	disc of the joint
postglenoid process	mandibular condyle	synovial fluid
temporal bone	joint capsule	poles
upper synovial cavity		

References

Chapter 5, Temporomandibular joint. In Fehrenbach MJ, Herring SW: *Illustrated anatomy of the head and neck,* ed 4, St. Louis, 2012, Saunders; and Chapter 19, Temporomandibular joint. In Bath-Balogh M, Fehrenbach MJ: *Illustrated dental embryology, histology, and anatomy,* ed 3, St. Louis, 2011, Saunders.

FIGURE 4-26 **Paranasal sinuses (anterior and lateral views)**

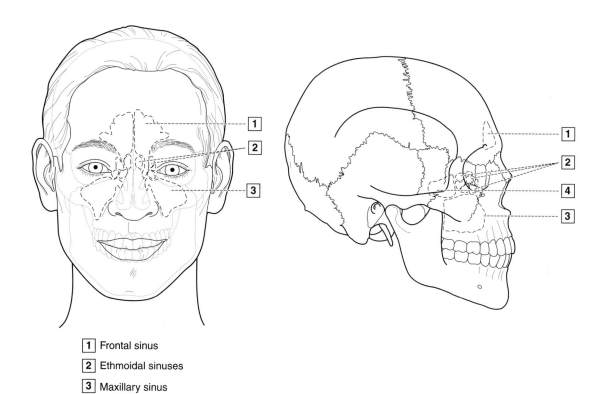

1 Frontal sinus
2 Ethmoidal sinuses
3 Maxillary sinus
4 Sphenoidal sinus

REVIEW QUESTIONS

Fill in the blanks by choosing the appropriate terms from the list below.

1. The _____ are paired, air-filled cavities in bone of the skull, which project laterally, superiorly, and posteriorly into surrounding bones and are lined with respiratory mucosa consisting of ciliated pseudostratified columnar epithelium that is continuous with the epithelial lining of the nasal cavity.

2. The paranasal sinuses communicate with the _____ through small ostia or openings in the lateral nasal wall; these openings mark the outpouchings from which the paranasal sinuses develop.

3. The paired _____ are located in the frontal bone just superior to the nasal cavity, with each one communicating with and draining into the nasal cavity by a constricted canal to the middle nasal meatus, the frontonasal duct; they are not present at birth but at approximately 2 years of age, the two anterior ethmoidal sinuses grow into the frontal bone, forming one on each side that are visible on radiographs by age 7.

4. The paired _____ are located in the body of the sphenoid bone and communicate with and drain into the nasal cavity through an opening superior to each superior nasal concha; they are not present at birth but at approximately 2 years of age, the two posterior ethmoidal sinuses grow into the sphenoid bone to form them.

5. The _____, or *ethmoid air cells,* are a variable number of small cavities in the lateral mass of each of the ethmoid bones; at birth only a few are present and they do not start to grow until 6 to 8 years of age.

6. The posterior ethmoid air cells open into the _____ of the nasal cavity, and the middle and anterior ethmoid air cells open into the middle meatus.

7. The _____ are paired paranasal sinuses located in each body of the maxillae, just posterior to the maxillary canine and premolars; they are small at birth and grow until puberty, and thus are not fully developed until all the permanent teeth have erupted in early adulthood.

8. The maxillary sinuses are the largest of the paranasal sinuses, and each one has a(n) _____, three walls, a roof, and a floor.

9. Each maxillary sinus is further divided into communicating compartments by inner bony walls, or _____.

10. The maxillary sinus drains into the _____ on each side.

middle meatus	superior meatus	nasal cavity
septa	sphenoidal sinuses	paranasal sinuses
apex	frontal sinuses	ethmoidal sinuses
maxillary sinuses		

References

Chapter 3, Skeletal system. In Fehrenbach MJ, Herring SW: *Illustrated anatomy of the head and neck,* ed 4, St. Louis, 2012, Saunders; and Chapter 11, Head and neck structures. In Bath-Balogh M, Fehrenbach MJ: *Illustrated dental embryology, histology, and anatomy,* ed 3, St. Louis, 2011, Saunders.

FIGURE 4-27   Temporal fossa and boundaries (lateral view)

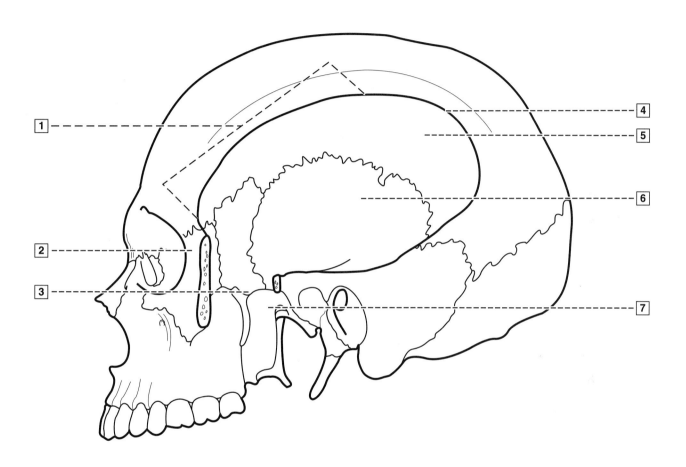

1	Temporal fossa	**5**	Parietal bone
2	Frontal process of zygomatic bone	**6**	Squamous part of temporal bone
3	Infratemporal crest of greater wing of sphenoid bone	**7**	Infratemporal fossa
4	Inferior temporal line		

REVIEW QUESTIONS

Fill in the blanks by choosing the appropriate terms from the list below.

1. There are three depressions, or fossae, present on the skull: _____, infratemporal, and pterygopalatine fossae.

2. The temporal fossa is a flat, fan-shaped paired depression on the lateral surface of the _____.

3. The temporal fossa is formed by parts of five bones: zygomatic, frontal, greater wing of the sphenoid, temporal, and _____ bones.

4. The boundaries of the temporal fossa include superiorly and posteriorly, the inferior temporal line; anteriorly, the _____ of the zygomatic bone; medially, the surface of the temporal bone; and laterally, the zygomatic arch.

5. Inferiorly, the boundary between the temporal fossa and the infratemporal fossa is the _____ on the greater wing of the sphenoid bone.

6. The temporal fossa includes a narrow strip of the parietal bone, the _____ of the temporal bone, the temporal surface of the frontal bone, and the temporal surface of the greater wing of the sphenoid bone.

7. The temporal fossa contains the body of the _____ and area blood vessels and nerves.

8. The temporal fossa is a shallow depression on the side of the skull bounded by the two _____.

9. At the superior border of the temporal fossa, a pair of temporal lines, the superior and _____ temporal lines, arch across the skull from the zygomatic process of the frontal bone to the supramastoid crest of the temporal bone.

10. Inferior to the anterior part of the temporal fossa on the lateral surface of the skull is the depression of the _____.

infratemporal crest	temporalis muscle	infratemporal fossa
squamous part	temporal	temporal lines
parietal	frontal process	inferior
skull		

Reference

Chapter 3, Skeletal system. In Fehrenbach MJ, Herring SW: *Illustrated anatomy of the head and neck,* ed 4, St. Louis, 2012, Saunders.

FIGURE 4-28   **Infratemporal fossa and boundaries (inferior view)**

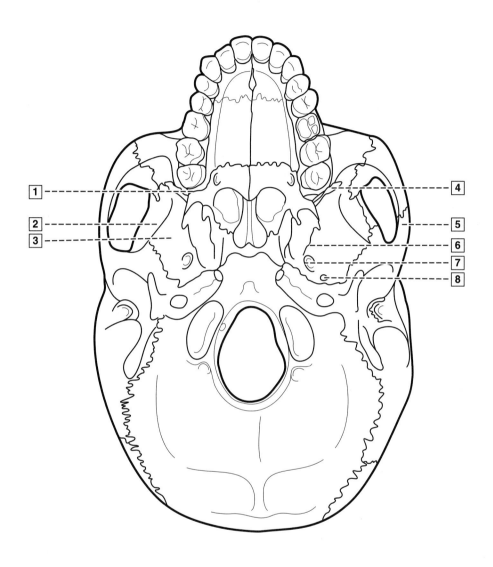

1 Maxillary tuberosity

2 Infratemporal crest of great wing of sphenoid bone

3 Infratemporal fossa

4 Inferior orbital fissure

5 Zygomatic arch

6 Lateral pterygoid plate of sphenoid bone

7 Foramen ovale

8 Foramen spinosum

REVIEW QUESTIONS

Fill in the blanks by choosing the appropriate terms from the list below.

1. The _____ is a paired depression on the external surface of the skull that is inferior to the anterior part of the temporal fossa.

2. A transverse ridge, the _____, on the greater wing of the sphenoid bone contributes to the adjoining temporal fossa and infratemporal fossa.

3. The boundaries of the infratemporal fossa include superiorly, the greater wing of the sphenoid bone; anteriorly, the maxillary tuberosity of the maxilla; medially, the _____ of the sphenoid bone; and laterally, the ramus of the mandible and zygomatic arch.

4. No bony inferior or _____ boundary exists for the infratemporal fossa; the fossa is bounded by only bone and soft tissue.

5. Many structures pass from the infratemporal fossa into the orbit through the _____, which is located at the anterior and superior end of the fossa.

6. Other structures pass into the infratemporal fossa from the _____ of the brain.

7. The infratemporal fossa contains the maxillary artery and its second part branches, that arise from here, including the middle meningeal artery, which goes into the cranial cavity through the _____; the inferior alveolar artery, which enters the mandible through the mandibular foramen; and the posterior alveolar artery, which enters the maxilla through the posterior superior alveolar foramina on the maxillary tuberosity.

8. The infratemporal fossa contains the _____ of veins and the pterygoid muscles.

9. The infratemporal fossa contains the mandibular nerve of the fifth cranial nerve, or trigeminal nerve (including the inferior alveolar and lingual nerves), which enters by way of the _____, passing between the cranial and oral cavities.

10. The depression of the _____ is deep to the infratemporal fossa.

pterygopalatine fossa	lateral pterygoid plate	infratemporal fossa
foramen spinosum	inferior orbital fissure	foramen ovale
posterior	infratemporal crest	pterygoid plexus
cranial cavity		

Reference

Chapter 3, Skeletal system. In Fehrenbach MJ, Herring SW: *Illustrated anatomy of the head and neck,* ed 4, St. Louis, 2012, Saunders.

FIGURE 4-29 Pterygopalatine fossa and boundaries (oblique lateral view)

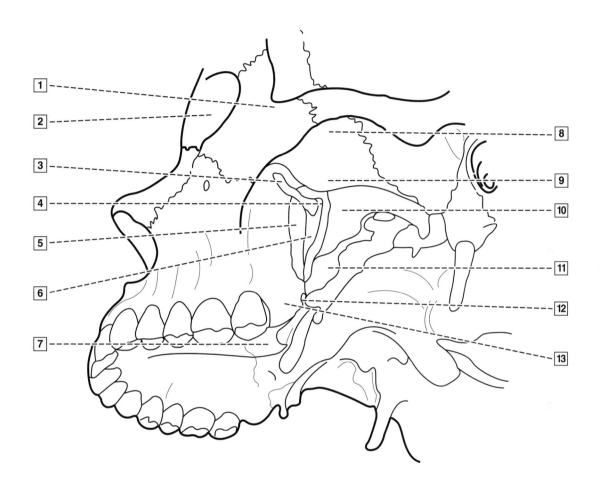

1 Zygomatic arch		**8** Temporal fossa
2 Orbit		**9** Infratemporal crest of the greater wing of sphenoid bone
3 Inferior orbital fissure		**10** Infratemporal fossa
4 Sphenopalatine foramen		**11** Lateral pterygoid plate of the sphenoid bone
5 Pterygopalatine fossa		**12** Pterygopalatine canal
6 Pterygomaxillary fissure		**13** Maxillary tuberosity
7 Palatine bone		

REVIEW QUESTIONS

Fill in the blanks by choosing the appropriate terms from the list below.

1. The _____ is a paired, cone-shaped depression deep to the infratemporal fossa and posterior to the maxilla on each side of the external surface of the skull.

2. The pterygopalatine fossa is located between the pterygoid process and the _____, close to the apex of the orbit.

3. The pterygopalatine fossa communicates via fissure and foramina in its walls with the following: the cranial cavity, the infratemporal fossa, the orbit, the nasal cavity, and the _____.

4. The boundaries of the pterygopalatine fossa include superiorly, the inferior surface of the body of the sphenoid bone; anteriorly, the maxillary tuberosity of the maxilla; medially, the _____ of the palatine bone.

5. The boundaries of the pterygopalatine fossa include laterally, the pterygomaxillary fissure; inferiorly, the _____; and posteriorly, the pterygoid process of the sphenoid bone.

6. The pterygopalatine fossa contains the _____ and its branches that arise here, including the infraorbital and sphenopalatine arteries.

7. The pterygopalatine fossa contains the _____ of the fifth cranial nerve or trigeminal nerve and its branches, as well as the pterygopalatine ganglion.

8. The _____ is the entrance route for the maxillary nerve; however, a second foramen in the pterygoid process, the pterygoid canal, transmits autonomic fibers to the pterygopalatine ganglion.

9. The pterygopalatine canal connects with openings of the greater and lesser _____ of the palatine bones of the posterior hard palate.

10. The pterygopalatine fossa is medial to the _____, a vertical gap between the lateral pterygoid plate of the pterygoid process and the maxilla as well as the most posterior point in the anterior contour of the maxillary tuberosity.

maxillary nerve	vertical plate	pterygopalatine fossa
pterygomaxillary fissure	oral cavity	pterygopalatine canal
foramen rotundum	maxillary tuberosity	palatine foramina
maxillary artery		

Reference

Chapter 3, Skeletal system. In Fehrenbach MJ, Herring SW: *Illustrated anatomy of the head and neck,* ed 4, St. Louis, 2012, Saunders.

FIGURE 4-30 Occipital bone with cervical vertebrae (posterior, superior, and posterosuperior views)

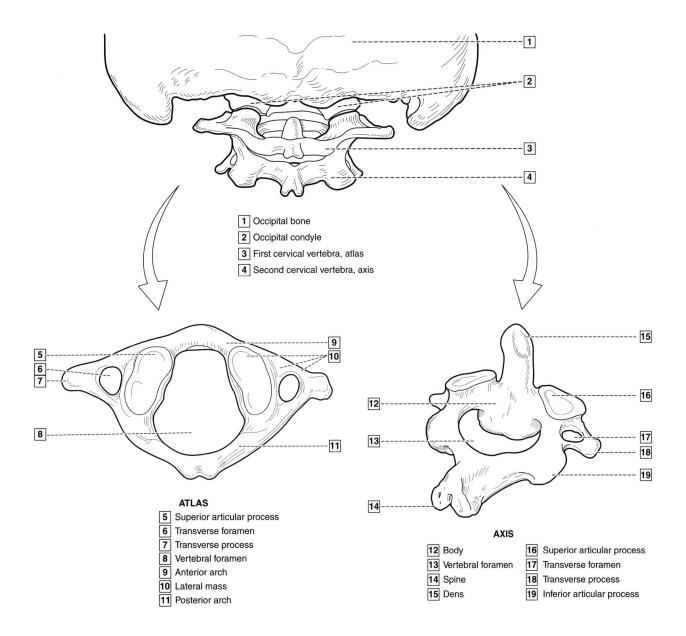

1 Occipital bone
2 Occipital condyle
3 First cervical vertebra, atlas
4 Second cervical vertebra, axis

ATLAS

5 Superior articular process
6 Transverse foramen
7 Transverse process
8 Vertebral foramen
9 Anterior arch
10 Lateral mass
11 Posterior arch

AXIS

12 Body
13 Vertebral foramen
14 Spine
15 Dens
16 Superior articular process
17 Transverse foramen
18 Transverse process
19 Inferior articular process

REVIEW QUESTIONS

Fill in the blanks by choosing the appropriate terms from the list below.

1. The _____ are located in the vertebral column between the skull and the thoracic vertebrae.

2. All seven cervical vertebrae have a central _____ for the spinal cord and associated tissue.

3. In contrast to most other vertebrae, the cervical vertebrae are characterized by the presence of a _____ in the transverse process on each side of the vertebral foramen, with the vertebral artery running through these structures.

4. The most superior, or first, cervical vertebra is the _____, which articulates superiorly with the skull at the occipital condyles of the occipital bone.

5. The atlas has the form of an irregular ring consisting of two _____ connected by a shorter anterior arch and a longer posterior arch; it has no body.

6. More medially, the lateral masses of the atlas present large concave _____ for the corresponding occipital condyles of the skull.

7. The second cervical vertebra, or _____, is characterized by having a dens, or *odontoid process*; it forms the pivot upon which the first cervical vertebra (the atlas), which carries the head, rotates.

8. The _____ of the axis articulates anteriorly with the anterior arch of the first cervical vertebra, the atlas.

9. The _____ of the axis is inferior to its dens.

10. The _____ of the axis is located posterior to its body.

atlas	transverse foramen	lateral masses
superior articular processes	body	vertebral foramen
axis	spine	cervical vertebrae
dens		

Reference

Chapter 3, Skeletal system. In Fehrenbach MJ, Herring SW: *Illustrated anatomy of the head and neck,* ed 4, St. Louis, 2012, Saunders.

FIGURE 4-31 Hyoid bone and associated landmarks (posterolateral and anterior views)

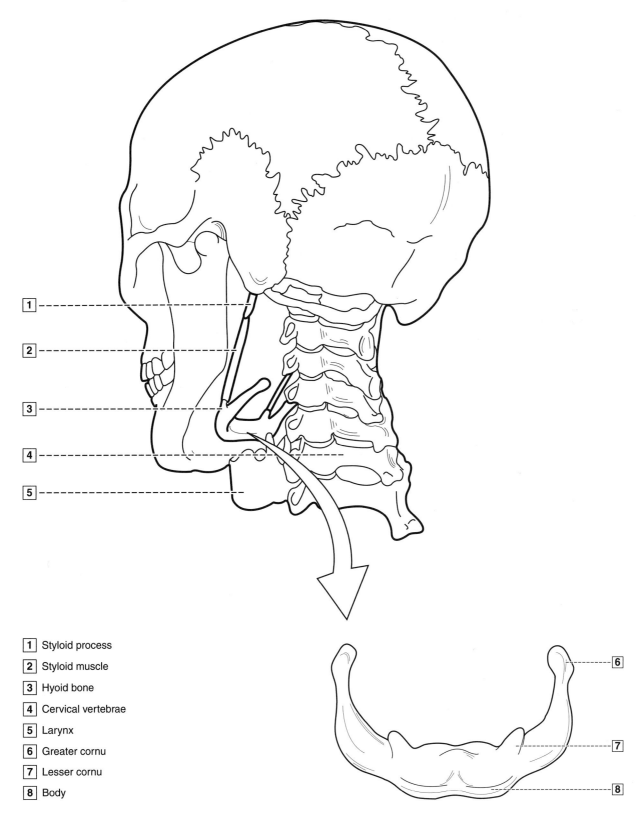

1 Styloid process
2 Styloid muscle
3 Hyoid bone
4 Cervical vertebrae
5 Larynx
6 Greater cornu
7 Lesser cornu
8 Body

REVIEW QUESTIONS

Fill in the blanks by choosing the appropriate terms from the list below.

1. The _____ is suspended in the neck from the styloid process of the temporal bone by the two stylohyoid ligaments.

2. At rest, the hyoid bone lies at the level of the base of the _____ anteriorly and the third cervical vertebra posteriorly.

3. The hyoid bone does not _____ with any other skull or vertebral bones, giving it its characteristic mobility, which is necessary for mastication, swallowing, and speech; instead, many muscles attach to the hyoid bone.

4. It is important to not confuse clinically the hyoid bone with the inferiorly placed _____, or *Adam's apple.*

5. The hyoid bone is superior and anterior to the thyroid cartilage of the larynx; it is usually at the level of the third _____ but raises during swallowing and other activities.

6. The hyoid bone is lowered by the broad _____, which connects it to the thyroid cartilage, thus raising the larynx.

7. The U-shaped hyoid bone consists of _____ parts as seen from an anterior view.

8. The anterior part of hyoid bone is the midline _____.

9. A pair of projections is located on each side of the hyoid bone, the _____ cornu and lesser cornu.

10. The cornu, or *horns,* on the hyoid bone serve as attachments for _____ and ligaments.

thyroid cartilage	hyoid bone	body of the hyoid bone
mandible	greater	thyrohyoid membrane
cervical vertebra	muscles	articulate
five		

Reference

Chapter 3, Skeletal system. In Fehrenbach MJ, Herring SW: *Illustrated anatomy of the head and neck,* ed 4, St. Louis, 2012, Saunders.

FIGURE 5-1 Sternocleidomastoid muscle (oblique view)

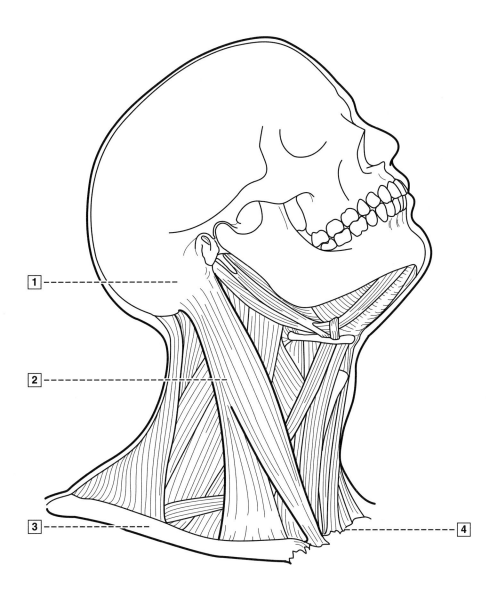

1 Mastoid process of temporal bone

2 Sternocleidomastoid

3 Clavicle

4 Sternum

277

REVIEW QUESTIONS

Fill in the blanks by choosing the appropriate terms from the list below.

1. The two superficial _____ are the sternocleidomastoid and trapezius muscles.

2. One of the largest and most superficial cervical muscles is the paired _____.

3. The sternocleidomastoid muscle is a thick cervical muscle and thus serves as a primary muscular landmark of the _____.

4. The sternocleidomastoid muscle divides the neck region into anterior and posterior _____, which helps define the location of other structures, such as the cervical lymph nodes.

5. The sternocleidomastoid muscle _____ from the medial part of the clavicle and the superior and lateral surfaces the sternum.

6. The sternocleidomastoid muscle passes posteriorly and superiorly to _____ on the mastoid process of the temporal bone.

7. The insertion of the sternocleidomastoid muscle is just posterior and inferior to the _____ of each ear.

8. If only one sternocleidomastoid muscle contracts when active, the head and neck _____ to the ipsilateral side, and the face and front of the neck rotate to the contralateral side.

9. If both sternocleidomastoid muscles contract when active, the head will _____ at the neck and extend at the junction between the neck and skull.

10. The sternocleidomastoid muscle is innervated by the eleventh cranial nerve, or the _____.

insert	cervical muscles	bend
accessory nerve	originates	external acoustic meatus
flex	sternocleidomastoid muscle	cervical triangles
neck		

Reference

Chapter 4, Muscular system. In Fehrenbach MJ, Herring SW: *Illustrated anatomy of the head and neck,* ed 4, St. Louis, 2012, Saunders.

FIGURE 5-2 Trapezius muscle (posterolateral view)

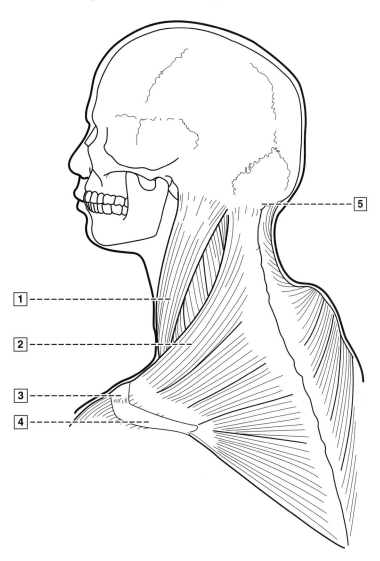

1	Sternocleidomastoid
2	Trapezius
3	Clavicle
4	Scapula
5	Occipital bone

REVIEW QUESTIONS

Fill in the blanks by choosing the appropriate terms from the list below.

1. The _____ is a paired superficial cervical muscle, which appears as a broad, flat, and triangular muscle that is superficial to both the lateral and posterior surfaces of the neck.

2. The trapezius muscle _____ from the external surface of the occipital bone and the posterior midline of the cervical and thoracic regions.

3. The trapezius muscle _____ on the lateral third of the clavicle and parts of the scapula.

4. The cervical fibers of the trapezius muscle act to _____ the clavicle and scapula when active, such as when the shoulders are shrugged.

5. The trapezius muscle is innervated by the eleventh cranial nerve, or the _____, as well as the third and fourth cervical nerves.

lift   trapezius muscle

originates   inserts

accessory nerve

Reference

Chapter 4, Muscular system. In Fehrenbach MJ, Herring SW: *Illustrated anatomy of the head and neck,* ed 4, St. Louis, 2012, Saunders.

FIGURE 5-3 Muscles of facial expression (frontal view)

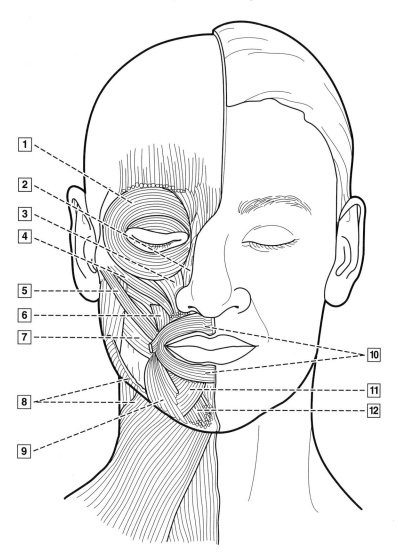

1	Orbicularis oculi	**7**	Buccinator
2	Levator labii superioris alaeque nasi	**8**	Platysma
3	Levator labii superioris	**9**	Depressor anguli oris
4	Zygomaticus minor	**10**	Orbicularis oris
5	Zygomaticus major	**11**	Depressor labii inferioris
6	Levator anguli oris	**12**	Mentalis

REVIEW QUESTIONS

Fill in the blanks by choosing the appropriate terms from the list below.

1. The muscles of facial expression are innervated by the seventh cranial nerve, or the _____, with each nerve serving one side of the face.

2. The _____, or *epicranius,* is located in the scalp region where it has two bellies: frontal and occipital bellies that are separated by a large, spread-out scalpal tendon, the epicranial aponeurosis; the bellies act together to raise the eyebrows and scalp as a muscle of facial expression, such as when a person shows surprise.

3. The _____ encircles the eye to close the eyelid when active as a muscle of facial expression.

4. The _____ is deep to the superior part of the orbicularis oculi muscle, and when active draws the skin of the eyebrow medially and inferiorly toward the nose as a muscle of facial expression, such as when a person frowns.

5. The _____ encircles the mouth between the skin and labial mucosa of the lips without any bony attachment, and with all its actions involves the lips as a muscle of facial expression.

6. The _____ forms the anterior part of the cheek or the lateral wall of the oral cavity and when active pulls each labial commissure laterally, shortening the cheek both vertically and horizontally as a muscle of facial expression.

7. The _____ as a muscle of facial expression serves to only elevate the upper lip when active.

8. The _____ elevates the upper lip and ala of the nose when active, thus also dilating each naris as a muscle of facial expression, such as with a sneering expression.

9. The _____ is lateral to the zygomaticus minor muscle and elevates the labial commissure of the upper lip and pulls it laterally when active as a muscle of facial expression, such as when a person smiles.

10. The _____ is a small muscle of facial expression in the oral region, medial to the zygomaticus major muscle and elevates the upper lip, assisting in smiling when active.

buccinator muscle	**zygomaticus major muscle**	**corrugator supercilii muscle**
levator labii superioris alaeque	**facial nerve**	**orbicularis oris muscle**
nasi muscle	**zygomaticus minor muscle**	**epicranial muscle**
orbicularis oculi muscle		
levator labii superioris muscle		

Reference

Chapter 4, Muscular system. In Fehrenbach MJ, Herring SW: *Illustrated anatomy of the head and neck,* ed 4, St. Louis, 2012, Saunders.

FIGURE 5-4 Muscles of facial expression (lateral view)

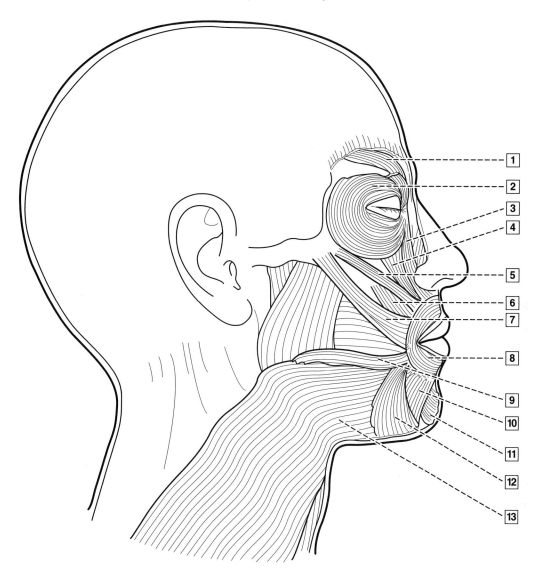

1	Corrugator supercilii	**6**	Levator anguli oris	**11**	Mentalis
2	Orbicularis oculi	**7**	Zygomaticus major	**12**	Depressor anguli oris
3	Levator labii superioris alaeque nasi	**8**	Orbicularis oris	**13**	Platysma
4	Levator labii superioris	**9**	Risorius		
5	Zygomaticus minor	**10**	Depressor labii inferioris		

REVIEW QUESTIONS

Fill in the blanks by choosing the appropriate terms from the list below.

1. The _____ as a muscle of facial expression acts to stretch the lips laterally when active, retracting the labial commissure and widening the mouth to produce a grimace.

2. The _____ as a muscle of facial expression depresses the labial commissure when active, such as when a person frowns.

3. Deep to the depressor anguli oris muscle is the _____, which depresses the lower lip when active as a muscle of facial expression, exposing the mandibular incisor teeth to express irony.

4. The _____ as a muscle of facial expression raises the chin when active, wrinkling the skin, causing the displaced lower lip to protrude, narrowing the oral vestibule as a muscle of facial expression to show the mood of thinking.

5. The _____ as a muscle of facial expression runs from the neck all the way to the mouth, superficial to the anterior cervical triangle, and acts to raise the skin of the neck when active as a muscle of facial expression.

platysma muscle

risorius muscle

depressor anguli oris muscle

depressor labii inferioris muscle

mentalis muscle

Reference

Chapter 4, Muscular system. In Fehrenbach MJ, Herring SW: *Illustrated anatomy of the head and neck,* ed 4, St. Louis, 2012, Saunders.

FIGURE 5-5   Muscles of facial expression: epicranial (lateral view)

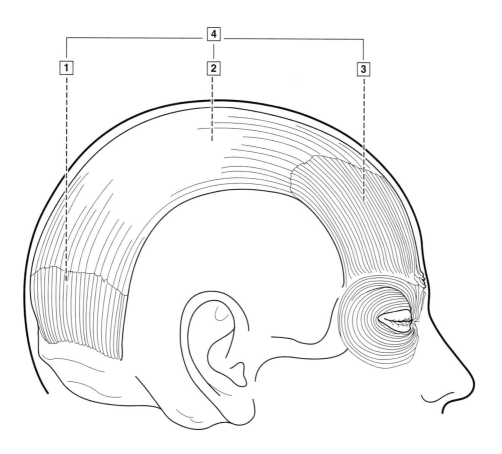

1 | Occipital belly
2 | Epicranial aponeurosis
3 | Frontal belly
4 | Epicranial

REVIEW QUESTIONS

Fill in the blanks by choosing the appropriate terms from the list below.

1. The epicranial muscle, or *epicranius,* is a muscle of facial expression where the muscle and its tendon are one of the layers that form the _____.

2. The epicranial muscle has two _____: the frontal and occipital bellies; when both are active they serve to raise the eyebrows and pulp the scalp posteriorly as a muscle of facial expression, such as when a person shows surprise.

3. The two bellies of the epicranial muscle are separated by a large, spread-out scalpel tendon, the _____, or *galea aponeurotica,* which is located at the most superior part of the skull.

4. The _____ of the epicranial muscle, or *frontalis,* arises from the epicranial aponeurosis and then inserts into the skin of the eyebrow and root of the nose.

5. The _____ of the epicranial muscle, or *occipitalis,* originates from the occipital bone and mastoid process of the temporal bone and then inserts in the epicranial aponeurosis.

epicranial aponeurosis	scalp
occipital belly	frontal belly
bellies	

Reference

Chapter 4, Muscular system. In Fehrenbach MJ, Herring SW: *Illustrated anatomy of the head and neck,* ed 4, St. Louis, 2012, Saunders.

FIGURE 5-6   Muscles of facial expression: buccinator (lateral view)

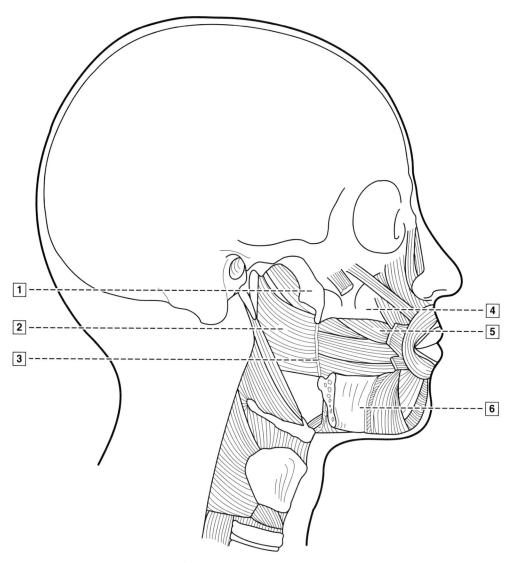

1. Pterygoid plate
2. Superior pharyngeal constrictor
3. Pterygomandibular raphe
4. Maxilla
5. Buccinator
6. Mandible (cut)

REVIEW QUESTIONS

Fill in the blanks by choosing the appropriate terms from the list below.

1. The _____ is a thin quadrilateral muscle of facial expression that assists the muscles of mastication.

2. The buccinator muscle forms the anterior part of the _____, or lateral wall of the oral cavity.

3. The buccinator muscle originates from three areas: the alveolar processes of both the maxilla and mandible, as well as a fibrous structure, the pterygomandibular raphe, which in the oral cavity is noted as the _____.

4. Many of the buccinator muscle fibers from the maxillary alveolar process and the superior part of the _____ travel obliquely downward toward the lower lip, whereas many of those fibers from the mandibular alveolar process and inferior part of the same fibrous structure travel obliquely upward toward the upper lip, creating an intersecting pattern at the labial commissures.

5. The action of buccinator muscle causes the muscle to compress the cheek to keep food pushed back on the _____ of the posterior teeth, such as when chewing.

occlusal surface   pterygomandibular fold

cheek   buccinator muscle

pterygomandibular raphe

Reference

Chapter 4, Muscular system. In Fehrenbach MJ, Herring SW: *Illustrated anatomy of the head and neck,* ed 4, St. Louis, 2012, Saunders.

FIGURE 5-7   Muscles of mastication: masseter (lateral view)

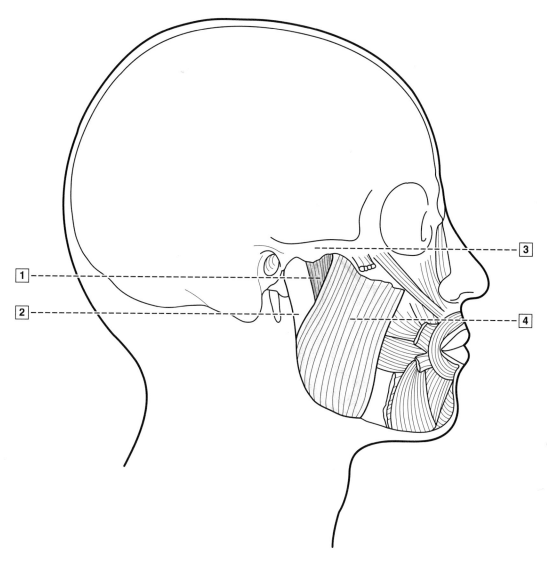

1 Deep head of masseter

2 Ramus of mandible

3 Zygomatic arch

4 Superficial head of masseter

REVIEW QUESTIONS

Fill in the blanks by choosing the appropriate terms from the list below.

1. The _____ are four pairs of muscles attached to the mandible and include the masseter, temporalis, medial pterygoid, and lateral pterygoid muscles.

2. The muscles of mastication work with the _____ to accomplish movements of the mandible.

3. The muscles of mastication are innervated by the _____ of the fifth cranial nerve, or trigeminal nerve, with each nerve serving one side of the face.

4. The _____ is a broad, thick, flat, rectangular muscle of mastication on each side of the face, anterior to the parotid salivary gland.

5. The masseter muscle has two _____ that differ in depth: the superficial and the deep.

6. The _____ of the masseter muscle originates from the zygomatic process of the maxilla, and from the anterior two thirds of the inferior border of the zygomatic arch.

7. The _____ of the masseter muscle originates from the posterior one third and the entire medial surface of the zygomatic arch, which is partly concealed by the superficial head.

8. Both heads of the masseter muscle pass inferiorly to insert on different parts of the external surface of the _____.

9. The superficial head of the masseter muscle inserts on the lateral surface of the _____, and the deep head of the muscle inserts on the mandibular ramus superior to the other head.

10. The action of the masseter muscle during bilateral contraction of the entire muscle is to _____ the mandible when active, raising the lower jaw.

mandibular nerve	elevate	superficial head
heads	masseter muscle	temporomandibular joint
deep head	mandible	muscles of mastication
angle of the mandible		

Reference

Chapter 4, Muscular system. In Fehrenbach MJ, Herring SW: *Illustrated anatomy of the head and neck,* ed 4, St. Louis, 2012, Saunders.

ANSWER KEY 1. muscles of mastication, 2. temporomandibular joint, 3. mandibular nerve, 4. masseter muscle, 5. heads, 6. superficial head, 7. deep head, 8. mandible, 9. angle of the mandible, 10. elevate.

FIGURE 5-8   Muscles of mastication: temporalis (lateral view)

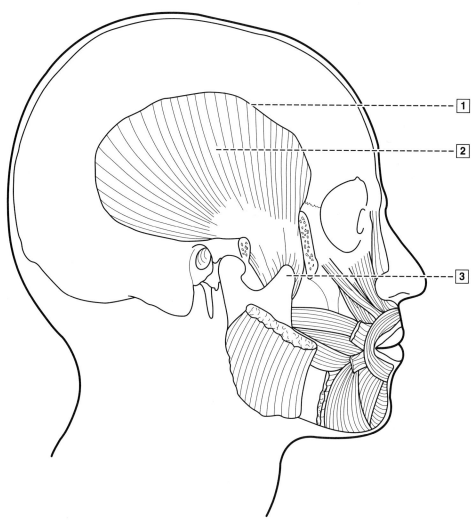

1 Inferior temporal line

2 Temporalis

3 Coronoid process of mandible

REVIEW QUESTIONS

Fill in the blanks by choosing the appropriate terms from the list below.

1.   The _____ is a broad, fan-shaped muscle of mastication on each side of the head that fills the temporal fossa and is located superior to the zygomatic arch.

2.   The temporalis muscle originates from the entire _____ on the temporal bone that is bound superiorly by the inferior temporal line and inferiorly by the infratemporal crest.

3.   The temporalis muscle passes inferiorly to insert onto the medial surface, apex, and anterior border of the coronoid process of the _____ at the anteromedial border of the ramus.

4.   If the entire temporalis muscle contracts, the main action is to _____ the mandible, raising the lower jaw.

5.   If only the posterior part of the temporalis muscle contracts, the muscle moves the lower jaw _____; moving the lower jaw backward causes retraction of the mandible.

temporalis muscle   temporal fossa

elevate   backward

mandible

Reference

Chapter 4, Muscular system. In Fehrenbach MJ, Herring SW: *Illustrated anatomy of the head and neck,* ed 4, St. Louis, 2012, Saunders.

FIGURE 5-9 Muscles of mastication: medial and lateral pterygoid (lateral view)

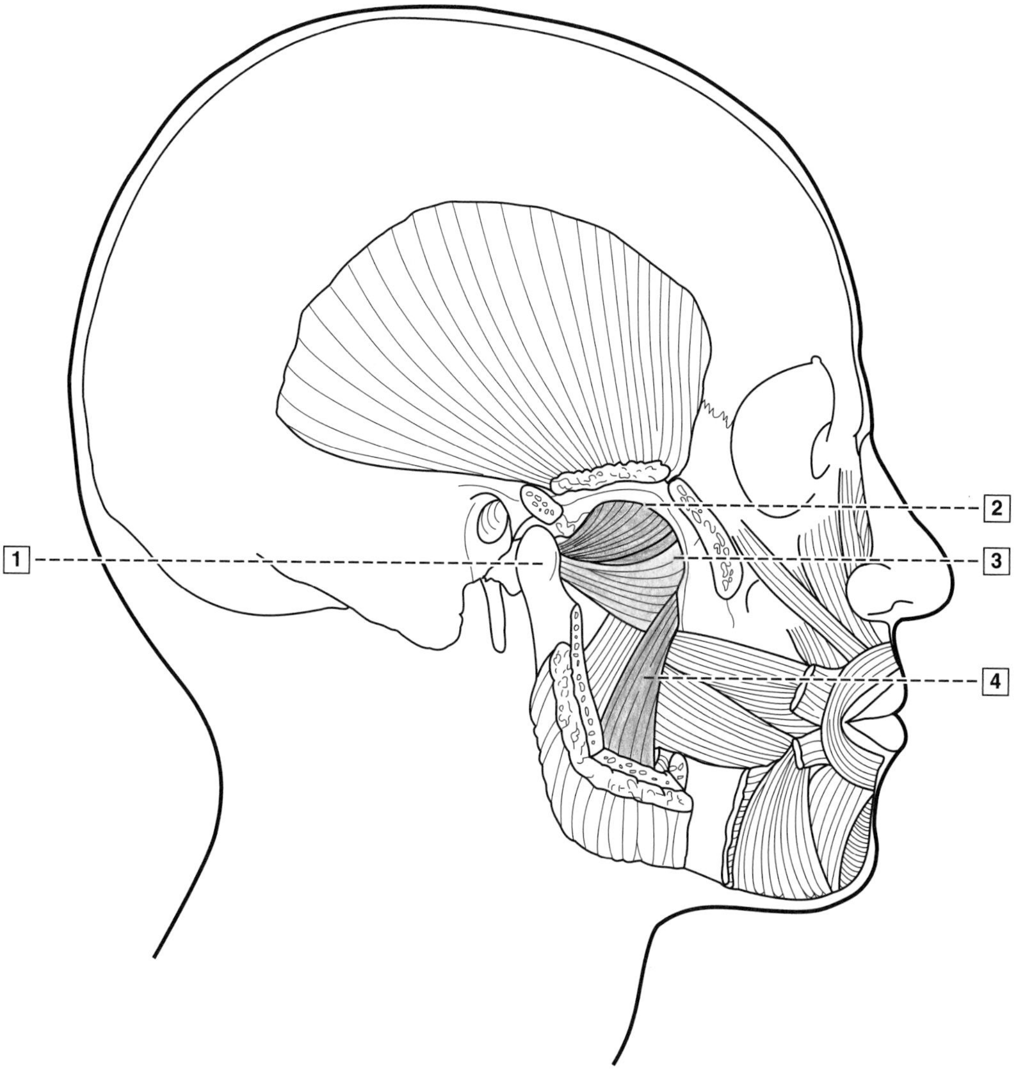

1. Mandibular condyle
2. Superior head of lateral pterygoid
3. Inferior head of lateral pterygoid
4. Medial pterygoid

REVIEW QUESTIONS

Fill in the blanks by choosing the appropriate terms from the list below.

1. Deeper, yet similar in form to the more superficial masseter muscle, another muscle of mastication is the _____.

2. The medial pterygoid muscle has two _____ of differing depth: the deep and the superficial, similar to the masseter muscle.

3. The larger _____ of the medial pterygoid muscle originates from the pterygoid fossa on the medial surface of the lateral pterygoid plate of the sphenoid bone.

4. The smaller _____ of the medial pterygoid muscle originates from the lateral surfaces of the pyramidal process of the palatine bone and maxillary tuberosity of the maxilla.

5. After their point of origin, both heads of the medial pterygoid muscle pass inferiorly, posteriorly, and laterally to insert on the _____, including the medial surface of the ramus as well as the angle of the mandible as far superior as the mandibular foramen, in a slinglike configuration.

6. The medial pterygoid muscle _____ the mandible when active, raising the lower jaw; it parallels the action of the masseter muscle but is weaker.

7. The _____ is a short, thick, almost conical muscle of mastication superior to the medial pterygoid muscle that lies within the infratemporal fossa, deep to the temporalis muscle.

8. The lateral pterygoid muscle has two separate heads of _____: the superior and the inferior; these two heads are separated anteriorly by a slight interval but fused together posteriorly.

9. The superior head of the lateral pterygoid muscle originates from the infratemporal surface and infratemporal crest of the greater wing of the _____ and passes inferiorly to insert on the anterior margin of both the temporomandibular joint disc and capsule; the inferior head originates from the lateral surface of the lateral pterygoid plate of the same bone and inserts on the anterior surface of the neck of the mandible at the pterygoid fovea.

10. Unlike the other three muscles of mastication, the lateral pterygoid muscle is the only muscle of mastication that assists in depressing the mandible, lowering the lower jaw; however, the main action when both muscles contract is to bring the lower jaw _____, thus causing the protrusion of the mandible; in contrast, when only one muscle is contracted, the lower jaw shifts to the contralateral side, causing lateral deviation of the mandible.

forward	heads	lateral pterygoid muscle
elevates	medial pterygoid muscle	origin
mandible	deep head	sphenoid bone
superficial head		

Reference

Chapter 4, Muscular system. In Fehrenbach MJ, Herring SW: *Illustrated anatomy of the head and neck,* ed 4, St. Louis, 2012, Saunders.

FIGURE 5-10   Hyoid muscles (anterior view)

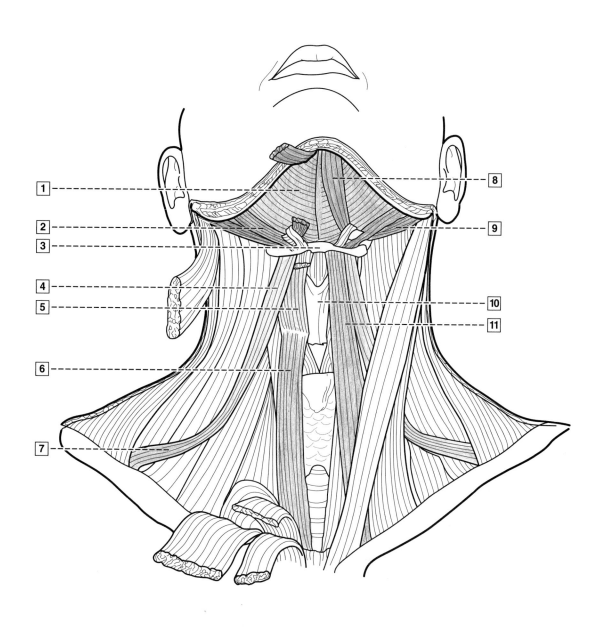

1 Mylohyoid	7 Inferior belly of omohyoid
2 Stylohyoid	8 Anterior belly of digastric
3 Hyoid bone	9 Posterior belly of digastric
4 Superior belly of omohyoid	10 Thyroid cartilage
5 Thyrohyoid	11 Sternohyoid
6 Sternothyroid	

REVIEW QUESTIONS

Fill in the blanks by choosing the appropriate terms from the list below.

1. The _____ assist in the actions of mastication and swallowing through their attachment to the hyoid bone; the muscles can be further grouped based on their vertical position in relationship to the hyoid bone: the suprahyoid muscles or the infrahyoid muscles.

2. The _____ are superior to the hyoid bone as well as its inferior hyoid muscles; these muscles may be further divided according to their horizontal position in relationship to the hyoid bone: anterior or posterior.

3. The _____ group includes the anterior belly of the digastric muscle, the mylohyoid muscle, and the geniohyoid muscle.

4. The _____ group includes the posterior belly of the digastric muscle and the stylohyoid muscle.

5. One action of both the anterior and posterior suprahyoid muscles is to cause the hyoid bone and larynx to _____ if the mandible is stabilized by contraction of the muscles of mastication, as occurs during swallowing.

6. The action of anterior suprahyoid muscles causes the mandible to _____ and the jaws to open.

7. The _____ is a suprahyoid muscle that has two separate bellies: anterior and posterior; one way these bellies differ is that the anterior belly is a part of the anterior suprahyoid muscle group and the posterior belly is a part of the posterior suprahyoid muscle group.

8. Each digastric muscle demarcates the superior part of the _____, forming (with the mandible) a submandibular triangle on each side of the neck; the right and left anterior bellies of the muscle also form a midline submental triangle.

9. The _____ of the digastric muscle originates on the intermediate tendon, which is loosely attached to the body and the greater cornu of the hyoid bone, and then passes superiorly and anteriorly to insert close to the symphysis on the medial surface of the mandible; its innervation is by the mylohyoid nerve, a branch of the mandibular nerve of the fifth cranial nerve, or trigeminal nerve.

10. The _____ of the digastric muscle arises from the mastoid notch, medial to the mastoid process of the temporal bone, and then passes anteriorly and inferiorly to insert on the intermediate tendon; it is innervated by the posterior digastric nerve, a branch of the seventh cranial nerve or facial nerve.

anterior belly	**anterior suprahyoid muscle**	**posterior belly**
digastric muscle	**hyoid muscles**	**suprahyoid muscles**
anterior cervical triangle	**posterior suprahyoid muscle**	**depress**
elevate		

Reference

Chapter 4, Muscular system. In Fehrenbach MJ, Herring SW: *Illustrated anatomy of the head and neck,* ed 4, St. Louis, 2012, Saunders.

FIGURE 5-11   Suprahyoid muscles (lateral view except for the geniohyoid)

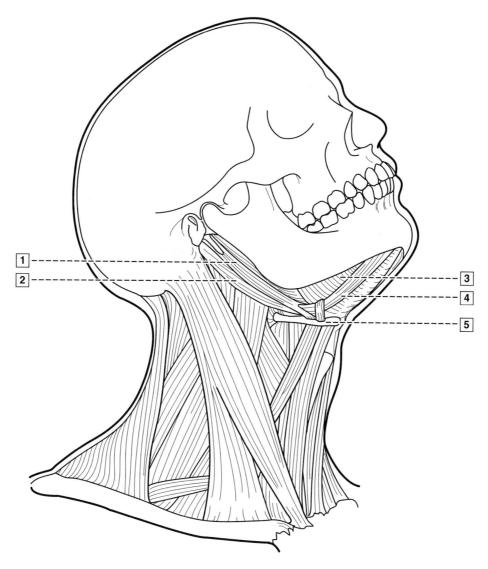

1	Stylohyoid
2	Posterior belly of digastric
3	Mylohyoid
4	Anterior belly of digastric
5	Hyoid bone

REVIEW QUESTIONS

Fill in the blanks by choosing the appropriate terms from the list below.

1. The _____ is an anterior suprahyoid muscle that is deep to the digastric muscle, with fibers running transversely between the rami of the mandible.

2. The mylohyoid muscle originates from the mylohyoid line on the medial surface of the _____.

3. The right and left muscles of the mylohyoid muscle pass inferiorly to unite medially, forming the _____, with the most posterior fibers of the muscle inserting on the body of the hyoid bone.

4. In addition to either elevating the hyoid bone or depressing the mandible, the mylohyoid muscle also _____ the floor of the mouth.

5. The mylohyoid muscle also helps _____ the tongue when active.

6. The mylohyoid muscle is innervated by the _____, a branch of the mandibular nerve of the fifth cranial nerve or trigeminal nerve.

7. The _____ is a thin posterior suprahyoid muscle that has two slips, superficial and deep, on either side of the intermediate tendon of the digastric muscle.

8. The stylohyoid muscle originates from the _____ of the temporal bone.

9. The stylohyoid muscle passes anteriorly and inferiorly to insert on the body of the _____.

10. The stylohyoid muscle is innervated by the _____, a branch of the seventh cranial nerve, or facial nerve.

stylohyoid nerve	floor of the mouth	stylohyoid muscle
mylohyoid muscle	mandible	hyoid bone
elevate	mylohyoid nerve	forms
styloid process		

Reference

Chapter 4, Muscular system. In Fehrenbach MJ, Herring SW: *Illustrated anatomy of the head and neck,* ed 4, St. Louis, 2012, Saunders.

ANSWER KEY 1. mylohyoid muscle, 2. mandible, 3. floor of the mouth, 4. forms, 5. elevate, 6. mylohyoid nerve, 7. stylohyoid muscle, 8. styloid process, 9. hyoid bone, 10. stylohyoid nerve.

FIGURE 5-12 Suprahyoid muscles: geniohyoid (anterior view)

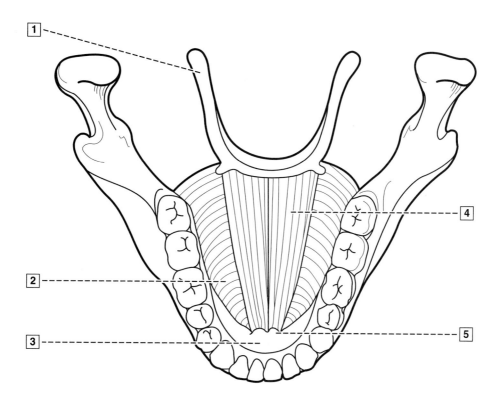

1 Hyoid bone
2 Mylohyoid
3 Mandible
4 Geniohyoid
5 Genial tubercles

REVIEW QUESTIONS

Fill in the blanks by choosing the appropriate terms from the list below.

1. The _____ is an anterior suprahyoid muscle that is superior to the medial border of the mylohyoid muscle.

2. The geniohyoid muscle originates from the medial surface of the mandible, near the mandibular symphysis at the _____.

3. At the point of origin until insertion, the geniohyoid muscles are in _____ with each other.

4. The geniohyoid muscle passes posteriorly and inferiorly to insert on the body of the _____.

5. The geniohyoid muscle is innervated by the first cervical nerve that is conducted by way of the twelfth cranial nerve, or _____.

genial tubercles   geniohyoid muscle

hyoid bone   hypoglossal nerve

contact

Reference

Chapter 4, Muscular system. In Fehrenbach MJ, Herring SW: *Illustrated anatomy of the head and neck,* ed 4, St. Louis, 2012, Saunders.

FIGURE 5-13 Infrahyoid muscles (lateral view)

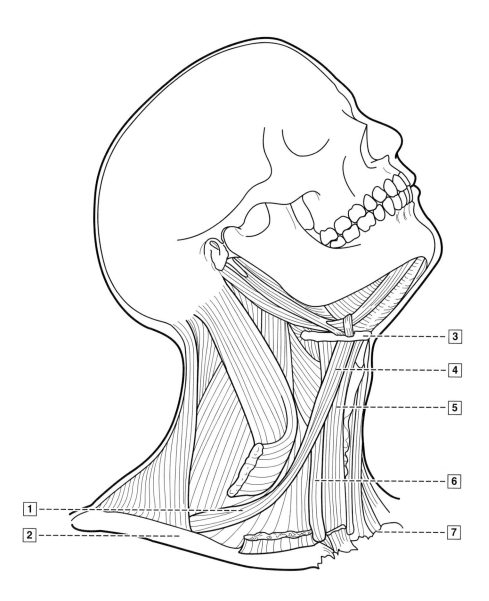

1 Inferior belly of omohyoid
2 Clavicle
3 Hyoid bone
4 Superior belly of omohyoid
5 Sternohyoid
6 Sternothyroid
7 Sternum

REVIEW QUESTIONS

Fill in the blanks by choosing the appropriate terms from the list below.

1. The _____ are four pairs of hyoid muscles inferior to the hyoid bone; they include the sternohyoid, sternothyroid, thyrohyoid, and omohyoid muscles.

2. Most of the infrahyoid muscles _____ the hyoid bone, with some exceptions, and they are innervated by the second and third cervical nerves.

3. The _____ is an infrahyoid muscle that is superficial to the thyroid gland and that originates from the posterior surface of the sternum, deep and medial to the sternohyoid muscle, at the level of the first rib. It then passes superiorly to insert on the thyroid cartilage.

4. The sternothyroid muscle depresses the _____ and larynx, yet does not directly depress the hyoid bone.

5. The _____ is an infrahyoid muscle that is superficial to the sternothyroid muscle as well as the thyroid cartilage and thyroid gland and that originates from the posterior and superior surfaces of the sternum, close to where the sternum joins each clavicle, and then later passes superiorly to insert on the body of the hyoid bone.

6. The _____ is an infrahyoid muscle that is located laterally to both the sternothyroid and thyrohyoid muscles; it has two separate bellies: superior and inferior.

7. The _____ of the omohyoid muscle divides the inferior part of the anterior cervical triangle into the carotid and muscular triangles; in the posterior cervical triangle, the inferior belly serves to demarcate the subclavian triangle inferiorly from the occipital triangle superiorly.

8. The _____ of the omohyoid muscle originates from the scapula and then passes anteriorly and superiorly, crossing the internal jugular vein deep to the sternocleidomastoid muscle where it then attaches by a short tendon to the superior belly; the superior belly originates from the short tendon attached to the inferior belly and then inserts on the lateral border of the body of the hyoid bone.

9. The _____ is located deep to both the omohyoid and sternohyoid muscles; it originates on the thyroid cartilage and inserts on the body and greater cornu of the hyoid bone, appearing as a continuation of the sternothyroid muscle.

10. In addition to depressing the hyoid bone, the thyrohyoid muscle _____ the thyroid cartilage and larynx.

superior belly	sternothyroid muscle	inferior belly
omohyoid muscle	infrahyoid muscles	thyroid cartilage
sternohyoid muscle	raises	thyrohyoid muscle
depress		

Reference

Chapter 4, Muscular system. In Fehrenbach MJ, Herring SW: *Illustrated anatomy of the head and neck,* ed 4, St. Louis, 2012, Saunders.

FIGURE 5-14 Tongue muscles (cross section)

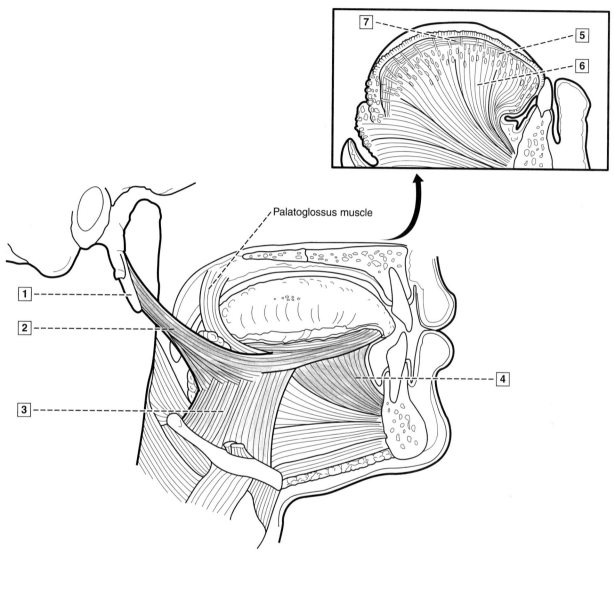

Palatoglossus muscle

EXTRINSIC

1 Styloid process
2 Styloglossus
3 Hyoglossus
4 Genioglossus

INTRINSIC

5 Transverse
6 Vertical
7 Longitudinal

REVIEW QUESTIONS

Fill in the blanks by choosing the appropriate terms from the list below.

1. The _____ is a thick vascular mass of voluntary muscle surrounded by a mucous membrane that is anchored to the floor of the mouth by the lingual frenum; it has complex movements during mastication, speaking, and swallowing that are a result of the combined action of its muscles.

2. The muscles of the tongue can be grouped according to their location: intrinsic and extrinsic, with both muscle groups intertwining; in addition, each half of the tongue has muscular groups within these two main groups that are separated by the _____, a deep fibrous structure in the midline that corresponds with the median lingual sulcus; all are innervated by the twelfth cranial or hypoglossal nerve.

3. The _____ are located inside the tongue; these muscles change the shape of the tongue.

4. The _____ is the most superficial of the intrinsic muscles and runs in an oblique and longitudinal direction in the dorsal surface from the base to the apex; deep to this muscle is the transverse muscle, which runs in a transverse direction from the median septum to pass outward toward the lateral surface.

5. The _____ runs in a vertical direction from the dorsal surface to the ventral surface in the body; in contrast, the inferior longitudinal muscle is in the ventral surface of the tongue and runs in a longitudinal direction from the base to the apex.

6. The superior and inferior longitudinal muscles act together to change the _____ of the tongue by shortening and thickening it and act singly to help it curl in various directions; the transverse and vertical muscles act together to make the tongue long and narrow.

7. The three pairs of _____ have different origins outside the tongue but all their insertions are inside the tongue; they include the styloglossus, genioglossus, and hyoglossus muscles, with each name indicating its location.

8. The _____ is an extrinsic tongue muscle that originates from the styloid process of the temporal bone and then passes inferiorly and anteriorly to insert into two parts of the lateral surface of the tongue: at the apex and at the border of the body and base; it serves to retract the tongue when active, moving it superiorly and posteriorly.

9. The _____ is a fan-shaped extrinsic tongue muscle superior to the geniohyoid, which arises from the genial tubercles on the medial surface of the mandible; a few of its most inferior fibers insert on the hyoid bone, but most insert into the tongue from its base almost to the apex, with right and left muscles separated by the tongue's median septum so that different parts of the muscle can protrude the tongue out of the oral cavity or depress parts of the tongue surface when active.

10. The _____ is an extrinsic tongue muscle that originates on both the greater cornu and a part of the body of the hyoid bone to then insert into the lateral surface of the body of the tongue; it depresses the tongue when active.

hyoglossus muscle	vertical muscle	median septum
superior longitudinal muscle	extrinsic tongue muscles	shape
tongue	styloglossus muscle	intrinsic tongue muscles
genioglossus muscle		

Reference

Chapter 4, Muscular system. In Fehrenbach MJ, Herring SW: *Illustrated anatomy of the head and neck,* ed 4, St. Louis, 2012, Saunders.

FIGURE 5-15   Muscles of the pharynx (posterior view)

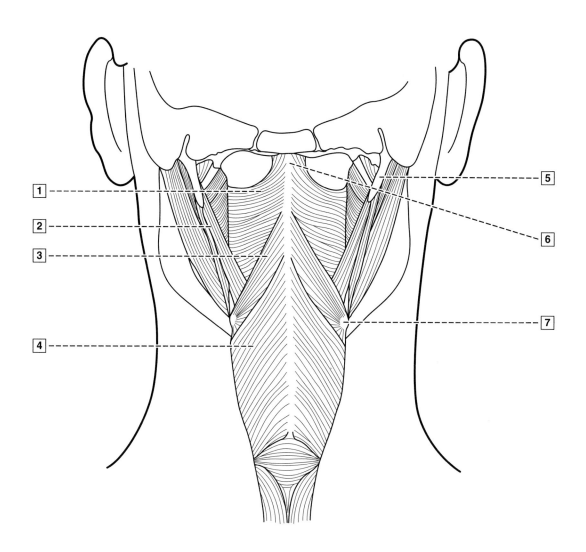

1 Superior pharyngeal constrictor
2 Stylopharyngeus
3 Middle pharyngeal constrictor
4 Inferior pharyngeal constrictor
5 Styloid process
6 Median pharyngeal raphe
7 Hyoid bone

REVIEW QUESTIONS

Fill in the blanks by choosing the appropriate terms from the list below.

1. The _____, or *throat,* is part of both the respiratory and digestive tracts.

2. The pharynx is connected to both the _____ and oral cavity.

3. The pharynx consists of _____ parts: the nasopharynx, oropharynx, and laryngopharynx.

4. The _____ are involved in producing the actions involved in speaking, swallowing, and middle ear function.

5. The muscles of the pharynx are responsible for initiating the _____ when food is taken into the oral cavity.

6. The muscles of the pharynx include the stylopharyngeus muscle, the pharyngeal constrictor muscles, and the _____.

7. The _____ is a paired longitudinal muscle of the pharynx that originates from the styloid process of the temporal bone.

8. The stylopharyngeus muscle inserts into the lateral and posterior _____.

9. The stylopharyngeus muscle serves to _____ the pharynx when active, as well as simultaneously widening the pharynx.

10. The stylopharyngeus muscle is innervated by the ninth cranial nerve, or the _____.

pharyngeal walls	elevate	stylopharyngeus muscle
swallowing process	pharynx	three
soft palate muscles	muscles of the pharynx	nasal cavity
glossopharyngeal nerve		

Reference

Chapter 4, Muscular system. In Fehrenbach MJ, Herring SW: *Illustrated anatomy of the head and neck,* ed 4, St. Louis, 2012, Saunders.

FIGURE 5-16 Muscles of the pharynx (lateral view)

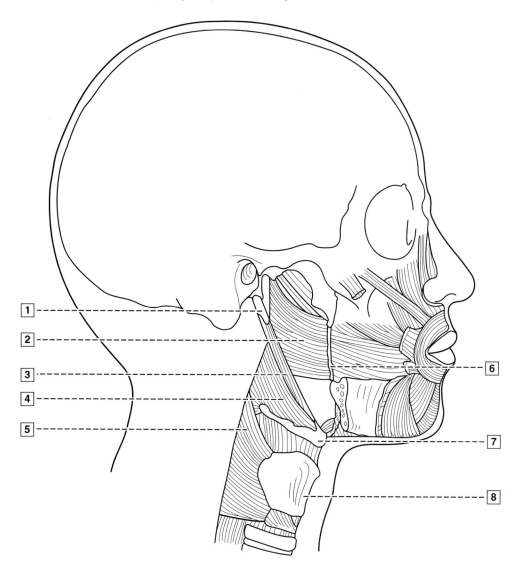

1 Styloid process

2 Superior pharyngeal constrictor

3 Stylopharyngeus

4 Middle pharyngeal constrictor

5 Inferior pharyngeal constrictor

6 Pterygomandibular raphe

7 Hyoid bone

8 Thyroid cartilage

REVIEW QUESTIONS

Fill in the blanks by choosing the appropriate terms from the list below.

1. The _____ form the lateral and posterior walls of the pharynx.

2. The pharyngeal constrictor muscles consist of _____ overlapping paired muscles based on their vertical relationship to the pharynx: the superior, middle, and inferior pharyngeal constrictor muscles.

3. The origin of each pharyngeal constrictor muscle is different, although the muscles overlap each other and also have similar _____.

4. The superior pharyngeal constrictor muscle originates from the pterygoid hamulus, the _____, and the pterygomandibular raphe.

5. The middle pharyngeal constrictor muscle originates on the _____ and stylohyoid ligament.

6. The inferior pharyngeal constrictor muscle originates from both the thyroid cartilage and cricoid cartilage of the _____.

7. The three pharyngeal constrictor muscles overlap each other from the point of insertion, causing the _____ to be the most superficial of the muscles.

8. The pharyngeal constrictor muscles insert into the _____, a midline fibrous band of the posterior wall of the pharynx that is itself attached to the base of the skull.

9. The pharyngeal constrictor muscles _____ both the pharynx and larynx and help drive food inferiorly into the esophagus during swallowing.

10. The pharyngeal constrictor muscles are innervated by the _____.

pharyngeal constrictor muscles	raise	larynx
inferior constrictor muscle	three	hyoid bone
pharyngeal plexus	median pharyngeal raphe	insertions
mandible		

Reference

Chapter 4, Muscular system. In Fehrenbach MJ, Herring SW: *Illustrated anatomy of the head and neck,* ed 4, St. Louis, 2012, Saunders.

ANSWER KEY 1. pharyngeal constrictor muscles, 2. three, 3. insertions, 4. mandible, 5. hyoid bone, 6. larynx, 7. inferior constrictor muscle, 8. median pharyngeal raphe, 9. raise, 10. pharyngeal plexus.

FIGURE 5-17 Muscles of the pharynx: muscle of the soft palate (posterior views)

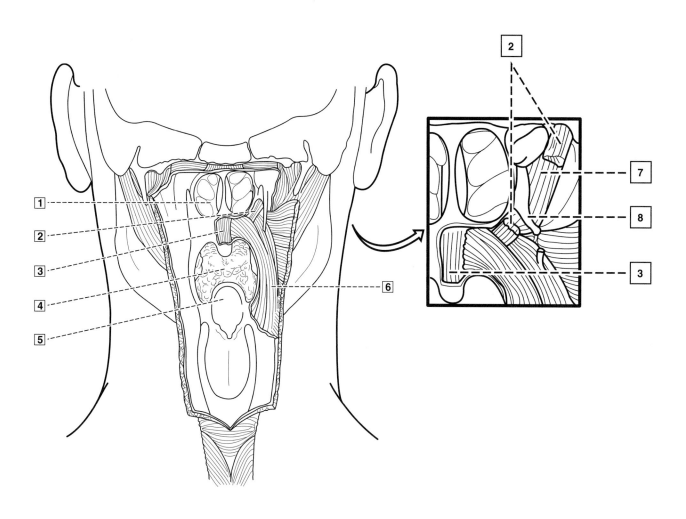

1	Nasal cavity	5	Epiglottis
2	Levator veli palatini	6	Palatopharyngeus
3	Muscle of uvula	7	Tensor veli palatini
4	Dorsal surface of tongue	8	Hamulus

REVIEW QUESTIONS

Fill in the blanks by choosing the appropriate terms from the list below.

1. The five paired _____ are all involved in speaking and swallowing and include: the palatoglossus muscle, the palatopharyngeus muscle, the levator veli palatini muscle, the tensor veli palatini muscle, and the muscle of the uvula.

2. When the muscles of the soft palate are relaxed, the soft palate extends posteriorly to the oropharynx, but the combined actions of several muscles of the soft palate move the _____ and uvula superiorly and posteriorly to contact the posterior pharyngeal wall that is being moved anteriorly; thus it is the movement of both the soft palate and pharyngeal wall between the nasopharynx and oral cavity during swallowing that prevents food from entering the nasal cavity.

3. The muscles of the soft palate are innervated by the pharyngeal plexus, except the tensor veli palatini muscle, which is supplied by the _____ of the fifth cranial nerve, or the trigeminal nerve.

4. The _____ forms the anterior faucial pillar in the oral cavity, a vertical fold anterior to each palatine tonsil that originates from the median palatine raphe and then inserts into the lateral surface of the tongue; it elevates the base of the tongue, arching the tongue against the soft palate, and depresses the soft palate toward the tongue when active so that the muscles on both sides form a sphincter, separating the oral cavity from the pharynx.

5. The _____ forms the posterior faucial pillar in the oral cavity, a vertical fold posterior to each palatine tonsil that originates in the soft palate and then inserts in the walls of the laryngopharynx and on the thyroid cartilage; it moves the palate posteroinferiorly and the posterior pharyngeal wall anterosuperiorly to help close off the nasopharynx during swallowing when active.

6. The _____ is located mainly superior to the soft palate, originates from the inferior surface of the temporal bone, and then inserts into the median palatine raphe, a midline fibrous band of the palate.

7. The levator veli palatini muscle _____ the soft palate and helps bring it into contact with the posterior pharyngeal wall to close off the nasopharynx during speech and swallowing when active.

8. The _____ is a special muscle that stiffens the soft palate and also slightly lowers the soft palate, with some of its fibers responsible for opening the auditory tube to allow air to flow between the pharynx and middle ear cavity.

9. The tensor veli palatine muscle originates from the _____ and the inferior surface of the sphenoid bone and then passes inferiorly between the medial pterygoid muscle and medial pterygoid plate; the muscle forms a tendon near the pterygoid hamulus, a tendon that winds around the hamulus, using it as a pulley, then spreads out to insert into the median palatine raphe.

10. The _____ is a muscle of the soft palate that lies entirely within the uvula of the palate, which is a midline tissue structure that hangs inferiorly from the posterior margin of the soft palate; it is important to note that this muscle shortens and broadens the uvula when active, changing the contour of the posterior part of the soft palate, with the change in contour allowing the soft palate to adapt closely to the posterior pharyngeal wall to help close off the nasopharynx during swallowing.

auditory tube area	soft palate	mandibular nerve
tensor veli palatini muscle	levator veli palatini muscle	palatopharyngeus muscle
raises	muscles of the soft palate	palatoglossus muscle
muscle of the uvula		

Reference

Chapter 4, Muscular system. In Fehrenbach MJ, Herring SW: *Illustrated anatomy of the head and neck,* ed 4, St. Louis, 2012, Saunders.

FIGURE 6-1 Pathways to and from the heart: arteries and veins (frontal view)

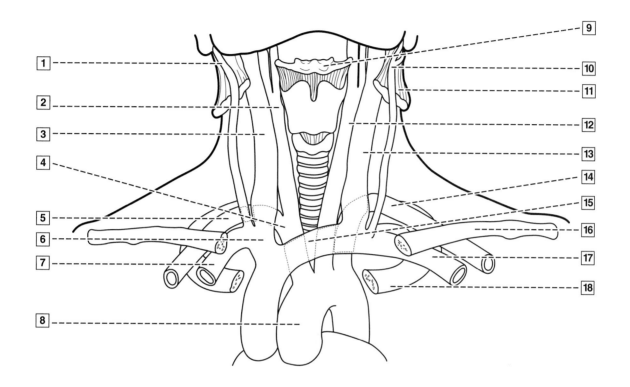

1	Right external jugular vein	10	Left external jugular vein
2	Right common carotid artery	11	Sternocleidomastoid muscle (cut)
3	Right internal jugular vein	12	Left common carotid artery
4	Brachiocephalic artery	13	Left internal jugular vein
5	Right subclavian artery	14	Left subclavian artery
6	Right brachiocephalic vein	15	Left brachiocephalic vein
7	Right subclavian vein	16	Clavicle (cut)
8	Aorta	17	Left subclavian vein
9	Hyoid bone	18	First rib (cut)

REVIEW QUESTIONS

Fill in the blanks by choosing the appropriate terms from the list below.

1. The basic origins from the _____ of the common carotid arteries and subclavian arteries that supply the head and neck are different for the right and left sides of the body.

2. For the left side of the body, the common carotid artery and subclavian artery arise directly from the _____.

3. For the right side of the body, the common carotid artery and subclavian artery are both branches from the _____, which is a direct branch of the aorta.

4. The _____ is branchless and travels superiorly along the neck, lateral to the trachea and larynx, to the superior border of the thyroid cartilage; later it travels in a sheath deep to the sternocleidomastoid muscle that also contains the internal jugular vein and tenth cranial or vagus nerve.

5. The _____ arises lateral to the common carotid artery, and gives rise to branches that supply both intracranial and extracranial structures, but its major destination is the upper extremity (arm).

brachiocephalic artery   **common carotid artery**

aorta   **heart**

subclavian artery

Reference

Chapter 6, Vascular system. In Fehrenbach MJ, Herring SW: *Illustrated anatomy of the head and neck,* ed 4, St. Louis, 2012, Saunders.

FIGURE 6-2 Common carotid artery: internal and external arteries (lateral view)

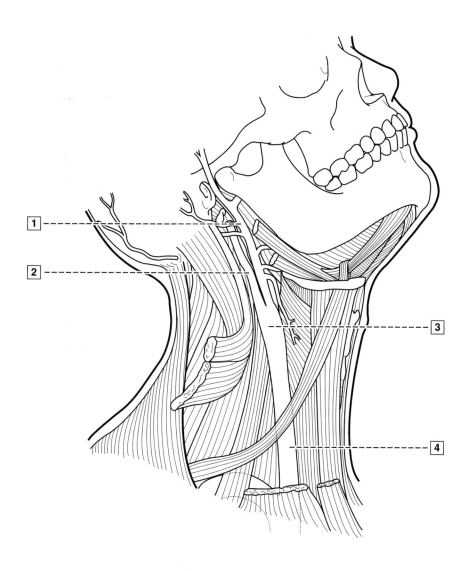

1 | External carotid
2 | Internal carotid
3 | Carotid sinus
4 | Common carotid

REVIEW QUESTIONS

Fill in the blanks by choosing the appropriate terms from the list below.

1. The _____ is an artery that ends by dividing into the internal and external carotid arteries at about the level of the larynx.

2. Just before the common carotid artery bifurcates into the internal and external carotid arteries, it exhibits a swelling, the _____.

3. The _____ travels superiorly in a slightly lateral position (in relationship to the external carotid artery) after leaving the common carotid artery; however, this artery has no branches in the neck but continues adjacent to the internal jugular vein within the carotid sheath to the skull base, where it enters the cranium to supply the intracranial structures and is the source of the ophthalmic artery, which supplies the eye, orbit, and lacrimal gland.

4. As with the internal carotid artery, the _____ begins at the superior border of the thyroid cartilage, at the termination of the common carotid artery and the carotid sheath, and then travels superiorly in a more medial position (in relationship to the internal carotid artery) after arising from the common carotid artery.

5. The external carotid artery supplies the _____ tissue of the head and neck, including the oral cavity, and has four sets of branches grouped according to their location to the main artery: anterior, medial, posterior, and terminal branches.

extracranial   external carotid artery

internal carotid artery   common carotid artery

carotid sinus

Reference

Chapter 6, Vascular system. In Fehrenbach MJ, Herring SW: *Illustrated anatomy of the head and neck,* ed 4, St. Louis, 2012, Saunders.

FIGURE 6-3 Common carotid artery: external carotid (lateral view)

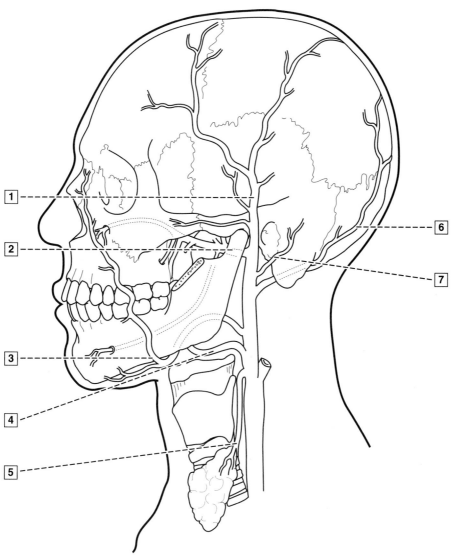

TERMINAL BRANCHES
- **1** Maxillary
- **2** Superficial temporal

ANTERIOR BRANCHES
- **3** Facial
- **4** Lingual
- **5** Superior thyroid

POSTERIOR BRANCHES
- **6** Occipital
- **7** Posterior auricular

MEDIAL BRANCH
Ascending pharyngeal
(not shown)

REVIEW QUESTIONS

Fill in the blanks by choosing the appropriate terms from the list below.

1. The _____ travels superiorly in a more medial position (in relationship to the internal carotid artery) after arising from the common carotid artery, having four sets of branches grouped according to their location to the main artery: anterior, medial, posterior, and terminal.

2. The _____ is an anterior branch from the external carotid artery.

3. The superior thyroid artery has _____ branches—the infrahyoid artery, the sternocleidomastoid branch, the superior laryngeal artery, and the cricothyroid branch—that supply the tissue inferior to the hyoid bone, including the infrahyoid muscles, the sternocleidomastoid muscle, the muscles of the larynx, and the thyroid gland.

4. The _____ is an anterior branch from the external carotid artery that arises superior to the superior thyroid artery at the level of the hyoid bone and anteriorly to the apex of the tongue by way of its inferior surface to supply the tissue superior to the hyoid bone, including the suprahyoid muscles and floor of the mouth by way of the dorsal lingual, deep lingual, sublingual, and suprahyoid branches, as well as branches to the tongue.

5. The _____, or *external maxillary artery,* is an anterior branch from the external carotid artery that arises slightly superior to the lingual artery as it branches off anteriorly; however, in some cases, the facial and lingual arteries share a common trunk.

6. There is only one medial branch off the external carotid artery, the small _____, which arises close to the origin of the external carotid artery.

7. The ascending pharyngeal artery has _____ small branches: the pharyngeal branch and meningeal branch, which supply the pharyngeal walls (where they anastomose with the ascending palatine artery), soft palate, and meninges, as well as tonsillar branches.

8. The _____ is a posterior branch of the external carotid artery that arises from the external carotid artery as it passes superiorly just deep to the ascending ramus of the mandible and then travels to the posterior part of the scalp to supply the suprahyoid and sternocleidomastoid muscles, as well as the scalp and meninges in the occipital region through its muscular branches, sternocleidomastoid branches, auricular branches, and meningeal branches.

9. The small _____ is a posterior branch of the external carotid artery that arises superior to the occipital artery and stylohyoid muscle at about the level of the tip of the styloid process to supply the internal ear by its auricular branch and the mastoid air cells by the stylomastoid artery.

10. The two terminal branches of the external carotid artery include the superficial temporal artery and maxillary artery, or *internal maxillary artery*; the external carotid artery splits into these terminal branches within the _____ on each side of the face.

posterior auricular artery	two	parotid salivary gland
four	external carotid artery	superior thyroid artery
occipital artery	facial artery	lingual artery
ascending pharyngeal artery		

Reference

Chapter 6, Vascular system. In Fehrenbach MJ, Herring SW: *Illustrated anatomy of the head and neck,* ed 4, St. Louis, 2012, Saunders.

FIGURE 6-4   External carotid artery: maxillary (lateral view)

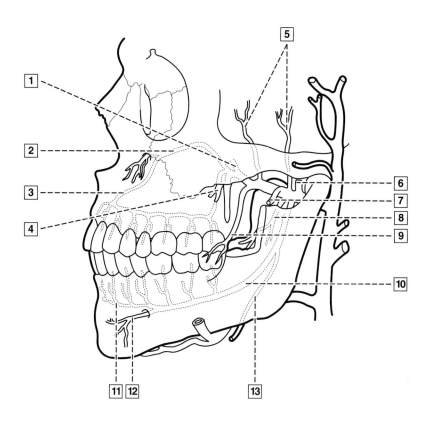

1 Sphenopalatine (cut)

2 Infraorbital

3 Anterior superior alveolar with its dental and alveolar branches (branch of infraorbital)

4 Posterior superior alveolar (part cut)

5 Deep temporals

6 Middle meningeal (cut)

7 Masseteric (cut)

8 Pterygoids

9 Buccal

10 Inferior alveolar

11 Incisive with its dental and alveolar branches

12 Mental

13 Mylohyoid

BRANCHES OF INFERIOR ALVEOLAR

Greater and lesser palatine
Nasal cavity branches
(not shown)

REVIEW QUESTIONS

Fill in the blanks by choosing the appropriate terms from the list below.

1. Within the infratemporal fossa, the _____, or *internal maxillary artery,* gives rise to many branches, including the middle meningeal and inferior alveolar arteries and several arteries to muscles; it is the larger terminal branch of the external carotid artery.

2. The _____ supplies the meninges of the brain by way of the foramen spinosum, located on the inferior surface of the skull, as well as the skull bones.

3. The _____ arises from the maxillary artery in the infratemporal fossa and then turns inferiorly to enter the mandibular foramen and then the mandibular canal along with the inferior alveolar nerve; within the canal it gives rise to dental and alveolar branches that supply the mandibular posterior teeth.

4. The _____ branches off from the inferior alveolar artery before it enters the mandibular canal by way of the mandibular foramen and then travels in the mylohyoid groove on the inner surface of the mandible to supply the floor of the mouth and the mylohyoid muscle.

5. The _____ arises from the inferior alveolar artery and exits the mandibular canal by way of the mental foramen, which is located on the outer surface of the mandible, usually deep to the apices of the mandibular first and second premolar teeth; after it exits the canal, the artery supplies the tissue of the chin and anastomoses with the inferior labial artery.

6. The _____ branches off the inferior alveolar artery, remaining within the mandibular canal to divide into dental and alveolar branches to supply the mandibular anterior teeth.

7. After traversing the infratemporal fossa, the maxillary artery enters the pterygopalatine fossa, which is deep and inferior to the eye. Just as the maxillary artery leaves the infratemporal fossa and enters the pterygopalatine fossa, it gives rise to the _____, which then enters the posterior superior alveolar foramina on the maxillary tuberosity, giving rise to dental branches and alveolar branches to supply the maxillary posterior teeth and anastomoses with the anterior superior alveolar artery.

8. The _____ branches off the maxillary artery in the pterygopalatine fossa and may share a common trunk with the posterior superior alveolar artery; later this artery then enters the orbit through the inferior orbital fissure and while in the orbit, the artery travels in the infraorbital canal to provide branches to the orbit as well as giving rise to the anterior superior alveolar artery.

9. After giving off branches in the infraorbital canal, the infraorbital artery emerges onto the face from the infraorbital foramen to supply parts of the infraorbital region of the face by its terminal branches and anastomose with the _____.

10. The _____ arises from the infraorbital artery and gives rise to dental and alveolar branches that supply the maxillary anterior teeth and anastomoses with the posterior superior alveolar artery.

middle meningeal artery	posterior superior alveolar artery	incisive artery
facial artery	mental artery	inferior alveolar artery
infraorbital artery	maxillary artery	mylohyoid artery
anterior superior alveolar artery		

Reference

Chapter 6, Vascular system. In Fehrenbach MJ, Herring SW: *Illustrated anatomy of the head and neck,* ed 4, St. Louis, 2012, Saunders.

FIGURE 6-5 Maxillary artery: palatal branches (sagittal section of nasal cavity)

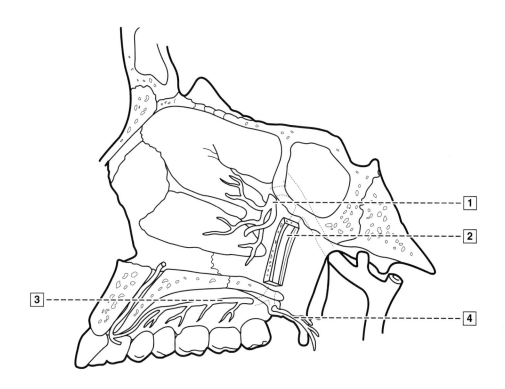

1. Sphenopalatine
2. Descending palatine
3. Greater palatine
4. Lesser palatine

REVIEW QUESTIONS

Fill in the blanks by choosing the appropriate terms from the list below.

1. In the pterygopalatine fossa, the maxillary artery gives rise to the _____, which travels to the palate through the pterygopalatine canal.

2. The descending palatine artery terminates in both the greater and lesser _____ by way of the greater and lesser palatine foramina to supply the hard and soft palates, respectively.

3. The maxillary artery ends by becoming the _____, its main terminal branch, which supplies the nasal cavity by way of the sphenopalatine foramen.

4. The sphenopalatine artery gives rise to the _____, as well as septal branches.

5. One of the arteries that branches off the sphenopalatine artery includes the _____ that accompanies the nasopalatine nerve through the incisive foramen on the maxillae.

nasopalatine branch   sphenopalatine artery

palatine arteries   descending palatine artery

posterior lateral nasal branches

Reference

Chapter 6, Vascular system. In Fehrenbach MJ, Herring SW: *Illustrated anatomy of the head and neck,* ed 4, St. Louis, 2012, Saunders.

FIGURE 6-6   External carotid artery: superficial temporal artery (lateral view)

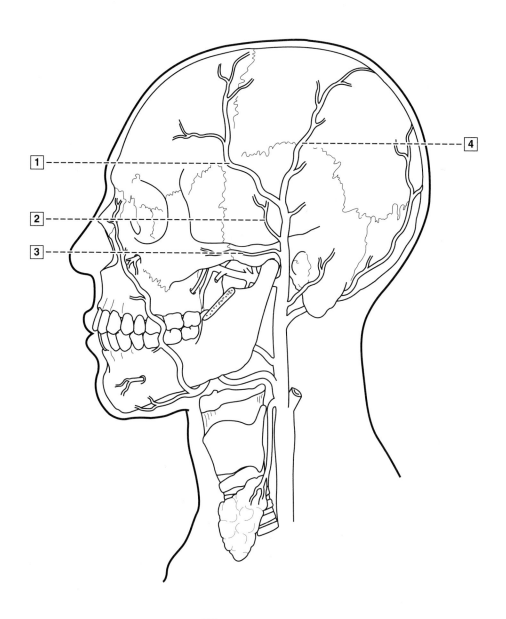

1	Frontal branch
2	Middle temporal
3	Transverse facial
4	Parietal branch

REVIEW QUESTIONS

Fill in the blanks by choosing the appropriate terms from the list below.

1. The _____ is the smaller terminal branch of the external carotid artery that arises within the parotid salivary gland.

2. The superficial temporal artery has _____ main branches, including the transverse facial artery, the middle temporal artery, the frontal branch, and the parietal branch.

3. The small _____ supplies the parotid salivary gland duct and nearby facial tissue.

4. The small _____ supplies the temporalis muscle.

5. The _____ and parietal branch supply in the frontal and parietal regions of the scalp, respectively.

superficial temporal artery   frontal branch

transverse facial artery   middle temporal branch

four

Reference

Chapter 6, Vascular system. In Fehrenbach MJ, Herring SW: *Illustrated anatomy of the head and neck,* ed 4, St. Louis, 2012, Saunders.

FIGURE 6-7   External carotid artery: anterior branches (sagittal section)

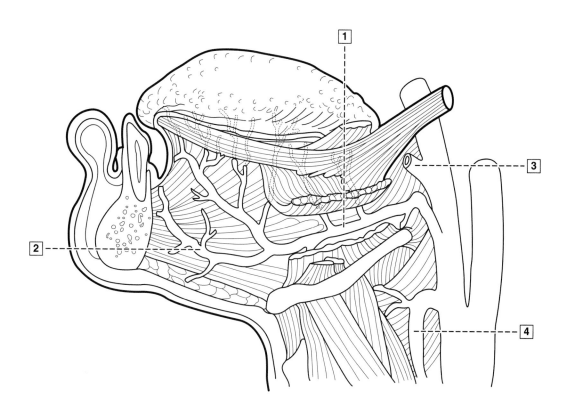

1	Lingual
2	Sublingual
3	Facial (cut)
4	Superior thyroid

REVIEW QUESTIONS

Fill in the blanks by choosing the appropriate terms from the list below.

1. There are _____ main anterior branches from the external carotid artery: the superior thyroid, the lingual, and the facial arteries.

2. The superior thyroid artery is an anterior branch from the _____.

3. The lingual artery is an anterior branch from the external carotid artery and arises _____ to the superior thyroid artery at the level of the hyoid bone.

4. The lingual artery travels anteriorly to the _____ by way of its inferior surface.

5. The lingual artery supplies the tissue superior to the_____, including the suprahyoid muscles and floor of the mouth by the dorsal lingual, deep lingual, sublingual, and suprahyoid branches.

6. The _____ is also supplied by branches of the lingual artery, including several small dorsal lingual branches to the base and body and the deep lingual artery, the terminal part of the lingual artery, to the apex; it also has tonsillar branches.

7. The _____ branches off the lingual artery to supply the mylohyoid muscle, sublingual salivary gland, and mucous membranes of the floor of the mouth.

8. The small _____ supplies the suprahyoid muscles.

9. The _____, or *external maxillary artery*, is the final anterior branch from the external carotid artery.

10. The facial artery arises slightly superior to the lingual artery as it branches off anteriorly; however, in some cases the facial and lingual arteries share a(n) _____.

facial artery	external carotid artery	sublingual artery
common trunk	tongue	three
hyoid bone	suprahyoid branch	apex of the tongue
superior		

Reference

Chapter 6, Vascular system. In Fehrenbach MJ, Herring SW: *Illustrated anatomy of the head and neck,* ed 4, St. Louis, 2012, Saunders.

ANSWER KEY   1. three, 2. external carotid artery, 3. superior, 4. apex of the tongue, 5. hyoid bone, 6. tongue, 7. sublingual artery, 8. suprahyoid branch, 9. facial artery, 10. common trunk.

FIGURE 6-8 External carotid artery: facial (lateral view)

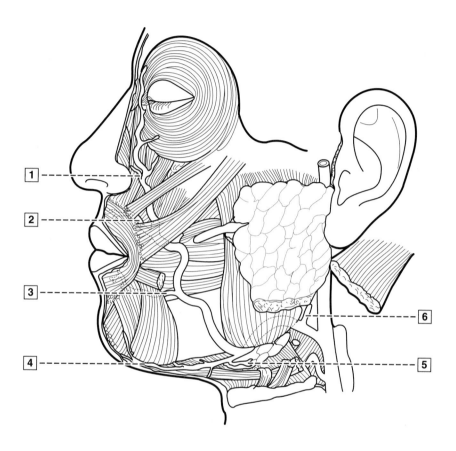

1 Angular

2 Superior labial

3 Inferior labial

4 Submental

5 Glandular branches

6 Ascending palatine

REVIEW QUESTIONS

Fill in the blanks by choosing the appropriate terms from the list below.

1. The _____, or *external maxillary artery,* is an anterior branch from the external carotid artery that arises slightly superior to the lingual artery as it branches off anteriorly; however, in some cases the facial and lingual arteries share a common trunk.

2. The facial artery has a complicated path that runs medial to the _____, over the submandibular salivary gland, and then around the bone's inferior border to its lateral side.

3. From the inferior border of the mandible, the facial artery runs anteriorly and superiorly near the angle of the mouth and along the side of the nose to terminate at the _____ so as to supply the face in the oral, buccal, zygomatic, nasal, infraorbital, and orbital regions.

4. The facial artery is mainly parallel to the _____ in the head area, although both blood vessels do not run adjacent to each other.

5. In the neck, the facial artery is _____ from the facial vein by the posterior belly of the digastric muscle, stylohyoid muscle, and submandibular salivary gland.

6. The facial artery has _____ major branches that include the ascending palatine branch, the glandular branches, the submental branch, the inferior labial branch, the superior labial branch, the angular branch, and the tonsillar branch.

7. The _____ is the first branch from the facial artery and supplies the soft palate, palatine muscles, and palatine tonsils.

8. Both the glandular branches and the _____ are branches from the facial artery that together supply the submandibular lymph nodes, submandibular salivary gland, and mylohyoid and digastric muscles.

9. The _____ is a branch from the facial artery that supplies the lower lip area, including the muscles of facial expression such as the depressor anguli oris muscle; additionally, the superior labial artery is a branch from the facial artery that supplies the upper lip tissue.

10. The _____ is the terminal branch of the facial artery and supplies the side of the nose.

ascending palatine artery	angular artery	submental artery
facial artery	separated	mandible
facial vein	seven	inferior labial artery
medial canthus		

Reference

Chapter 6, Vascular system. In Fehrenbach MJ, Herring SW: *Illustrated anatomy of the head and neck,* ed 4, St. Louis, 2012, Saunders.

FIGURE 6-9   External carotid artery: posterior branches (lateral view)

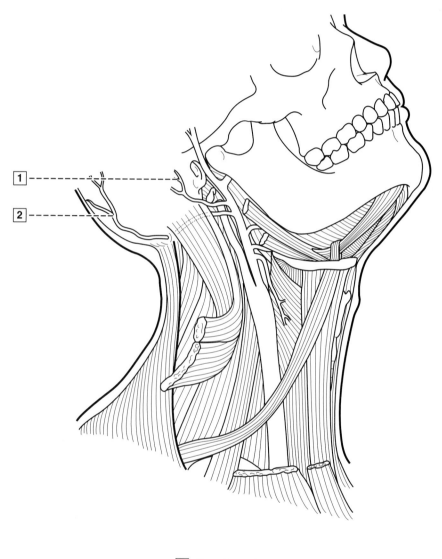

1   Posterior auricular
2   Occipital

REVIEW QUESTIONS

Fill in the blanks by choosing the appropriate terms from the list below.

1.   There are _____ posterior branches of the external carotid artery: the occipital and posterior auricular arteries.

2.   The occipital artery is a posterior branch of the _____.

3.   The occipital artery arises from the external carotid artery as it passes superiorly just deep to the ascending ramus of the _____ and then travels to the posterior part of the scalp.

4.   At its origin, the occipital artery is adjacent to the twelfth cranial nerve, or the _____.

5.   The occipital artery supplies the suprahyoid and sternocleidomastoid muscles, as well as the scalp and meninges in the _____.

6.   The occipital artery supplies the occipital region through the _____, as well as the sternocleidomastoid branches, auricular branches, and meningeal branches.

7.   The small posterior auricular artery is also a(n) _____ of the external carotid artery.

8.   The posterior auricular artery arises superior to the occipital artery and stylohyoid muscle at about the level of the tip of the _____.

9.   The posterior auricular artery supplies the internal ear by its _____.

10. The posterior auricular artery supplies the mastoid air cells by the _____.

stylomastoid artery	auricular branch	external carotid artery
two	hypoglossal nerve	occipital region
styloid process	posterior branch	mandible
muscular branches		

Reference

Chapter 6, Vascular system. In Fehrenbach MJ, Herring SW: *Illustrated anatomy of the head and neck,* ed 4, St. Louis, 2012, Saunders.

FIGURE 6-10   Vascular system: internal jugular and facial veins plus vessel anastomoses (lateral view)

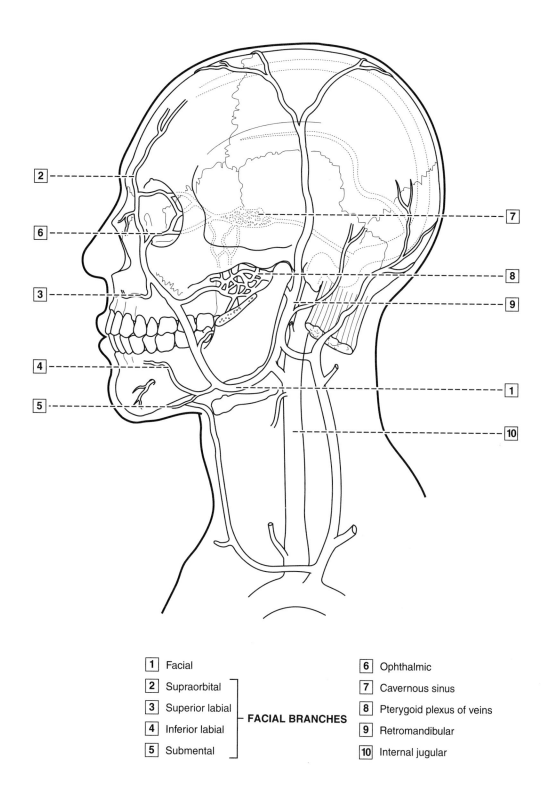

1 Facial	**6** Ophthalmic
2 Supraorbital	**7** Cavernous sinus
3 Superior labial	**8** Pterygoid plexus of veins
4 Inferior labial	**9** Retromandibular
5 Submental	**10** Internal jugular

FACIAL BRANCHES (brackets grouping items 2–5)

REVIEW QUESTIONS

Fill in the blanks by choosing the appropriate terms from the list below.

1. The _____ drains the brain as well as most of the other tissue of the head and neck, whereas the external jugular vein drains only a small part of the extracranial tissue; however, the two veins have many anastomoses.

2. The internal jugular vein originates in the cranial cavity and leaves the skull through the _____; along the way it receives many tributaries, including the veins from the lingual, sublingual, and pharyngeal areas, as well as the facial vein.

3. The internal jugular vein runs with the common carotid artery and its branches, as well as the vagus nerve in the _____, as it descends in the neck to merge with the subclavian vein.

4. The _____ drains into the internal jugular vein after it begins at the medial corner of the eye with the junction of two veins from the frontal region: the supratrochlear and supraorbital veins.

5. The supraorbital vein also anastomoses with the ophthalmic veins; the ophthalmic veins drain the tissue of the orbit, and this anastomosis provides a communication with the _____.

6. The facial vein receives branches from the same areas of the face that are supplied by the _____.

7. The facial vein anastomoses with the deep veins such as the _____ in the infratemporal fossa and with the large retromandibular vein before joining the internal jugular vein at the level of the hyoid bone.

8. The facial vein has some important tributaries in the oral region, such as the _____ that drains the upper lip.

9. The _____ drains the lower lip in the oral region as a tributary of the facial vein.

10. A facial vein tributary, the _____, drains the tissue of the chin as well as the submandibular region.

inferior labial vein	internal jugular vein	cavernous sinus
jugular foramen	carotid sheath	facial artery
submental vein	facial vein	pterygoid plexus
superior labial vein		

Reference

Chapter 6, Vascular system. In Fehrenbach MJ, Herring SW: *Illustrated anatomy of the head and neck,* ed 4, St. Louis, 2012, Saunders.

FIGURE 6-11 Vascular system: external jugular and retromandibular veins plus vessel anastomoses (lateral view)

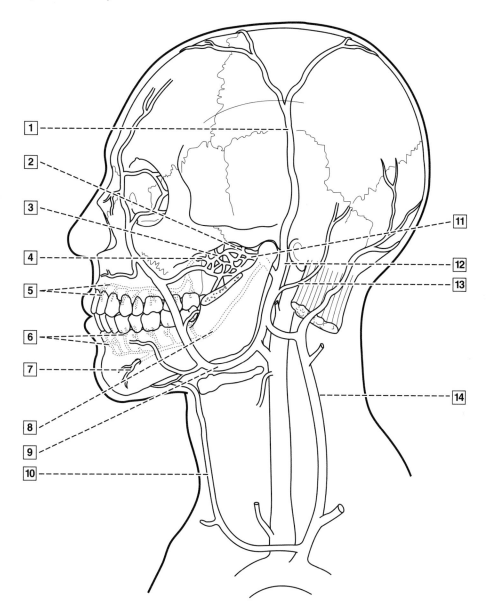

1	Superficial temporal	8	Inferior alveolar
2	Middle meningeal	9	Facial
3	Pterygoid plexus of veins	10	Anterior jugular
4	Posterior superior alveolar	11	Maxillary
5	Alveolar and dental branches of posterior superior alveolar	12	Retromandibular
6	Alveolar and dental branches of inferior alveolar	13	Posterior auricular
7	Mental branch of inferior alveolar	14	External jugular

REVIEW QUESTIONS

Fill in the blanks by choosing the appropriate terms from the list below.

1. The _____ forms the external jugular vein from a part of its route, having been initially formed from the merger of the superficial temporal vein and maxillary vein and having drained those areas by those veins; the vein then emerges from the parotid salivary gland and courses inferiorly.

2. Inferior to the parotid salivary gland, the retromandibular vein usually divides, with the anterior division joining the facial vein, and the posterior division continuing its inferior course on the surface of the sternocleidomastoid muscle; later is joined by the _____, which drains the lateral scalp posterior to the ear, the posterior division of the retromandibular veins now becomes the external jugular vein.

3. The superficially located _____ drains the lateral scalp and goes on to drain into and form the retromandibular vein, along with the deeper maxillary vein.

4. The _____, or *internal maxillary vein,* is deeper than the superficial temporal vein and begins in the infratemporal fossa by collecting blood from the pterygoid plexus, accompanying the maxillary artery, as well as the middle meningeal, posterior superior alveolar, inferior alveolar, and other veins such as those from the nasal cavity and palate; after then receiving these veins, it merges with the superficial temporal vein to drain into and form the retromandibular vein.

5. The _____ is a collection of small anastomosing vessels located around the pterygoid muscles and surrounding the maxillary artery on each side of the face within the infratemporal fossa; it anastomoses with both the facial and retromandibular veins as it drains the veins from the deep parts of the face and then drains into the maxillary vein.

6. The _____ also drains the blood from both the dura mater of the meninges (not the arachnoid or pia mater) and the bones of the vault into the pterygoid plexus of veins.

7. The pterygoid plexus of veins also drains the _____, which is formed by the merging of its dental and alveolar branches of the maxillary teeth.

8. The _____ forms from the merging of its dental branches and alveolar branches of the mandibular teeth, where they also drain into the pterygoid plexus; additionally, the mental branches of this vein enter the mental foramen after draining the chin area on the outer surface of the mandible, where they anastomose with branches of the facial vein.

9. The _____ drains into the external jugular vein (or directly into the subclavian vein) before it joins the subclavian vein after its beginning inferior to the chin, communicates with veins in the area, and descends near the midline within the superficial fascia, receiving branches from the superficial cervical structures; however, only one of these veins may be present, but if two veins are present, they end up anastomosing with each other through a jugular venous arch.

10. On each side of the body, the external jugular vein joins the subclavian vein from the arm, and then the internal jugular vein merges with the subclavian vein to form the brachiocephalic vein, which then unites to form the superior vena cava to travel ultimately to the _____.

pterygoid plexus of veins	**posterior superior alveolar vein**	**posterior auricular vein**
superficial temporal vein	**inferior alveolar vein**	**anterior jugular vein**
maxillary vein	**retromandibular vein**	**heart**
middle meningeal vein		

Reference

Chapter 6, Vascular system. In Fehrenbach MJ, Herring SW: *Illustrated anatomy of the head and neck,* ed 4, St. Louis, 2012, Saunders.

FIGURE 7-1 Lacrimal apparatus (frontal and deep views)

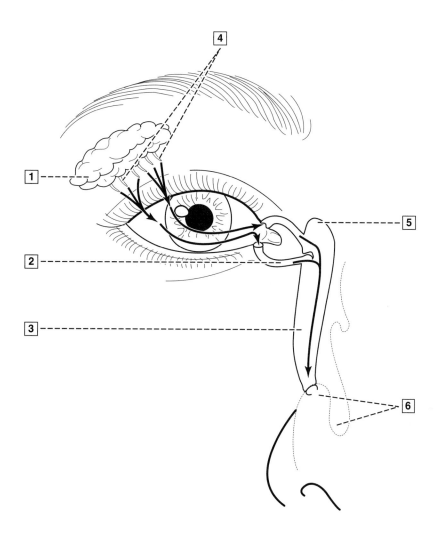

1. Lacrimal gland
2. Lacrimal canal
3. Nasolacrimal duct
4. Lacrimal ducts
5. Lacrimal sac
6. Inferior meatus and turbinate

REVIEW QUESTIONS

Fill in the blanks by choosing the appropriate terms from the list below.

1. The _____ are paired exocrine glands that secrete lacrimal fluid, or *tears*, which is a watery fluid that lubricates the conjunctiva lining the inside of the eyelids and the front of each eyeball.

2. Each lacrimal gland is located in the depression of the _____ of the frontal bone, which is located just inside the lateral part of the supraorbital ridge within the orbit.

3. The larger orbital part of the lacrimal gland contains the _____ that drain the gland, because it is an exocrine gland.

4. The lacrimal fluid, or *tears,* secreted from the lacrimal gland collect in the fornix conjunctiva of the upper eyelid and pass over the eye surface to the _____, which are small holes found at each medial canthus.

5. Any _____, or *tears,* secreted from the lacrimal gland that passes over the eye surface ends up in the nasolacrimal sac, a thin-walled structure behind each medial canthus.

6. From the nasolacrimal sac, the lacrimal fluid secreted by the lacrimal gland continues into the nasolacrimal duct, ultimately draining into the _____.

7. The nasolacrimal duct is formed at the junction of the lacrimal bones and _____ bone of the face.

8. The lacrimal gland is innervated by parasympathetic fibers from the _____, a branch of the seventh cranial nerve or facial nerve; these preganglionic fibers synapse at the pterygopalatine ganglion, and postganglionic fibers reach the gland through branches of the trigeminal nerve and the lacrimal nerve also serves as an afferent nerve for the gland.

9. The lacrimal gland drains into the _____ of the lymphatic system.

10. The lacrimal gland is supplied by the _____, a branch of the ophthalmic artery of the internal carotid artery.

lacrimal artery	lacrimal fossa	lacrimal puncta
superficial parotid lymph nodes	lacrimal ducts	lacrimal fluid
lacrimal glands	greater petrosal nerve	maxillary
inferior nasal meatus		

Reference

Chapter 7, Glandular tissue. In Fehrenbach MJ, Herring SW: *Illustrated anatomy of the head and neck,* ed 4, St. Louis, 2012, Saunders.

FIGURE 7-2 Major salivary glands and ducts (ventral and frontal aspects with internal views)

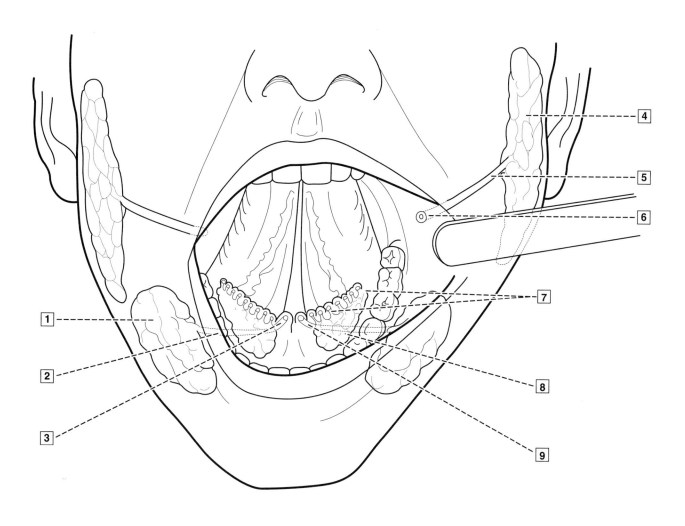

1	Submandibular gland	5	Parotid duct (Stenson duct)
2	Submandibular duct (Wharton duct)	6	Parotid papilla
3	Sublingual caruncle with duct openings from submandibular and sublingual glands	7	Sublingual ducts
		8	Sublingual gland
4	Parotid gland	9	Sublingual duct (Bartholin duct)

REVIEW QUESTIONS

Fill in the blanks by choosing the appropriate terms from the list below.

1. The _____ produce saliva, which is part of the immune system as well as the digestive system; saliva lubricates and cleanses the oral cavity and helps in digestion.

2. The salivary glands are controlled by the _____ nervous system, which is not subject to voluntary control.

3. The salivary glands are divided by size into major and minor glands; both the major and minor salivary glands are _____ and thus have ducts associated with them that help drain the saliva directly into the oral cavity where the saliva can function.

4. The _____ are large paired salivary glands that have named ducts associated with them.

5. The _____ is the largest encapsulated major salivary gland.

6. The named duct associated with the parotid salivary gland is the _____, or *Stensen duct*, which opens up into the oral cavity on the inner surface of the cheek, usually opposite the maxillary second molar as marked by the parotid papilla.

7. The _____ is the second largest encapsulated major salivary gland.

8. The named duct associated with the submandibular salivary gland is the _____, or *Wharton duct*, which travels along the anterior floor of the mouth and then opens into the oral cavity at the sublingual caruncle.

9. The _____ is the smallest, most diffuse, and only unencapsulated major salivary gland.

10. The short ducts associated with the sublingual salivary gland in some cases combine to form the duct named the _____, or *Bartholin duct*, which then opens directly into the oral cavity through the same opening as the submandibular duct, the sublingual caruncle.

major salivary glands	submandibular duct	parotid salivary gland
sublingual duct	autonomic	salivary glands
submandibular salivary gland	sublingual salivary gland	exocrine glands
parotid duct		

References

Chapter 7, Glandular tissue. In Fehrenbach MJ, Herring SW: *Illustrated anatomy of the head and neck,* ed 4, St. Louis, 2012, Saunders; and Chapter 11, Head and neck structures. In Bath-Balogh M, Fehrenbach MJ: *Illustrated dental embryology, histology, and anatomy,* ed 3, St. Louis, 2011, Saunders.

FIGURE 7-3 Salivary gland (microanatomic view)

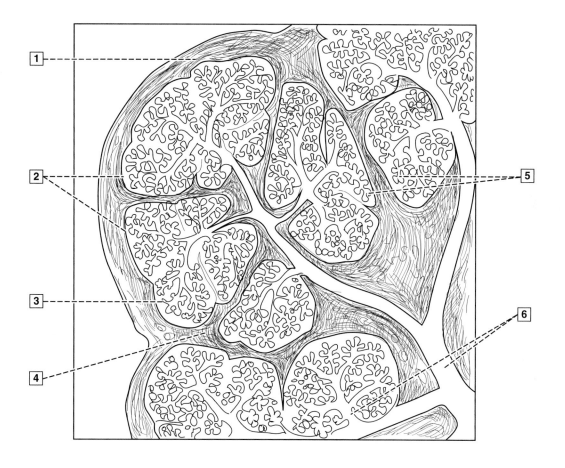

1 Capsule

2 Lobes

3 Lobule

4 Septum

5 Acini

6 Ductal system

REVIEW QUESTIONS

Fill in the blanks by choosing the appropriate terms from the list below.

1. The connective tissue of the salivary gland is divided into the outer _____, which surrounds the entire gland, as well as the inner dividing septa.

2. Each _____ helps divide the inner part of the salivary gland into the larger lobes and smaller lobules.

3. The epithelial cells of the salivary gland that produce saliva are the _____.

4. The secretory cells of the salivary gland are found in a group, or a(n) _____; each group is located at the terminal part of the gland connected to the ductal system, with many groups within each lobule of the gland.

5. The _____ of salivary glands consists of hollow tubes connected initially with the acinus and then with other ducts as the ducts progressively grow larger from the inner to the outer parts of the salivary gland.

6. The _____ are smaller than the larger major salivary glands but are more numerous; they are innervated by the seventh cranial nerve, or the facial nerve.

7. The minor salivary glands are scattered in the tissue of the buccal, labial, and lingual mucosa, the soft palate, the lateral parts of the hard palate, and the _____.

8. The minor salivary glands, the _____, are specific glands that are associated with the base of the large circumvallate lingual papillae on the posterior part of the dorsal surface of the tongue; they flush out the trough surrounding each circumvallate lingual papillae with the saliva they produce.

9. Most minor salivary glands secrete a mainly _____ type of salivary product, because they have mainly mucous acini, with some serous secretion and serous acini present; however, the von Ebner glands secrete only a serous type of salivary product, because these glands have only serous acini.

10. The minor salivary glands are also _____ like the major salivary glands, but their unnamed ducts are shorter than those of the major ones and open directly onto the mucosal surface.

exocrine glands	von Ebner glands	septum
floor of the mouth	mucous	ductal system
secretory cells	acinus	minor salivary glands
capsule		

References

Chapter 7, Glandular tissue. In Fehrenbach MJ, Herring SW: *Illustrated anatomy of the head and neck,* ed 4, St. Louis, 2012, Saunders; and Chapter 11, Head and neck structures. In Bath-Balogh M, Fehrenbach MJ: *Illustrated dental embryology, histology, and anatomy,* ed 3, St. Louis, 2011, Saunders.

FIGURE 7-4   Salivary glands: acini and ducts (microanatomic view)

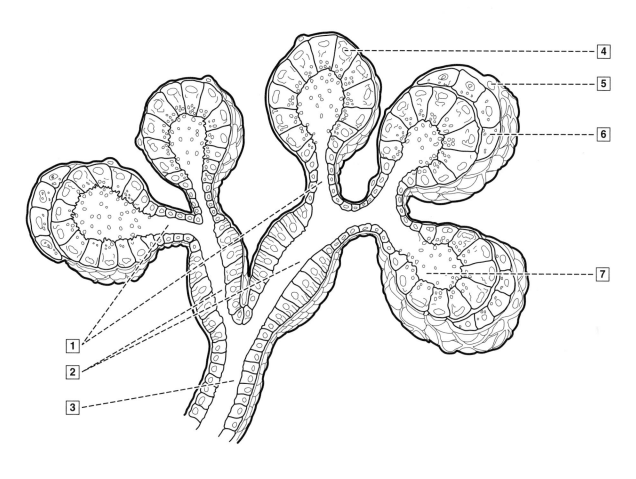

1 Intercalated ducts	**5** Myoepithelial cell
2 Striated ducts	**6** Serous demilune
3 Excretory duct	**7** Lumen of acinus
4 Mucous cell	

REVIEW QUESTIONS

Fill in the blanks by choosing the appropriate terms from the list below.

1. The two types of _____ of the salivary glands that compose the inner part of the glands are classified as either mucous or serous cells, depending on the type of secretion produced.

2. Each _____ of the salivary gland consists of a single layer of cuboidal epithelial cells surrounding a lumen, a central opening where the saliva is deposited after being produced by the secretory cells.

3. The _____ have a cloudier-looking cytoplasm and produce a mucous secretory product; the mucous acini are composed of these cells that produce a mucous secretory product and have wide lumens.

4. The _____ have a clear cytoplasm and produce a serous secretory product; the serous acini are composed of these cells that produce a serous secretory product and have narrow lumens.

5. The mucoserous acini have either a group of mucous cells surrounding the lumen and a(n) _____, or a group of serous cells located superficial to the group of mucous secretory cell layer.

6. To facilitate the flow of saliva out of each lumen of the salivary gland into the connecting ducts, _____ are located on the surface of some of the acini, as well as on parts of the ductal system, namely the intercalated ducts; each one consists of a cell body with four to eight cytoplasmic processes radiating outward.

7. The duct associated with an acinus or terminal part of the salivary gland is the _____, which is attached to the acinus and consists of a hollow tube lined with a single layer of cuboidal epithelial cells; many of these types of ducts are found in each lobule of the gland.

8. The larger _____ is a part of the ductal system that is connected to the intercalated ducts in the lobules of the salivary gland; it consists of a hollow tube lined with a single layer of columnar epithelial cells characterized by what appear to be *basal striations.*

9. The final part of the salivary gland ductal system is the large _____, which is located in the septum of the salivary gland and is the duct whereby saliva exits into the oral cavity; this duct consists of a hollow tube lined with a variety of epithelial cells.

10. The cells lining the excretory duct initially consist of _____, which then undergoes a transition to stratified cuboidal epithelium as the duct moves to the outer part of the salivary gland, and then becomes stratified squamous epithelium, blending with surrounding oral mucosa at the ductal opening.

striated duct	mucous cells	acinus
excretory duct	pseudostratified columnar epithelium	intercalated duct
myoepithelial cells	serous demilune	secretory cells
serous cells		

Reference

Chapter 11, Head and neck structures. In Bath-Balogh M, Fehrenbach MJ: *Illustrated dental embryology, histology, and anatomy,* ed 3, St. Louis, 2011, Saunders.

FIGURE 7-5 Major salivary glands: parotid gland (lateral view)

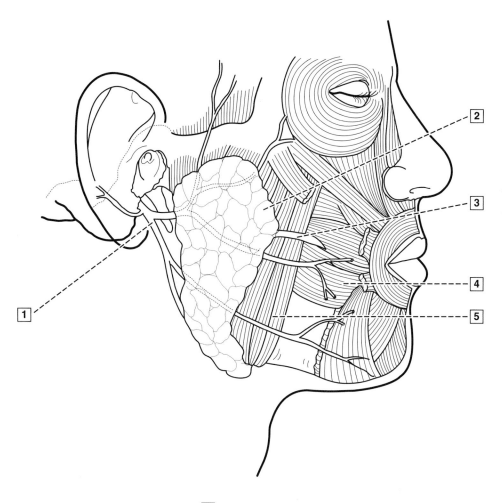

1 Facial nerve (VII)

2 Parotid gland

3 Parotid duct (Stenson duct)

4 Buccinator muscle

5 Masseter muscle

REVIEW QUESTIONS

Fill in the blanks by choosing the appropriate terms from the list below.

1. The _____ is the largest encapsulated major salivary gland.

2. The salivary product from the parotid salivary gland is a mainly _____ type of secretion from mainly serous acini.

3. The parotid salivary gland is divided into _____ lobes: the superficial and the deep.

4. The parotid salivary gland occupies the _____, an area posterior to the mandibular ramus, as well as anterior and inferior to the ear.

5. The parotid salivary gland extends irregularly from the _____ to the angle of the mandible.

6. The named duct associated with the parotid salivary gland is the _____, or *Stensen duct*; the gland is associated with mainly long intercalated ducts and short striated ducts; the duct emerges from the anterior border of the parotid salivary gland, superficial to the masseter muscle, and then pierces the buccinator muscle, to open up into the oral cavity on the inner surface of the cheek, usually opposite the maxillary second molar.

7. The _____ is a small elevation of tissue that marks the opening of the parotid duct on the inner surface of the cheek.

8. The parotid salivary gland is innervated by the motor or efferent (parasympathetic) nerves of the _____ of the ninth cranial nerve, or glossopharyngeal nerve, as well as by the afferent nerves from the auriculotemporal branch of the fifth cranial nerve, or trigeminal nerve; however, the seventh cranial nerve, or facial nerve, and its branches travel through the gland between its superficial and deep lobes to serve as a divider but are not involved in its innervation.

9. The parotid salivary gland drains into the _____ of the lymphatic system.

10. The parotid salivary gland is supplied by branches of the _____ of the vascular system.

otic ganglion	parotid fascial space	external carotid artery
parotid papilla	two	deep parotid lymph nodes
serous	parotid duct	zygomatic arch
parotid salivary gland		

References

Chapter 7, Glandular tissue. In Fehrenbach MJ, Herring SW: *Illustrated anatomy of the head and neck,* ed 4, St. Louis, 2012, Saunders; and Chapter 11, Head and neck structures. In Bath-Balogh M, Fehrenbach MJ: *Illustrated dental embryology, histology, and anatomy,* ed 3, St. Louis, 2011, Saunders.

ANSWER KEY 1. parotid salivary gland, 2. serous, 3. two, 4. parotid fascial space, 5. zygomatic arch, 6. parotid duct, 7. parotid papilla, 8. otic ganglion, 9. deep parotid lymph nodes, 10. external carotid artery.

FIGURE 7-6 Major salivary glands: submandibular gland (lateral view)

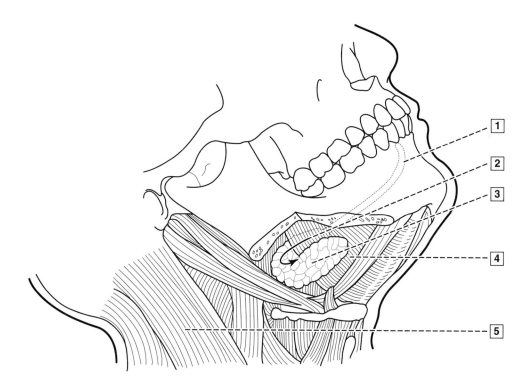

1 Submandibular duct (Wharton duct)

2 Deep lobe, submandibular gland

3 Superficial lobe, submandibular gland

4 Mylohyoid muscle

5 Sternocleidomastoid muscle

REVIEW QUESTIONS

Fill in the blanks by choosing the appropriate terms from the list below.

1. The _____ is the second largest encapsulated major salivary gland.

2. The saliva from the submandibular salivary gland is a(n) _____ salivary product that has both serous and mucous secretions from both serous and mucoserous acini; the gland also contains serous demilunes.

3. The submandibular salivary gland occupies the _____ in the submandibular fascial space, mainly in its posterior part.

4. Most of the submandibular salivary gland is a larger lobe superficial to the _____, but a smaller and deeper lobe wraps around the posterior border of the muscle.

5. The submandibular salivary gland is located _____ to the sublingual salivary gland.

6. The named duct associated with the submandibular salivary gland is the _____, or *Wharton duct*; the gland is associated with mainly short intercalated ducts and long striated ducts.

7. The submandibular duct arises from the deep lobe of the submandibular salivary gland and remains medial to the mylohyoid muscle; the duct then travels along the anterior floor of the mouth and opens into the oral cavity at the _____, a small papilla near the midline of the floor of the mouth on each side of the lingual frenum.

8. The submandibular salivary gland is innervated by the efferent (parasympathetic) fibers of the _____ and the submandibular ganglion of the seventh cranial nerve, or facial nerve.

9. The submandibular salivary gland drains into the _____ of the lymphatic system.

10. The submandibular salivary gland is supplied by branches of the _____ and lingual arteries.

facial	submandibular fossa	posterior
submandibular salivary gland	submandibular duct	submandibular lymph nodes
mixed	mylohyoid muscle	sublingual caruncle
chorda tympani		

References

Chapter 7, Glandular tissue. In Fehrenbach MJ, Herring SW: *Illustrated anatomy of the head and neck,* ed 4, St. Louis, 2012, Saunders; and Chapter 11, Head and neck structures. In Bath-Balogh M, Fehrenbach MJ: *Illustrated dental embryology, histology, and anatomy,* ed 3, St. Louis, 2011, Saunders.

FIGURE 7-7 Major salivary glands: sublingual gland (ventral and frontal aspects with internal views)

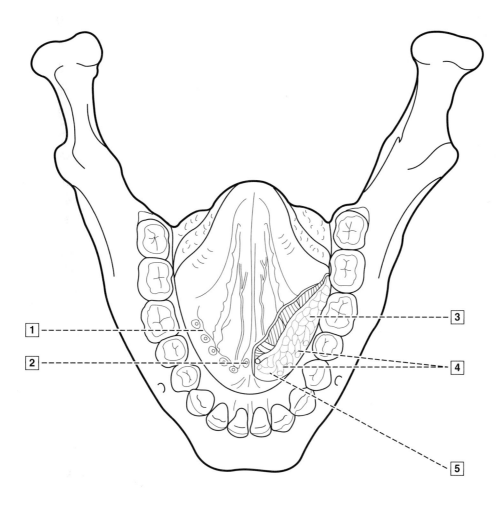

1   Sublingual fold

2   Sublingual caruncle

3   Sublingual gland

4   Sublingual ducts

5   Sublingual duct (Bartholin duct)

REVIEW QUESTIONS

Fill in the blanks by choosing the appropriate terms from the list below.

1. The _____ is the smallest, most diffuse, and only unencapsulated major salivary gland.

2. The saliva from the sublingual salivary gland is a(n) _____ salivary product, but with the mucous secretion predominating; the gland has mainly mucous acini with some mucoserous acini.

3. The sublingual salivary gland occupies the _____ in the sublingual fascial space at the floor of the mouth.

4. The sublingual salivary gland is located _____ to the mylohyoid muscle and medial to the body of the mandible.

5. The sublingual salivary gland is located _____ to the submandibular salivary gland.

6. The short named ducts associated with the sublingual gland in some cases combine to form the _____, or *Bartholin duct*; the gland is associated with mainly absent intercalated ducts and rare or absent striated ducts.

7. The sublingual duct opens directly into the oral cavity through the same opening as the _____, the sublingual caruncle; other small ducts of the gland open along the sublingual fold, a fold of tissue on each side of the floor of the mouth.

8. The sublingual salivary gland is innervated by the efferent (parasympathetic) fibers of the _____ and the submandibular ganglion of the seventh cranial nerve or facial nerve.

9. The sublingual salivary gland drains into the _____ of the lymphatic system.

10. The sublingual salivary gland is supplied by the _____ of the vascular system.

sublingual fossa	submandibular lymph nodes	sublingual salivary gland
anterior	submandibular duct	chorda tympani
sublingual duct	superior	sublingual artery
mixed		

References

Chapter 7, Glandular tissue. In Fehrenbach MJ, Herring SW: *Illustrated anatomy of the head and neck,* ed 4, St. Louis, 2012, Saunders; and Chapter 11, Head and neck structures. In Bath-Balogh M, Fehrenbach MJ: *Illustrated dental embryology, histology, and anatomy,* ed 3, St. Louis, 2011, Saunders.

FIGURE 7-8   Thyroid and parathyroid glands (anterior and posterior views)

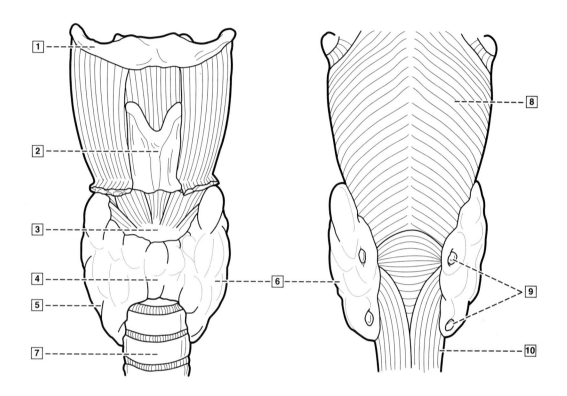

1	Hyoid bone	**6**	Left lobe of thyroid gland
2	Thyroid cartilage	**7**	Trachea
3	Cricoid cartilage	**8**	Interior pharyngeal constrictor muscle
4	Isthmus	**9**	Parathyroid glands
5	Right lobe of thyroid gland	**10**	Esophagus

REVIEW QUESTIONS

Fill in the blanks by choosing the appropriate terms from the list below.

1. The _____ is the largest endocrine gland; because it is ductless, the gland produces and secretes thyroxine directly into the vascular system to stimulate the metabolic rate.

2. The thyroid gland consists of two _____, right and left, connected anteriorly by an isthmus at the midline.

3. The thyroid gland is located in the anterior and lateral regions of the _____, inferior to the thyroid cartilage, at the junction between the larynx and trachea; the gland is encased in previsceral fascia, which is firmly adherent to the upper part of the trachea.

4. The thyroid gland is _____ when swallowing occurs because of its fascial encasement; when a person swallows, the gland moves superiorly, as does the whole larynx.

5. The thyroid gland is supplied by the _____ of the vascular system.

6. The parathyroid glands usually consist of _____ small endocrine glands, two on each side; because the glands are ductless, they produce and secrete parathyroid hormone directly into the vascular system to regulate calcium and phosphorus levels.

7. The parathyroid glands are usually adjacent to or within the thyroid gland on its

    _____.

8. Both the thyroid gland and parathyroid glands are innervated by _____ through the cervical ganglia.

9. Both the thyroid gland and parathyroid glands drain into the _____ of the lymphatic system.

10. The parathyroid glands are supplied primarily by the _____ of the vascular system.

thyroid gland	sympathetic nerves	lateral lobes
superior and inferior thyroid arteries	neck	inferior thyroid arteries
four	posterior surface	superior deep cervical lymph nodes
mobile		

Reference

Chapter 7, Glandular tissue. In Fehrenbach MJ, Herring SW: *Illustrated anatomy of the head and neck,* ed 4, St. Louis, 2012, Saunders; and Chapter 11, Head and neck structures. In Bath-Balogh M, Fehrenbach MJ: *Illustrated dental embryology, histology, and anatomy,* ed 3, St. Louis, 2011, Saunders.

ANSWER KEY 1. thyroid gland, 2. lateral lobes, 3. neck, 4. mobile, 5. superior and inferior thyroid arteries, 6. four, 7. posterior surface, 8. sympathetic nerves, 9. superior deep cervical lymph nodes, 10. inferior thyroid arteries.

FIGURE 7-9   Thyroid gland (microanatomic view)

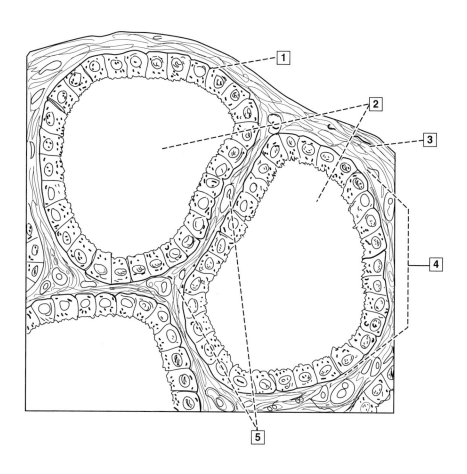

1 | Thyroid epithelium
2 | Colloid
3 | Capsule
4 | Follicle
5 | Septum

REVIEW QUESTIONS

Fill in the blanks by choosing the appropriate terms from the list below.

1. The thyroid gland is covered by an outer _____ composed of connective tissue that extends into the inner gland by way of septa.

2. Each _____ divides the inner thyroid gland into larger lobes and smaller lobules.

3. Each _____ is composed of follicles in the thyroid gland, irregularly shaped spheroidal masses that are embedded in a meshwork of reticular fibers.

4. Each _____ consists of a layer of simple cuboidal epithelium enclosing a cavity that is usually filled with colloid in the thyroid gland.

5. The _____ is a stiff material, which is reserved for the future production of thyroxine by the thyroid gland.

lobule	capsule
colloid	septum
follicle	

Reference

Chapter 11, Head and neck structures. In Bath-Balogh M, Fehrenbach MJ: *Illustrated dental embryology, histology, and anatomy,* ed 3, St. Louis, 2011, Saunders.

FIGURE 7-10   **Thyroid gland development**

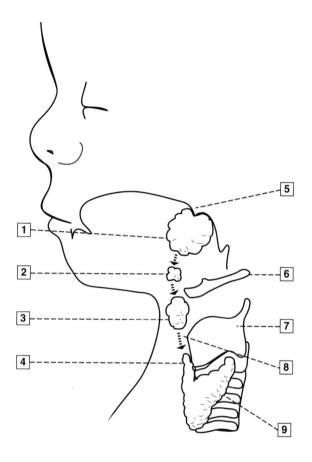

1	Lingual thyroid	**6**	Hyoid bone
2	Accessory thyroid tissue	**7**	Thyroid cartilage
3	Cervical thyroid	**8**	Tract of thyroglossal duct
4	Pyramidal thyroid	**9**	Normal position of thyroid
5	Foramen cecum		

REVIEW QUESTIONS

Fill in the blanks by choosing the appropriate terms from the list below.

1. The thyroid gland is the first _____ to appear in embryonic development, and it develops from endoderm invaded by mesenchyme.

2. At approximately the 24th day of _____, the thyroid gland develops.

3. The thyroid gland forms from a median downgrowth at the _____, connected by a thyroglossal duct, a narrow tube that later becomes obliterated.

4. The _____ shows the origin of the thyroid gland and the migration pathway of the thyroid gland into the neck region.

5. The _____, which is the opening of the thyroglossal duct associated with the development of the thyroid gland, is a small, pitlike depression located where the sulcus terminalis points backward toward the oropharynx.

endocrine gland	base of the tongue
thyroglossal duct	prenatal development
foramen cecum	

Reference

Chapter 11, Head and neck structures. In Bath-Balogh M, Fehrenbach MJ: *Illustrated dental embryology, histology, and anatomy,* ed 3, St. Louis, 2011, Saunders.

ANSWER KEY 1. endocrine gland, 2. prenatal development, 3. base of the tongue, 4. thyroglossal duct, 5. foramen cecum.

FIGURE 7-11 **Thymus gland (anterior view)**

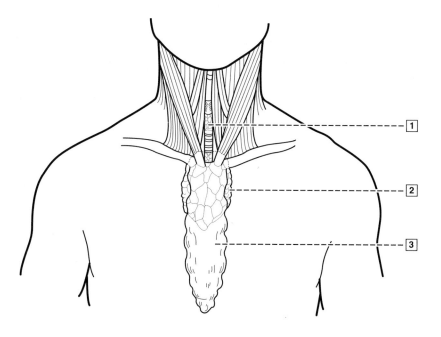

1 Thyroid gland

2 Thymus

3 Sternum

REVIEW QUESTIONS

Fill in the blanks by choosing the appropriate terms from the list below.

1. The thymus gland is a(n) _____ and therefore ductless; the gland is made of many lobules, with each lobule having an outer cortex and an inner medulla and separated by connective tissue septa.

2. The thymus gland is part of the _____ that fights disease processes; within the gland the T-cell lymphocytes, white blood cells of the immune system, mature in the gland in response to stimulation by thymus hormones.

3. The gland grows from birth to puberty while performing this task; after puberty the thymus gland stops growing and starts to shrink, undergoing thymic _____ through the process of atrophy.

4. In adulthood the thymus gland has almost _____ and returned to its low birth weight, making it mainly a temporary structure.

5. The adult thymus gland consists of two _____, right and left, connected by an isthmus at the midline.

6. The thymus gland is located in the thorax and the anterior region of the base of the neck, _____ to the thyroid gland.

7. The thymus gland is _____ and lateral to the trachea and deep to the sternum and the sternohyoid and sternothyroid muscles, as well as anterior to the heart.

8. The thymus gland is innervated by branches of the tenth cranial nerve, or the _____, as well as the cervical nerves.

9. The lymphatic system of the thymus gland arises within the substance of the gland and terminates in the _____.

10. The thymus gland is supplied by the _____ and the internal thoracic artery.

immune system	involution	disappeared
superficial	vagus nerve	endocrine gland
inferior thyroid artery	inferior	internal jugular vein
lateral lobes		

Reference

Chapter 7, Glandular tissue. In Fehrenbach MJ, Herring SW: *Illustrated anatomy of the head and neck,* ed 4, St. Louis, 2012, Saunders.

ANSWER KEY 1. endocrine gland, 2. immune system, 3. involution, 4. disappeared, 5. lateral lobes, 6. inferior, 7. superficial, 8. vagus nerve, 9. internal jugular vein, 10. inferior thyroid artery.

FIGURE 8-1 Brain (ventral view)

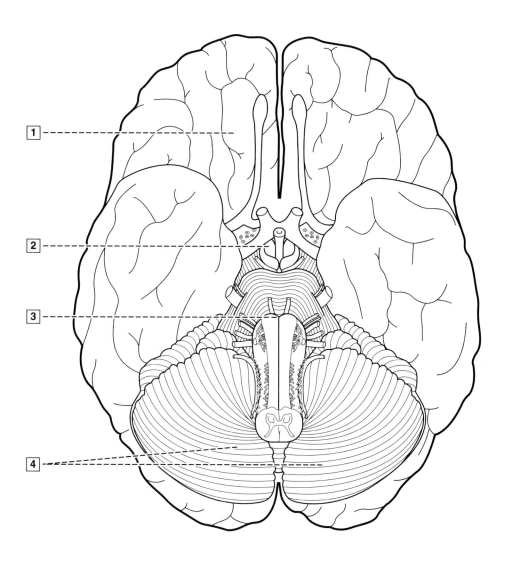

1	Cerebral hemisphere
2	Diencephalon
3	Brainstem
4	Cerebellum

REVIEW QUESTIONS

Fill in the blanks by choosing the appropriate terms from the list below.

1. The _____ is an extensive, intricate network of neural structures that activates, coordinates, and controls all functions of the body; it has two main divisions: the central and the peripheral nervous systems.

2. One of the major divisions of the nervous system, the _____ includes both the brain and spinal cord.

3. The central nervous system is surrounded by bone, either the skull or vertebrae, and a system of membranes containing _____, a protective nourishing fluid that circulates around the brain and spinal cord of the central nervous system.

4. Both the bones of the skull and vertebrae and the system of membranes serve to _____ the central nervous system.

5. The major divisions of the _____ of the central nervous system include the cerebrum, the cerebellum, the brainstem, and the diencephalon.

6. The _____ is the largest division of the brain.

7. The cerebrum of the brain consists of two _____.

8. The cerebrum of the brain _____ sensory data and motor functions and governs many aspects of intelligence and reasoning, learning, and memory.

9. The _____ is the second largest division of the brain, after the cerebrum.

10. The cerebellum of the brain functions to _____ muscle coordination and maintains normal muscle tone and posture, as well as coordinating balance.

brain	cerebellum	cerebrum
produce	protect	coordinates
central nervous system	cerebrospinal fluid	cerebral hemispheres
nervous system		

Reference

Chapter 8, Nervous system. In Fehrenbach MJ, Herring SW: *Illustrated anatomy of the head and neck,* ed 4, St. Louis, 2012, Saunders.

FIGURE 8-2 Brain and spinal cord (lateral sagittal view)

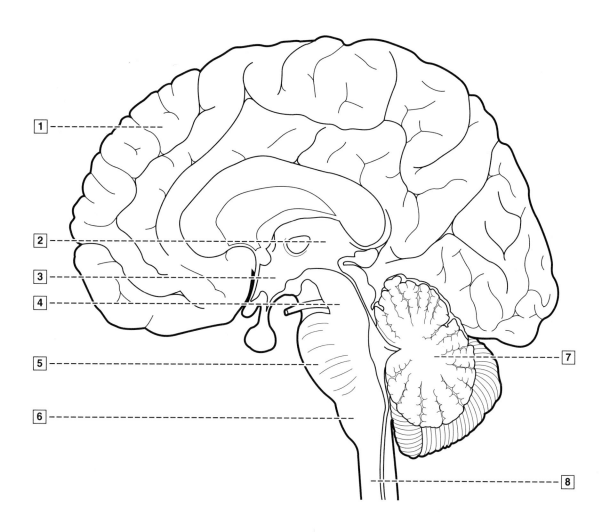

1	**CEREBRAL HEMISPHERE**	**BRAINSTEM**	7	**CEREBELLUM**
	DIENCEPHALON	4 Midbrain	8	**SPINAL CORD**
2	Thalamus	5 Pons		
3	Hypothalamus	6 Medulla		

REVIEW QUESTIONS

Fill in the blanks by choosing the appropriate terms from the list below.

1. The _____ of the brain has a number of divisions including the medulla, pons, and midbrain.

2. The _____ of the brainstem is closest to the spinal cord and is involved with the regulation of heartbeat, breathing, vasoconstriction (blood pressure), and reflex centers for vomiting, coughing, sneezing, swallowing, and hiccupping; the cell bodies of the motor neurons for the tongue are located there.

3. The _____ of the brainstem connects the medulla with the cerebellum and with higher brain centers; the cell bodies for fifth (trigeminal) and seventh (facial) cranial nerves are found there.

4. The _____ of the brainstem includes relay stations for hearing, vision, and motor pathways.

5. Superior to the brainstem, the _____ of the brain primarily includes the thalamus and hypothalamus.

6. The _____ of the diencephalon serves as a central relay point for incoming nerve impulses.

7. The _____ of the diencephalon regulates homeostasis; it has regulatory areas for thirst, hunger, body temperature, water balance, and blood pressure, linking the nervous system to the endocrine system.

8. The other component of the central nervous system besides the brain, the _____, runs along the dorsal side of the body and links the brain to the rest of the body; it is composed of two types of brain substance, gray matter and white matter, and in adults is encased in a series of bony vertebrae that make up the vertebral column.

9. The inner _____ of the spinal cord consists mostly of unmyelinized cell bodies and dendrites, with the surrounding white matter made up of tracts of axons, insulated in sheaths of myelin and formed from a combination of lipids and proteins.

10. Some tracts of axons in the white matter of the spinal cord are _____, because they carry messages to the brain, and others are descending, because they carry messages from the brain; the spinal cord is also involved in reflexes that do not immediately involve the brain.

pons	hypothalamus	midbrain
diencephalon	ascending	medulla
gray matter	brainstem	thalamus
spinal cord		

Reference

Chapter 8, Nervous system. In Fehrenbach MJ, Herring SW: *Illustrated anatomy of the head and neck,* ed 4, St. Louis, 2012, Saunders.

FIGURE 8-3   Meninges with associated structures (sagittal section)

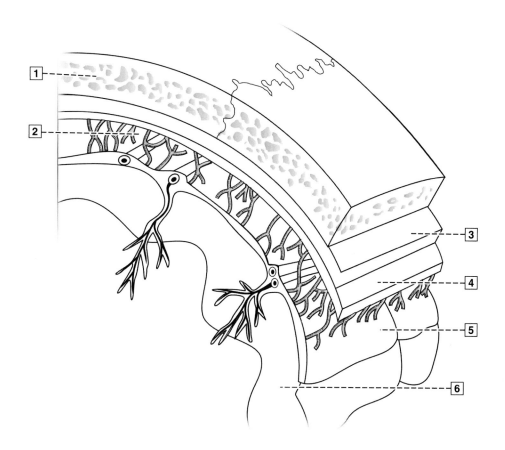

1 Skull
2 Subarachnoid space
3 Dura mater
4 Arachnoid
5 Pia mater
6 Cerebral cortex

REVIEW QUESTIONS

Fill in the blanks by choosing the appropriate terms from the list below.

1. The central nervous system is surrounded by bone, either the skull or vertebrae, and a system of _____; all of these structures serve to protect it.

2. The system of membranes surrounding the central nervous system is the _____.

3. The meninges contains the _____, a protective nourishing fluid that circulates around the brain and spinal cord of the central nervous system.

4. The meninges of the central nervous system has _____ layers: dura mater, arachnoid mater, and pia mater.

5. The tough outer layer of the meninges, the _____, surrounds and supports the brain and spinal cord of the central nervous system as well as lining the inner surface of the skull.

6. The delicate middle layer of the meninges is the _____; it lines, but is not adherent to, the inner surface of the dura mater.

7. From the inner surface of arachnoid matter of the meninges, thin processes, or _____, extend downward, crossing the subarachnoid space, and becoming continuous with the pia mater.

8. The inner layer of the meninges that is firmly attached to the surface of the brain is the _____; it closely invests the surface of the brain.

9. The pia matter of the meninges follows the contours of the brain, entering the grooves and fissures on its surface, and is closely applied to the roots of the _____ at their origins.

10. The dura mater of the meninges also surrounds and supports the large _____, or dural sinuses, carrying blood from the brain toward the heart.

cranial nerves	dura mater	meninges
pia mater	membranes	three
venous channels	arachnoid mater	cerebrospinal fluid
trabeculae		

References

Chapter 8, Nervous system. In Fehrenbach MJ, Herring SW: *Illustrated anatomy of the head and neck,* ed 4, St. Louis, 2012, Saunders; and Chapter 8, Head and neck. In Drake R, Vogl AW, Mitchell AWM: *Gray's anatomy for students,* ed 2, Philadelphia, 2010, Churchill Livingstone.

FIGURE 8-4 Brain and cranial nerves (ventral surface showing nerve attachment)

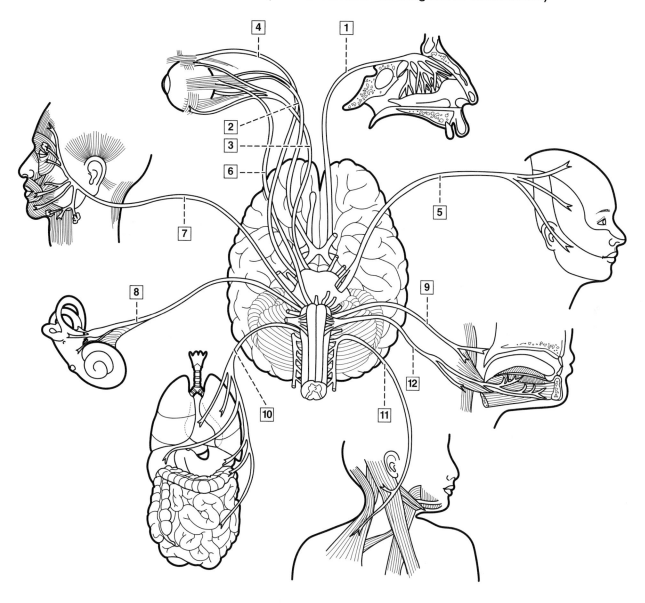

1 Olfactory nerve (I)	**7** Facial nerve (VII)
2 Optic nerve (II)	**8** Vestibulocochlear nerve (VIII)
3 Oculomotor nerve (III)	**9** Glossopharyngeal nerve (IX)
4 Trochlear nerve (IV)	**10** Vagus nerve (X)
5 Trigeminal nerve (V)	**11** Accessory nerve (XI)
6 Abducens nerve (VI)	**12** Hypoglossal nerve (XII)

REVIEW QUESTIONS

Fill in the blanks by choosing the appropriate terms from the list below.

1. The _____ are an important part of the peripheral nervous system; all twelve pairs are connected to the brain at its base and pass through the skull by way of fissures or foramina.

2. The first cranial nerve (I), or _____, transmits smell from the nasal mucosa to the brain and thus functions as an afferent nerve; the nerve enters the skull through the perforations in the cribriform plate of the ethmoid bone to join the olfactory bulb in the brain.

3. The second cranial nerve (II), or _____, transmits sight from the retina of the eye to the brain and thus functions as an afferent nerve; the nerve enters the skull through the optic canal of the sphenoid bone on its way from the retina.

4. In the skull, both the right and left optic nerves join at the _____, where many of the fibers cross to the contralateral side before continuing into the brain as the optic tracts.

5. The third cranial nerve (III), or _____, serves as an efferent nerve to some of the eye muscles that move the eyeball; the nerve also carries preganglionic parasympathetic fibers to the ciliary ganglion near the eyeball, and the postganglionic fibers innervate small muscles inside the eyeball.

6. The oculomotor nerve lies in the lateral wall of the cavernous sinus and exits the skull through the superior orbital fissure of the _____ on its way to the orbit.

7. The small fourth cranial nerve (IV), or _____, serves as an efferent nerve for one eye muscle, as well as proprioception, similar to the oculomotor nerve but without any parasympathetic fibers.

8. Similar to the oculomotor nerve, the trochlear nerve runs in the lateral wall of the cavernous sinus and exits the skull through the _____ of the sphenoid bone on its way to the orbit.

9. The fifth cranial nerve (V), or _____, has both an efferent component for the muscles of mastication, as well as some other cranial muscles, and an afferent component for the teeth, tongue, and oral cavity, as well as most of the skin of the face and head; additionally it has no preganglionic parasympathetic fibers, although many postganglionic parasympathetic fibers travel along with its branches.

10. The trigeminal nerve is the largest cranial nerve and has two _____: sensory and motor.

trigeminal nerve	optic chiasma	olfactory nerve
cranial nerves	oculomotor nerve	superior orbital fissure
trochlear nerve	sphenoid bone	roots
optic nerve		

Reference

Chapter 8, Nervous system. In Fehrenbach MJ, Herring SW: *Illustrated anatomy of the head and neck,* ed 4, St. Louis, 2012, Saunders.

FIGURE 8-5 Cranial nerves and skull (internal view of the skull base)

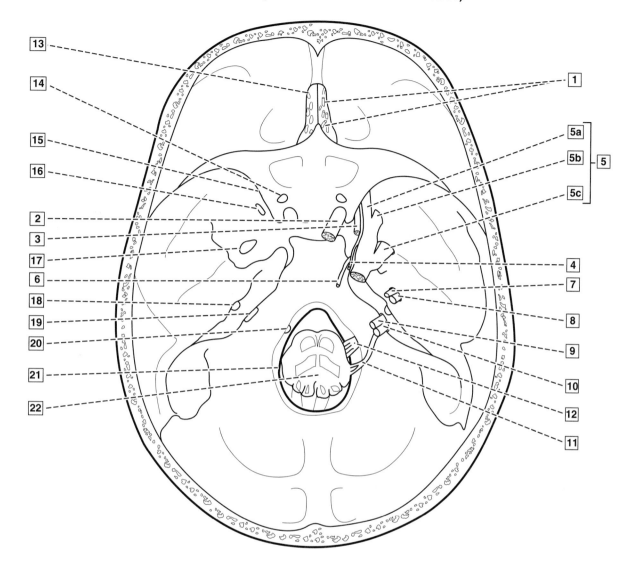

CRANIAL NERVES

1	Olfactory nerve (I)
2	Optic nerve (II)
3	Oculomotor nerve (III)
4	Trochlear nerve (IV)
5	**Trigeminal nerve (V)**
5a	Ophthalmic nerve
5b	Maxillary nerve
5c	Mandibular nerve

6	Abducens nerve (VI)
7	Facial nerve (VII)
8	Vestibulocochlear nerve (VIII)
9	Glossopharyngeal nerve (IX)
10	Vagus nerve (X)
11	Accessory nerve (XI)
12	Hypoglossal nerve (XII)

ASSOCIATED STRUCTURES

13	Cribriform plate
14	Optic canal
15	Superior orbital fissure
16	Foramen rotundum
17	Foramen ovale
18	Internal acoustic meatus
19	Jugular foramen
20	Hypoglossal canal
21	Foramen magnum
22	Spinal cord

REVIEW QUESTIONS

Fill in the blanks by choosing the appropriate terms from the list below.

1. The sixth cranial nerve (VI), or _____ or *abducent nerve,* serves as an efferent nerve to one of the muscles that moves the eyeball, similar to the oculomotor and trochlear nerves; similar to both of those cranial nerves, the nerve exits the skull through the superior orbital fissure of the sphenoid bone on its way to the orbit.

2. The seventh cranial nerve (VII), or _____, carries both efferent and afferent components; the nerve carries an efferent component for the muscles of facial expression and for the preganglionic parasympathetic innervation of the lacrimal gland (relaying in the pterygopalatine ganglion), as well as the submandibular and sublingual salivary glands (relaying in the submandibular ganglion).

3. The facial nerve leaves the cranial cavity by passing through the _____, which leads to the facial canal inside the temporal bone; finally, the nerve exits the skull by way of the stylomastoid foramen of the temporal bone.

4. The eighth cranial nerve (VIII), or _____, serves as an afferent nerve for hearing and balance, because it conveys signals from the inner ear of the temporal bone to the brain; it then enters the cranial cavity through the internal acoustic meatus of the temporal bone and then supplies the two major parts of the inner ear: the cochlea and semicircular canals.

5. The ninth cranial nerve (IX), or _____, carries an efferent component for the pharyngeal muscle, the stylopharyngeus muscle, and the preganglionic gland parasympathetic innervation for the parotid salivary gland (relaying the otic ganglion); the nerve also carries an afferent component for the oropharynx and for taste and general sensation from the base of the tongue, and thus is the afferent limb of the gag reflex.

6. The glossopharyngeal nerve passes through the skull by way of the _____ between the occipital and temporal bones; the tympanic branch, with sensory fibers for the middle ear and preganglionic parasympathetic fibers for the parotid gland, arises here and reenters the skull.

7. After supplying the ear, parasympathetic fibers of the glossopharyngeal nerve leave the skull through the _____ of the sphenoid bone as the lesser petrosal nerve; its preganglionic fibers then terminate in the otic ganglion, which is located near the medial surface of the mandibular nerve of the trigeminal nerve, just inferior to the foramen ovale, so as to supply the inferior branches of the nerve supply the carotid artery, oropharynx, and base of the tongue (afferent component), as well as the stylopharyngeus muscle.

8. The tenth cranial nerve (X), or _____, carries a large efferent component for the muscles of the soft palate, pharynx, and larynx and for parasympathetic fibers to many organs in the thorax and abdomen including the thymus gland, heart, and stomach; it also carries a smaller afferent component for a small amount of skin around the ear and for taste sensation for the epiglottis; the nerve passes through the skull by way of the jugular foramen, between the occipital and temporal bones.

9. The eleventh cranial nerve (XI), or _____, functions as an efferent nerve for the trapezius and sternocleidomastoid muscles, as well as for muscles of the soft palate and pharynx, and exits the skull through the jugular foramen between the occipital and temporal bones; the nerve is only partly a cranial nerve and consists of two roots, one from the brain and one from the spinal cord.

10. The twelfth cranial nerve (XII), or _____, functions as an efferent nerve for both the intrinsic and extrinsic muscles of the tongue; the nerve exits the skull through the hypoglossal canal in the occipital bone.

facial nerve	vagus nerve	accessory nerve
abducens nerve	glossopharyngeal nerve	internal acoustic meatus
hypoglossal nerve	vestibulocochlear nerve	jugular foramen
foramen ovale		

Reference

Chapter 8, Nervous system. In Fehrenbach MJ, Herring SW: *Illustrated anatomy of the head and neck,* ed 4, St. Louis, 2012, Saunders.

FIGURE 8-6 Cranial nerve supply to the oral cavity

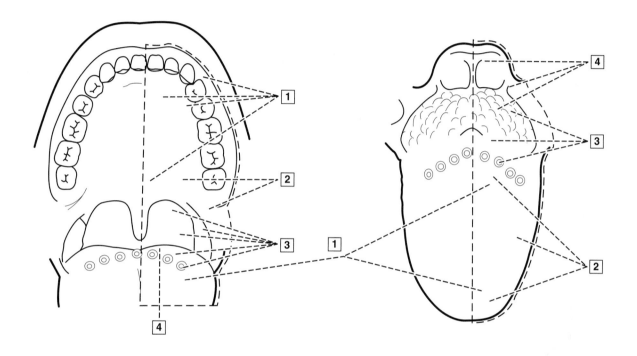

1 Trigeminal nerve (V)

2 Facial nerve (VII)

3 Glossopharyngeal nerve (IX)

4 Vagus nerve (X)

REVIEW QUESTIONS

Fill in the blanks by choosing the appropriate terms from the list below.

1. The fifth cranial nerve (V), or _____, has an afferent component for the teeth, tongue, and oral cavity.

2. The seventh cranial nerve (VII), or _____, carries an efferent component for the preganglionic parasympathetic innervation of both the submandibular and sublingual salivary glands (relaying in the submandibular ganglion) as well as the anterior two-thirds of the tongue.

3. The ninth cranial nerve (IX), or _____, carries an efferent component for the preganglionic gland parasympathetic innervation for the parotid salivary gland (relaying the otic ganglion); the nerve also carries an afferent component for the oropharynx and for taste by way of the circumvallate lingual papillae and general sensation from the base of the tongue and thus is the afferent limb of the gag reflex.

4. The _____ of the glossopharyngeal nerve has preganglionic parasympathetic fibers for the parotid salivary gland.

5. The tenth cranial nerve (X), or _____, carries a large efferent component for the muscles of the soft palate.

glossopharyngeal nerve   **trigeminal nerve**

vagus nerve   **tympanic branch**

facial nerve

Reference

Chapter 8, Nervous system. In Fehrenbach MJ, Herring SW: *Illustrated anatomy of the head and neck,* ed 4, St. Louis, 2012, Saunders.

FIGURE 8-7 Trigeminal nerve (V): ganglion and divisions (lateral view)

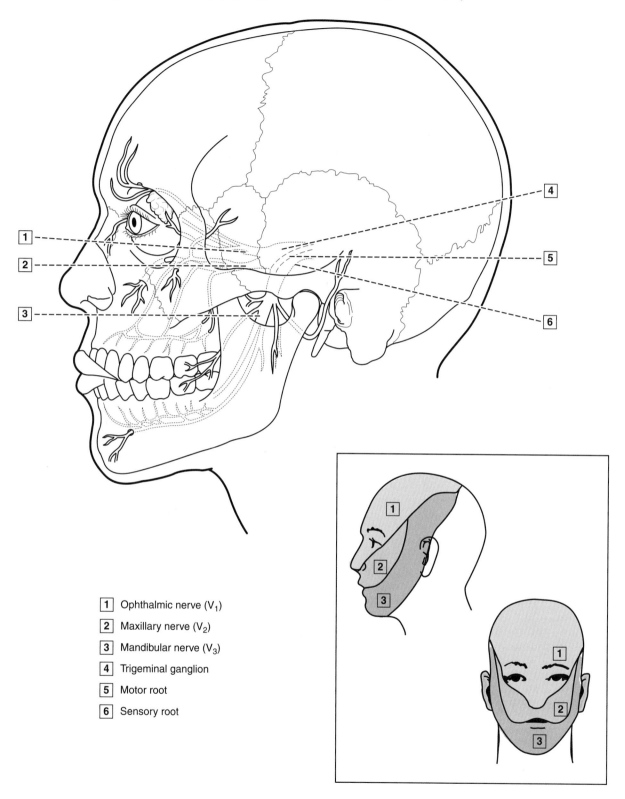

1 Ophthalmic nerve (V₁)

2 Maxillary nerve (V₂)

3 Mandibular nerve (V₃)

4 Trigeminal ganglion

5 Motor root

6 Sensory root

REVIEW QUESTIONS

Fill in the blanks by choosing the appropriate terms from the list below.

1. Within the skull, a bulge can be noted in the sensory root of the trigeminal nerve; the bulge is the _____, which is located on the anterior surface of the petrous part of the temporal bone.

2. Anterior to the trigeminal ganglion, the _____ arises from three nerves or divisions.

3. The sensory root's three nerves, or _____, include the ophthalmic, maxillary, and mandibular nerves.

4. The _____ of the sensory root provides sensation to the upper face and scalp.

5. The _____ of the sensory root provides sensation to the middle face and its deeper regions such as the oral cavity.

6. The _____ of the sensory root provides sensation to the lower face and its deeper regions such as the oral cavity.

7. The ophthalmic nerve and maxillary nerve of the sensory root carry only _____.

8. In contrast, the mandibular nerve of the sensory root runs together with the motor root and thus carries both afferent nerves and _____.

9. Each of the three nerves of the thicker sensory root of the trigeminal nerve enters the skull in one of three different locations in the _____: the ophthalmic nerve enters through the superior orbital fissure; the maxillary nerve enters by way of the foramen rotundum; and the mandibular nerve passes through the skull by way of the foramen ovale.

10. The thinner _____ of the trigeminal nerve exits the skull through the foramen ovale of the sphenoid bone and then travels with the mandibular nerve of the sensory root of the trigeminal nerve to supply the efferent nerves for the muscles of mastication.

afferent nerves	sphenoid bone	efferent nerves
trigeminal ganglion	sensory root	maxillary nerve
motor root	divisions	ophthalmic nerve
mandibular nerve		

Reference

Chapter 8, Nervous system. In Fehrenbach MJ, Herring SW: *Illustrated anatomy of the head and neck,* ed 4, St. Louis, 2012, Saunders.

FIGURE 8-8 Trigeminal nerve (V): ophthalmic (V₁) (lateral cutaway view)

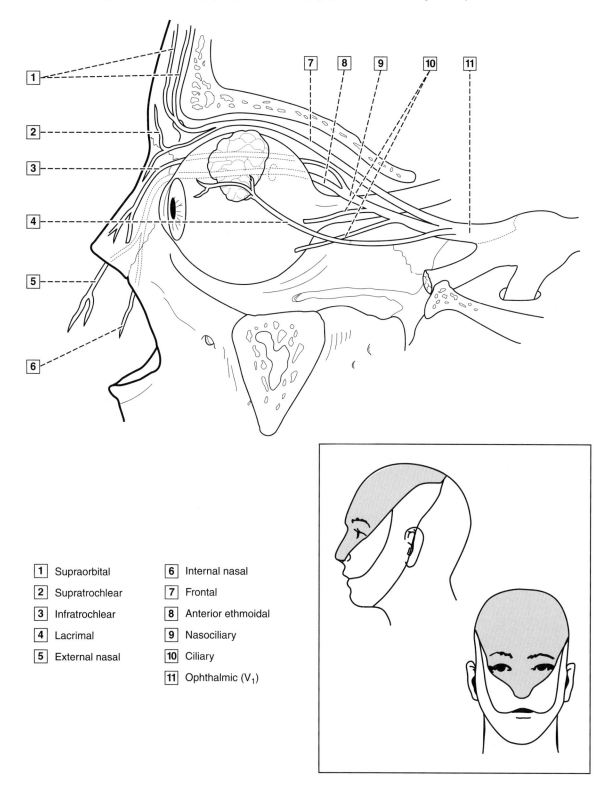

1 Supraorbital		**6** Internal nasal	
2 Supratrochlear		**7** Frontal	
3 Infratrochlear		**8** Anterior ethmoidal	
4 Lacrimal		**9** Nasociliary	
5 External nasal		**10** Ciliary	
		11 Ophthalmic (V₁)	

REVIEW QUESTIONS

Fill in the blanks by choosing the appropriate terms from the list below.

1. The first nerve division (V_1) of the sensory root of the trigeminal nerve is the _____.

2. The ophthalmic nerve is the smallest division of the _____ of the trigeminal nerve and serves as an afferent nerve for the conjunctiva, cornea, eyeball, orbit, forehead, and ethmoidal and frontal sinuses, plus a part of the dura mater.

3. The ophthalmic nerve carries sensory information toward the brain by way of the _____ of the sphenoid bone; other nerves that traverse this passageway include the third, fourth, and sixth cranial nerves.

4. The ophthalmic nerve arises from _____ major nerves: the frontal, lacrimal, and nasociliary nerves.

5. The _____ is an afferent nerve located in the orbit and is composed of a merger of the supraorbital nerve from the forehead and anterior scalp and the supratrochlear nerve from the bridge of the nose and medial parts of the upper eyelid and forehead.

6. The frontal nerve courses along the roof of the _____ toward the superior orbital fissure of the sphenoid bone where it is joined by the lacrimal and nasociliary nerves to form V_1.

7. The _____ serves as an afferent nerve for the lateral part of the upper eyelid, conjunctiva, and lacrimal gland, as well as delivering postganglionic parasympathetic nerves to the lacrimal gland, because the nerve is also responsible for the production of lacrimal fluid, or *tears*.

8. The lacrimal nerve runs posteriorly along the lateral roof of the orbit and then joins the frontal and nasociliary nerves near the superior orbital fissure of the _____ to form V_1.

9. Several afferent nerve branches converge to form the _____, including the infratrochlear nerve from the skin of the medial part of the eyelids and the side of the nose, ciliary nerves to and from the eyeball, and anterior ethmoidal nerve from the nasal cavity and paranasal sinuses; in contrast, the anterior ethmoidal nerve is formed by the external nasal nerve from the skin of the ala and apex of the nose and the internal nasal nerves from the anterior part of the nasal septum and lateral wall of the nasal cavity.

10. The nasociliary nerve is a(n) _____ that runs within the orbit, superior to the second cranial nerve or optic nerve, to join the frontal and lacrimal nerves near the superior orbital fissure of the sphenoid bone to form V_1.

lacrimal nerve	nasociliary nerve	ophthalmic nerve
sphenoid bone	superior orbital fissure	sensory root
frontal nerve	orbit	afferent nerve
three		

Reference

Chapter 8, Nervous system. In Fehrenbach MJ, Herring SW: *Illustrated anatomy of the head and neck,* ed 4, St. Louis, 2012, Saunders.

FIGURE 8-9 Trigeminal nerve (V): maxillary (V$_2$) (lateral view)

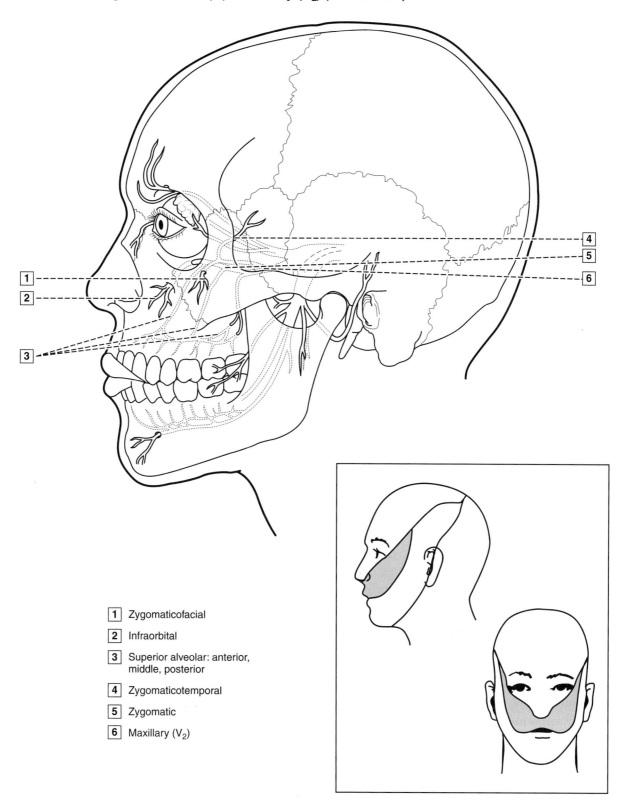

1 Zygomaticofacial

2 Infraorbital

3 Superior alveolar: anterior,
   middle, posterior

4 Zygomaticotemporal

5 Zygomatic

6 Maxillary (V$_2$)

REVIEW QUESTIONS

Fill in the blanks by choosing the appropriate terms from the list below.

1. The second nerve division (V_2) from the sensory root of the trigeminal nerve is the _____; the afferent nerve branches of the nerve carry sensory information for the maxillae and overlying skin, maxillary sinuses, nasal cavity, palate, nasopharynx, and part of the dura mater.

2. The maxillary nerve is a nerve trunk formed in the _____ by the convergence of many nerves; the largest contributor is the infraorbital nerve.

3. Tributaries of the infraorbital or maxillary nerve trunk include the zygomatic, the anterior, middle, and posterior superior alveolar, the greater and lesser palatine, and the nasopalatine nerves; after all these branches come together in the pterygopalatine fossa to form the maxillary nerve, the nerve enters the skull through the _____ of the sphenoid bone.

4. The _____ is an afferent nerve composed of the merger of the zygomaticofacial nerve and the zygomaticotemporal nerve in the orbit nerve and also conveys the postganglionic parasympathetic fibers for the lacrimal gland to the lacrimal nerve; later, the nerve courses posteriorly along the lateral orbit floor and enters the pterygopalatine fossa through the inferior orbital fissure between the sphenoid bone and maxilla to finally join V_2.

5. The small _____ serves as an afferent nerve for the skin of the cheek as the nerve pierces the frontal process of the zygomatic bone at the zygomaticofacial foramen and enters the orbit through its lateral wall; the nerve then turns posteriorly to join with the zygomaticotemporal nerve.

6. The _____ serves as an afferent nerve for the skin of the temporal region by piercing the temporal surface of the zygomatic bone at the zygomaticotemporal foramen; the nerve then traverses the lateral wall of the orbit to join the zygomaticofacial nerve, forming the zygomatic nerve.

7. The _____ is an afferent nerve formed from the merger of cutaneous branches from the upper lip, the medial part of the cheek, the lower eyelid, and the side of the nose.

8. The infraorbital nerve then passes into the infraorbital foramen of the maxilla to travel posteriorly through the infraorbital canal, along with the infraorbital blood vessels where it is joined by the _____.

9. From the infraorbital canal and groove, the infraorbital nerve passes into the pterygopalatine fossa through the inferior orbital fissure and after it leaves the infraorbital groove and within the pterygopalatine fossa, the infraorbital nerve receives the _____; this latter nerve originates from dental branches of the maxillary molar teeth.

10. The anterior superior alveolar nerve originates from dental branches of the maxillary anterior teeth and then ascends along the anterior wall of the maxillary sinus to join the infraorbital nerve within the infraorbital canal, along with the _____ that serves the maxillary premolar teeth through its dental branches, if present.

posterior superior alveolar nerve

infraorbital nerve

zygomatic nerve

anterior superior alveolar nerve

pterygopalatine fossa

zygomaticofacial nerve

foramen rotundum

maxillary nerve

zygomaticotemporal nerve

middle superior alveolar nerve

Reference

Chapter 8, Nervous system. In Fehrenbach MJ, Herring SW: *Illustrated anatomy of the head and neck,* ed 4, St. Louis, 2012, Saunders.

FIGURE 8-10   Maxillary nerve (V₂): major branches (lateral view)

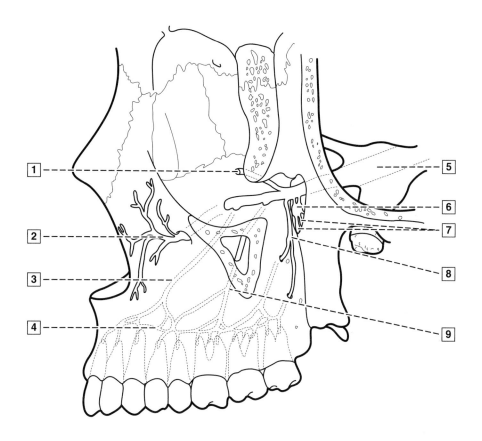

1 Zygomatic		**6** Pterygopalatine ganglion	
2 Infraorbital		**7** Greater and lesser palatine	
3 Anterior superior alveolar		**8** Posterior superior alveolar	
4 Dental plexus		**9** Middle superior alveolar	
5 Maxillary (V₂)			

373

REVIEW QUESTIONS

Fill in the blanks by choosing the appropriate terms from the list below.

1. The _____ serves as an afferent nerve of sensation (including pain) for the maxillary central incisors, lateral incisors, and canine, as well as their associated tissue.

2. The anterior superior alveolar nerve originates from dental branches in the pulp of the maxillary anterior teeth, which exit through the apical foramina; this nerve also receives interdental branches from the surrounding periodontium and innervates the overlying facial gingiva, forming a(n) _____, or nerve network, in the maxilla for the region, which is an important landmark for the anterior superior alveolar nerve block.

3. The anterior superior alveolar nerve then ascends along the _____ of the maxillary sinus to join the infraorbital nerve within the infraorbital canal.

4. The _____ serves as an afferent nerve of sensation (including pain), usually for the maxillary premolar teeth and mesiobuccal root of the maxillary first molar and their associated periodontium and overlying buccal gingiva, if present.

5. The middle superior alveolar nerve originates from dental branches in the pulp that exit the teeth it serves through the apical foramina, as well as interdental and interradicular branches from the periodontium if present; the nerve, like the posterior superior alveolar and anterior superior alveolar nerves, forms the dental plexus, or nerve network, in the _____, which are important landmarks for the middle superior alveolar nerve block.

6. The middle superior alveolar nerve then ascends to join the infraorbital nerve by running in the _____ of the maxillary sinus, if present; there is communication between the middle superior alveolar nerve and both the anterior superior alveolar nerve and posterior superior alveolar nerve.

7. The middle superior alveolar nerve is not always _____; and if that is what occurs, the area is innervated by both the anterior superior alveolar nerve and posterior superior alveolar nerve, but mainly by the anterior superior alveolar nerve.

8. The _____ joins the infraorbital nerve (or maxillary nerve directly in some cases) in the pterygopalatine fossa; then the nerve serves as an afferent nerve of sensation (including pain) for most parts of the maxillary molar teeth and their periodontium and buccal gingiva, as well as the maxillary sinus, because some afferent nerve branches of the nerve originate from dental branches in the pulp of each of the maxillary molar teeth that exit the teeth by way of the apical foramina, which are later then joined by interdental branches and interradicular branches from the periodontium to form a dental plexus or a nerve network in the maxilla for the region.

9. The internal branches of the posterior superior alveolar nerve exit from several _____ on the maxillary tuberosity of the maxilla, along with the posterior superior alveolar arteries (from the maxillary artery), which are important landmarks for the posterior superior alveolar nerve block; some branches of the nerve remain external to the posterior surface of the maxilla, which provide afferent innervation for the buccal gingiva that overlies the maxillary molars.

10. Both the external and internal branches of the posterior superior alveolar nerve move superiorly together along the maxillary tuberosity, which forms the _____ of the maxillary sinus, to join either the infraorbital nerve or maxillary nerve; the nerve usually provides afferent innervation for the maxillary second and third molars and the palatal and distal buccal root of the maxillary first molar, as well as the maxillary sinus mucous membranes.

present	maxilla	lateral wall
middle superior alveolar nerve	posterior superior alveolar foramina	posterior superior alveolar nerve
anterior wall	anterior superior alveolar nerve	posterolateral wall
dental plexus		

Reference

Chapter 8, Head and neck. In Drake R, Vogl AW, Mitchell AWM: *Gray's anatomy for students,* ed 2, Philadelphia, 2010, Churchill Livingstone.

FIGURE 8-11   Maxillary nerve (V₂): palatine branches (medial view of the nasal wall)

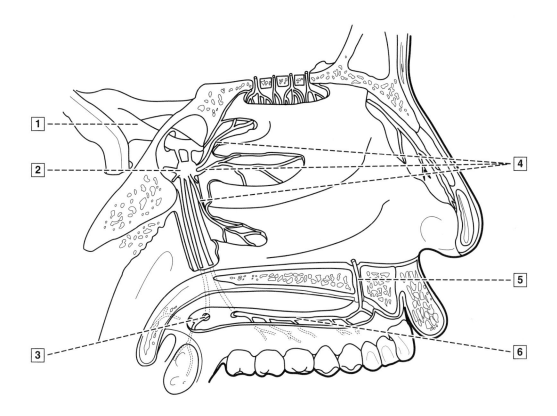

1	Maxillary (V₂)	**4**	Lateral nasal branches
2	Pterygopalatine ganglion	**5**	Nasopalatine (cut)
3	Lesser palatine	**6**	Greater palatine

REVIEW QUESTIONS

Fill in the blanks by choosing the appropriate terms from the list below.

1. Both palatine nerves join with the _____, or V$_2$, from the palate.

2. The _____, or *anterior palatine nerve,* is located between the mucoperiosteum and bone of the posterior hard palate; the nerve serves as an afferent nerve for the posterior hard palate and posterior lingual gingiva, with communication occurring with the terminal fibers of the nasopalatine nerve in the anterior hard palate, lingual to the maxillary canines.

3. Posteriorly, the greater palatine nerve enters the _____ in the horizontal plate of palatine bone near the maxillary second or third molar to travel within the pterygopalatine canal along with the greater palatine blood vessels, serving as important landmarks for the greater palatine nerve block.

4. The _____, or *posterior palatine nerve,* serves as an afferent nerve for the soft palate and palatine tonsils.

5. The lesser palatine nerve enters the _____ in the palatine bone near its junction with the pterygoid process of the sphenoid bone, along with the lesser palatine blood vessels; the lesser palatine nerve then joins the greater palatine nerve within the pterygopalatine canal.

6. Both palatine nerves move superiorly through the _____ toward the maxillary nerve in the pterygopalatine fossa; on the way the palatine nerves are joined by lateral nasal branches, which are afferent nerves from the posterior nasal cavity.

7. The _____ originates in the mucosa of the anterior hard palate, lingual to the maxillary central incisors.

8. Both the right and left nasopalatine nerves enter the _____ by way of the incisive foramen, deep to the incisive papilla, thus exiting the oral cavity, serving as important landmarks for the nasopalatine nerve block.

9. After traveling in the incisive canal upon entering by way of the _____, both nasopalatine nerves then travel along the nasal septum.

10. The nasopalatine nerve serves as an afferent nerve for the _____ and the lingual gingiva of the maxillary anterior teeth, as well as the nasal septal tissue; communication also occurs with the greater palatine nerve in the area that is located lingual to the maxillary canines.

greater palatine nerve	incisive foramen	lesser palatine nerve
lesser palatine foramen	anterior hard palate	greater palatine foramen
incisive canal	nasopalatine nerve	pterygopalatine canal
maxillary nerve		

Reference

Chapter 8, Nervous system. In Fehrenbach MJ, Herring SW: *Illustrated anatomy of the head and neck,* ed 4, St. Louis, 2012, Saunders.

FIGURE 8-12   Trigeminal nerve (V): mandibular (V₃) (lateral view)

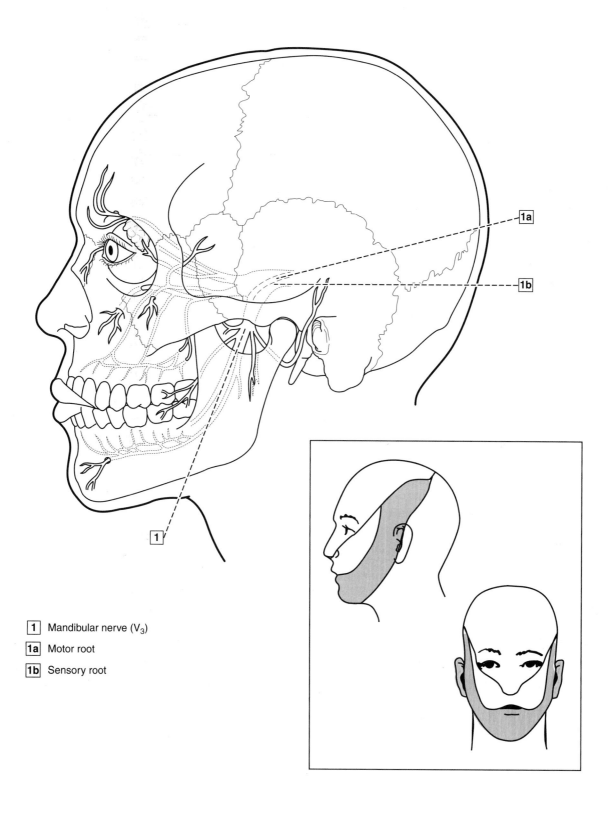

1	Mandibular nerve (V₃)
1a	Motor root
1b	Sensory root

REVIEW QUESTIONS

Fill in the blanks by choosing the appropriate terms from the list below.

1. The third nerve division (V₃) of the trigeminal nerve is the _____, which is a short main trunk formed by the merger of a smaller anterior trunk and a larger posterior trunk within the infratemporal fossa deep to the base of the skull before the nerve passes through the foramen ovale of the sphenoid bone; it is derived from both the sensory root and motor root of the cranial nerve.

2. The mandibular nerve then joins with the ophthalmic nerve and maxillary nerve to form the _____ of the trigeminal nerve.

3. The mandibular nerve is a(n) _____ nerve with both afferent nerves and efferent nerves and contains the entire efferent part of the trigeminal nerve.

4. A few small branches arise from the V₃ trunk before its separation into two _____: anterior and posterior; these branches from the undivided mandibular nerve include the meningeal branches, which are afferent nerves for parts of the dura mater.

5. Coming from the undivided mandibular nerve are the _____, which are efferent nerves for the medial pterygoid, tensor tympani, and tensor veli palatini muscles.

mixed	**mandibular nerve**
trigeminal ganglion	**trunks**
muscular branches	

Reference

Chapter 8, Nervous system. In Fehrenbach MJ, Herring SW: *Illustrated anatomy of the head and neck,* ed 4, St. Louis, 2012, Saunders.

FIGURE 8-13   Mandibular nerve (V₃): anterior trunk (lateral view)

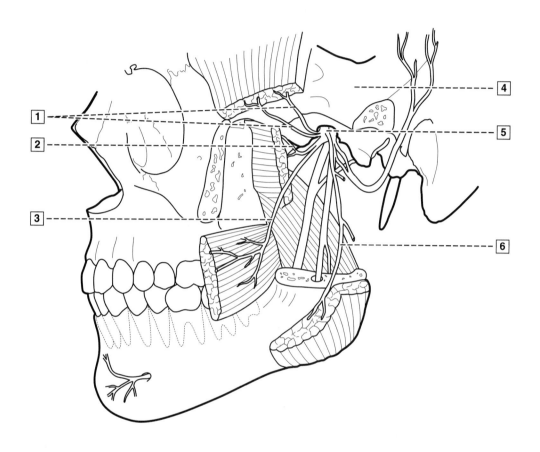

1 Anterior and posterior deep temporal
2 Lateral pterygoid
3 Buccal
4 Trigeminal ganglion location
5 Mandibular (V₃)
6 Masseteric

REVIEW QUESTIONS

Fill in the blanks by choosing the appropriate terms from the list below.

1. The _____, or anterior division of the mandibular nerve, is formed by the merger of the buccal nerve and additional nearby muscular nerve branches.

2. The anterior trunk of the mandibular nerve has both _____ and efferent nerves.

3. The _____, or *long buccal nerve,* serves as an afferent nerve for the skin of the cheek, buccal mucous membranes, and buccal gingiva of the mandibular posterior teeth.

4. The buccal nerve is located on the surface of the _____ and travels posteriorly in the cheek, deep to the masseter muscle.

5. At the level of the _____ of the most distal molar of the mandibular arch, the buccal nerve crosses anteriorly to the anterior border of the ramus and goes between the two heads of the lateral pterygoid muscle to join the anterior trunk of V_3, an important landmark for the buccal nerve block.

6. Several _____ are part of the anterior trunk of V_3; they arise from the motor root of the trigeminal nerve.

7. The _____, usually two, anterior and posterior, are efferent nerves that pass between the sphenoid bone and the superior border of the lateral pterygoid muscle and turn around the infratemporal crest of the sphenoid bone to terminate in the deep surface of the temporalis muscle that they innervate.

8. The _____ may arise in common with the masseteric nerve, and the anterior temporal nerve may be associated at its origin with the buccal nerve.

9. The _____ is an efferent nerve that passes between the sphenoid bone and the superior border of the lateral pterygoid muscle; the nerve then accompanies the masseteric blood vessels through the mandibular notch to innervate the masseter muscle.

10. A small sensory branch from the anterior trunk of the mandibular nerve also goes to the temporomandibular joint; the _____, after a short course, enters the deep surface of the lateral pterygoid muscle between the muscle's two heads of origin and serves as an efferent nerve for that muscle.

masseteric nerve	**muscular branches**	**afferent nerves**
buccal nerve	**posterior temporal nerve**	**buccinator muscle**
anterior trunk	**lateral pterygoid nerve**	**occlusal plane**
deep temporal nerves		

Reference

Chapter 8, Nervous system. In Fehrenbach MJ, Herring SW: *Illustrated anatomy of the head and neck,* ed 4, St. Louis, 2012, Saunders.

FIGURE 8-14 Mandibular nerve (V$_3$): anterior trunk (medial view)

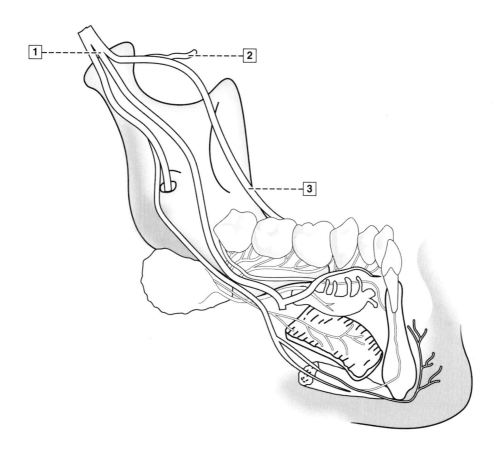

1   Mandibular nerve (V$_3$)

2   Anterior deep temporal nerve

3   Buccal nerve

REVIEW QUESTIONS

Fill in the blanks by choosing the appropriate terms from the list below.

1. The anterior trunk, or anterior division of the mandibular nerve, is formed by the merger of the _____ and additional nearby muscular nerve branches.

2. The anterior trunk of the mandibular nerve has both afferent nerves and _____.

3. The buccal nerve, or *long buccal nerve,* serves as a(n) _____ for the skin of the cheek, buccal mucous membranes, and buccal gingiva of the mandibular posterior teeth.

4. The buccal nerve is located on the surface of the buccinator muscle and travels posteriorly in the cheek, deep to the _____.

5. At the level of the occlusal plane of the most distal molar of the mandibular arch, the buccal nerve crosses anteriorly to the anterior border of the _____ and goes between the two heads of the lateral pterygoid muscle to join the anterior trunk of V$_3$, an important landmark for the buccal nerve block.

6. Several muscle branches are part of the anterior trunk of V$_3$; they arise from the _____ of the trigeminal nerve.

7. The deep temporal nerves, usually two, anterior and posterior, are efferent nerves that pass between the sphenoid bone and the superior border of the lateral pterygoid muscle and turn around the infratemporal crest of the sphenoid bone to terminate in the deep surface of the _____ that they innervate.

8. The posterior temporal nerve may arise in common with the masseteric nerve, and the _____ may be associated at its origin with the buccal nerve.

9. The masseteric nerve is an efferent nerve that passes between the sphenoid bone and the superior border of the lateral pterygoid muscle; the nerve then accompanies the masseteric blood vessels through the _____ to innervate the masseter muscle.

10. A small sensory branch from the anterior trunk of the mandibular nerve also goes to the temporomandibular joint; the lateral pterygoid nerve, after a short course, enters the deep surface of the _____ between the muscle's two heads of origin and serves as an efferent nerve for that muscle.

motor root	mandibular notch	masseter muscle
buccal nerve	ramus	anterior temporal nerve
efferent nerves	afferent nerve	lateral pterygoid muscle
temporalis muscle		

Reference

Chapter 8, Nervous system. In Fehrenbach MJ, Herring SW: *Illustrated anatomy of the head and neck,* ed 4, St. Louis, 2012, Saunders.

FIGURE 8-15 Mandibular nerve (V₃): posterior trunk (lateral view)

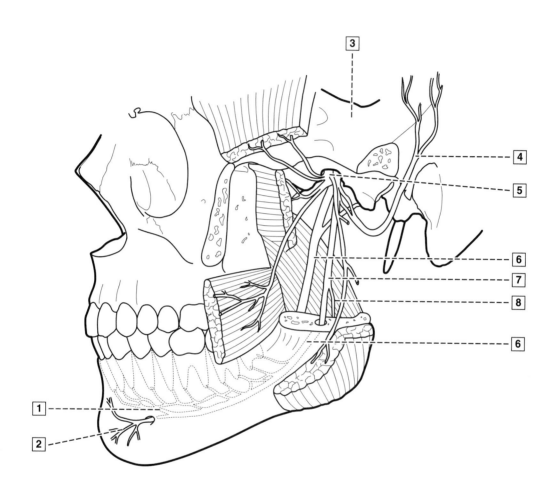

1 Incisive	**5** Mandibular (V₃)
2 Mental	**6** Lingual
3 Location of trigeminal ganglion	**7** Inferior alveolar
4 Auriculotemporal	**8** Mylohyoid

REVIEW QUESTIONS

Fill in the blanks by choosing the appropriate terms from the list below.

1. The merger of the auriculotemporal, lingual, and inferior alveolar nerves forms the _____, or posterior division of the mandibular nerve; the final nerve formed has both afferent nerves and efferent nerves.

2. The _____ travels with the superficial temporal artery and vein and serves as an afferent nerve for the external ear and scalp; the nerve also carries postganglionic parasympathetic nerve fibers to the parotid salivary gland.

3. Communication of the auriculotemporal nerve with the _____ near the ear occurs later; the auriculotemporal nerve courses deep to the lateral pterygoid muscle and neck of the mandible, then splits to encircle the middle meningeal artery, and finally joins the posterior trunk of V_3, an important landmark for the Gow-Gates mandibular nerve block.

4. The _____ is an afferent nerve formed from the merger of the mental and incisive nerves; after forming, the nerve continues to travel posteriorly through the mandibular canal, along with the inferior alveolar artery and vein; the nerve is then joined by dental branches such as both interdental and interradicular branches from the mandibular posterior teeth, forming a dental plexus, or nerve network, in the region.

5. The inferior alveolar nerve exits the mandible through the mandibular foramen after traveling the mandibular canal where it is joined by the _____; the mandibular foramen is an opening of the mandibular canal on the medial surface of the ramus, three fourths the distance from the coronoid notch to the posterior border of the ramus within the pterygomandibular space, an important landmark for the inferior alveolar nerve block.

6. The _____ is composed of external branches that serve as an afferent nerve for the chin, lower lip, and labial mucosa of the mandibular premolars and anterior teeth; the nerve then enters the mental foramen on the lateral surface of the mandible, usually between the apices of the mandibular first and second premolars, important landmarks for the mental nerve block, with the incisive nerve block administered at the same site with deeper anesthesia by using a more local anesthetic agent.

7. Either the inferior alveolar nerve block or Gow-Gates mandibular nerve block can be used to anesthetize the mental nerve along with other branches of the _____ from other target injection sites.

8. After entering via the mental foramen and traveling a distance within the mandibular canal, the mental nerve merges with the _____ to form the inferior alveolar nerve within the mandibular canal and before the newly formed nerve exits the canal.

9. The incisive nerve is an afferent nerve composed of dental branches from the mandibular premolar and anterior teeth that originate in the pulp, exit the teeth through the apical foramina, and join with interdental branches from the surrounding periodontium, forming a(n) _____ in the region.

10. The incisive nerve serves as an afferent nerve for the mandibular premolars and anterior teeth; the nerve then merges with the mental nerve just posterior to the mental foramen and goes on next to form the inferior alveolar nerve within the _____ before it exits.

inferior alveolar nerve	mandibular canal	dental plexus
posterior trunk	facial nerve	incisive nerve
auriculotemporal nerve	mandibular nerve	mental nerve
mylohyoid nerve		

Reference

Chapter 8, Nervous system. In Fehrenbach MJ, Herring SW: *Illustrated anatomy of the head and neck,* ed 4, St. Louis, 2012, Saunders.

FIGURE 8-16 Mandibular nerve (V₃): posterior trunk (medial view)

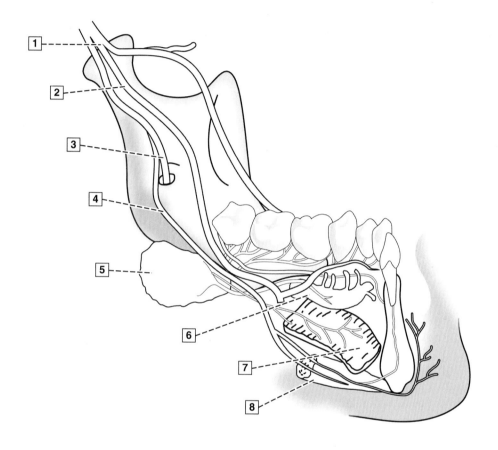

1	Mandibular nerve (V₃)	**5**	Submandibular salivary gland
2	Lingual nerve	**6**	Sublingual salivary gland
3	Inferior alveolar nerve	**7**	Mylohyoid muscle
4	Mylohyoid nerve	**8**	Anterior belly of digastric muscle

REVIEW QUESTIONS

Fill in the blanks by choosing the appropriate terms from the list below.

1. The _____ travels lateral to the medial pterygoid muscle, between the sphenomandibular ligament and ramus of the mandible; the nerve is posterior and slightly lateral to the lingual nerve and then joins the posterior trunk. It carries the afferent innervation for the mandibular teeth.

2. In some cases there are two nerves present on the one side, creating _____ inferior alveolar nerves; this situation can occur unilaterally or bilaterally and can be detected on a radiograph by the presence of a double mandibular canal.

3. The _____ is formed from afferent branches from the body of the tongue that travel along the lateral surface of the tongue; the nerve then passes posteriorly, passing from the medial to the lateral side of the duct of the submandibular salivary gland by going inferior to the duct.

4. The parasympathetic efferent innervation for the sublingual and submandibular salivary glands arises from the _____, more specifically, a branch of the nerve, the chorda tympani, but this nerve does travel along with the lingual nerve.

5. At the base of the tongue, the lingual nerve ascends and runs between the medial pterygoid muscle and the mandible, where it is positioned _____ and slightly medial to the inferior alveolar nerve; thus, the lingual nerve is also anesthetized when administering an inferior alveolar nerve block through diffusion of the local anesthetic agent.

6. The lingual nerve then continues to travel _____ to join the posterior trunk of V₃; the lingual nerve serves as an afferent nerve for general sensation for the body of the tongue, the floor of the mouth, and the lingual gingiva of the mandibular teeth.

7. After the inferior alveolar nerve exits the mandibular foramen, a small branch occurs, the _____.

8. The mylohyoid nerve pierces the sphenomandibular ligament and runs inferiorly and anteriorly in the mylohyoid groove and then onto the inferior surface of the _____, which it innervates.

9. The mylohyoid nerve serves as an efferent nerve to the mylohyoid muscle and _____ of the digastric muscle; however, the posterior belly of the digastric muscle is innervated by a branch from the facial nerve.

10. The mylohyoid nerve may in some cases also serve as an afferent nerve for the _____, which needs to be considered when the inferior alveolar nerve block fails; the mylohyoid nerve can then be anesthetized by local infiltration or by the Gow-Gates mandibular nerve block, which then also anesthetizes other branches of the mandibular nerve such as the inferior alveolar nerve, lingual nerve, and buccal nerve.

superiorly	**lingual nerve**	**inferior alveolar nerve**
mandibular first molar	**bifid**	**facial nerve**
anterior	**anterior belly**	**mylohyoid nerve**
mylohyoid muscle		

Reference

Chapter 8, Nervous system. In Fehrenbach MJ, Herring SW: *Illustrated anatomy of the head and neck,* ed 4, St. Louis, 2012, Saunders.

FIGURE 8-17 Mandibular nerve (V₃): motor and sensory branches (medial view)

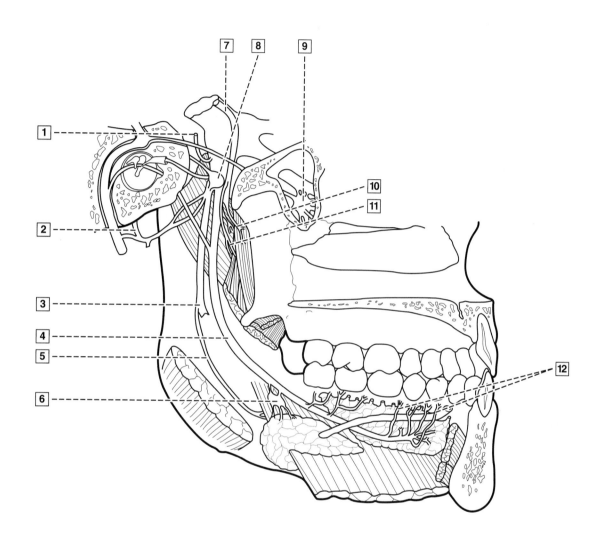

1 Middle meningeal		**7** Motor root of trigeminal nerve
2 Auriculotemporal		**8** Otic ganglion
3 Inferior alveolar		**9** Pterygopalatine ganglion
4 Lingual		**10** Nerve to tensor veli palatini muscle
5 Mylohyoid		**11** Nerve to medial pterygoid muscle
6 Submandibular ganglion		**12** Branches to tongue

REVIEW QUESTIONS

Fill in the blanks by choosing the appropriate terms from the list below.

1. The fifth cranial nerve (V), or _____, has both an efferent component for the muscles of mastication, as well as some other cranial muscles, and an afferent component for the teeth, tongue, and oral cavity, as well as most of the skin of the face and head; although the trigeminal nerve has no preganglionic parasympathetic fibers, many postganglionic parasympathetic fibers travel along with its branches.

2. The _____ (V_3) is the largest of the three nerve divisions that form the trigeminal nerve.

3. The mandibular nerve is derived from both the sensory and motor _____ of the cranial nerve; it has both afferent nerves and efferent nerves as well as containing the entire efferent part of the trigeminal nerve.

4. The _____ of the trigeminal nerve accompanies the mandibular nerve of the sensory root and also exits the skull through the foramen ovale of the sphenoid bone.

5. The mandibular nerve has a short main trunk formed by the merger of a smaller anterior and a larger posterior _____.

6. Coming from the undivided mandibular nerve are the _____, which are efferent nerves for the medial pterygoid, tensor tympani, and tensor veli palatini muscles.

7. The merger of the auriculotemporal, lingual, and inferior alveolar nerves forms the _____, or posterior division of the mandibular nerve; the final nerve formed has both afferent nerves and efferent nerves.

8. After the inferior alveolar nerve exits the mandibular foramen, a small branch occurs, the _____.

9. The seventh cranial nerve (VII), or _____, carries both efferent and afferent components; the nerve carries an efferent component for the preganglionic parasympathetic innervation of the lacrimal gland (relaying in the pterygopalatine ganglion) as well as the submandibular and sublingual salivary glands (relaying in the submandibular ganglion).

10. The ninth cranial nerve (IX), or _____, carries an efferent component for the pharyngeal muscle, the stylopharyngeus muscle, and the preganglionic gland parasympathetic innervation for the parotid salivary gland (relaying the otic ganglion).

mandibular nerve	**motor root**	**muscular branches**
posterior trunk	**facial nerve**	**trunk**
glossopharyngeal nerve	**mylohyoid nerve**	**trigeminal nerve**
roots		

Reference

Chapter 8, Nervous system. In Fehrenbach MJ, Herring SW: *Illustrated anatomy of the head and neck,* ed 4, St. Louis, 2012, Saunders.

ANSWER KEY   1. trigeminal nerve, 2. mandibular nerve, 3. roots, 4. motor root, 5. trunk, 6. muscular branches, 7. posterior trunk, 8. mylohyoid nerve, 9. facial nerve, 10. glossopharyngeal nerve.

FIGURE 8-18 Facial (VII) and trigeminal (V) nerves (medial view)

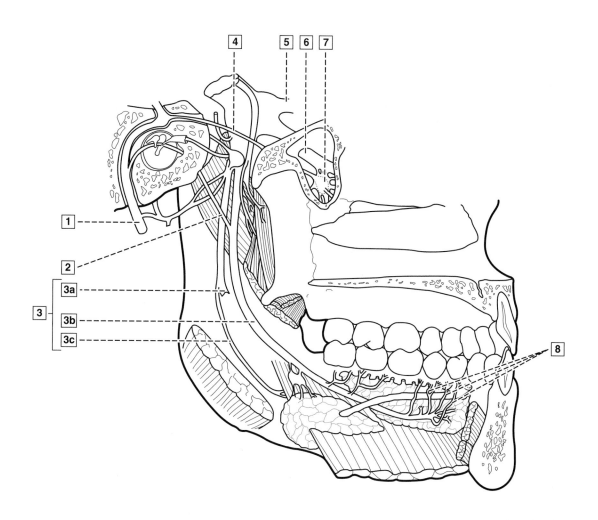

1 Facial (VII)	**4**	Greater petrosal
2 Chorda tympani	**5**	Ophthalmic (V₁)
3 **Mandibular nerve (V₃)**	**6**	Maxillary (V₂)
3a Inferior alveolar	**7**	Pterygopalatine ganglion
3b Lingual	**8**	Sensory fibers from tongue
3c Mylohyoid		

REVIEW QUESTIONS

Fill in the blanks by choosing the appropriate terms from the list below.

1. The seventh cranial nerve (VII), or _____, emerges from the brain and enters the internal acoustic meatus in the petrous part of the temporal bone. Within the bone, the nerve gives off a small efferent branch to the muscle in the middle ear (stapedius) and two larger branches, the greater petrosal and chorda tympani nerves, both of which carry parasympathetic fibers.

2. The main trunk of the facial nerve emerges from the skull through the _____ of the temporal bone and gives off two branches, the posterior auricular nerve and a branch to the posterior belly of the digastric and stylohyoid muscles.

3. The facial nerve then passes into the _____ and divides into numerous branches to supply the muscles of facial expression, but not the gland itself.

4. The _____ is a branch off the facial nerve before it exits the skull.

5. The greater petrosal nerve carries efferent nerve fibers: preganglionic parasympathetic fibers to the _____ in the pterygopalatine fossa.

6. The postganglionic fibers arising in the pterygopalatine ganglion from the greater petrosal nerve join with branches of the _____ (V_2) of the trigeminal nerve to be carried to the lacrimal gland (via the zygomatic and lacrimal nerves), nasal cavity, and minor salivary glands of the hard and soft palate; the greater petrosal nerve also carries afferent nerve fibers for taste sensation in the palate.

7. The _____ is a small branch of the facial nerve that is a parasympathetic efferent nerve for the submandibular and sublingual salivary glands and also serves as an afferent nerve for taste sensation for the body of the tongue.

8. After branching off the facial nerve within the petrous part of the temporal bone, the chorda tympani nerve crosses the medial surface of the tympanic membrane, or *eardrum*, and thereby exits the skull by the _____, located immediately posterior to the temporomandibular joint.

9. The chorda tympani nerve then travels with the _____ along the floor of the mouth in the same nerve bundle.

10. In the submandibular triangle, the chorda tympani nerve, appearing as part of the lingual nerve, has communication with the _____; the submandibular ganglion is located superior to the deep lobe of the submandibular salivary gland, for which it supplies parasympathetic efferent innervation.

petrotympanic fissure	parotid salivary gland	chorda tympani nerve
lingual nerve	submandibular ganglion	facial nerve
greater petrosal nerve	maxillary nerve	pterygopalatine ganglion
stylomastoid foramen		

Reference

Chapter 8, Nervous system. In Fehrenbach MJ, Herring SW: *Illustrated anatomy of the head and neck,* ed 4, St. Louis, 2012, Saunders.

FIGURE 8-19   Facial (VII) nerve (lateral view)

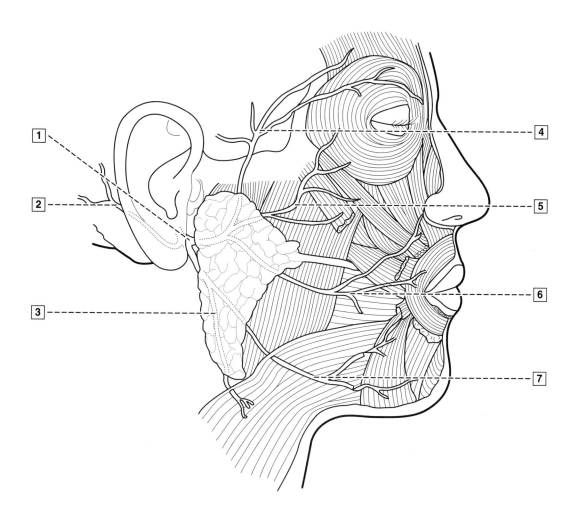

1 Facial nerve (VII)
2 Posterior auricular
3 Cervical branch
4 Temporal branches
5 Zygomatic branches
6 Buccal branches
7 Mandibular branch

REVIEW QUESTIONS

Fill in the blanks by choosing the appropriate terms from the list below.

1. The posterior auricular nerve, stylohyoid nerve, and posterior digastric nerve are branches of the
_____ (VII) after it exits the stylomastoid foramen; all the branches after the nerve
exits from the skull are efferent nerves.

2. The _____ supplies the occipital belly of the epicranial muscle.

3. The _____ supplies the stylohyoid muscle.

4. The _____ supplies the posterior belly of the digastric muscle.

5. Efferent nerve branches of the facial nerve originate within the parotid salivary gland and pass to
the _____ that they innervate; these branches include the temporal, zygomatic,
buccal, mandibular, and cervical branches.

6. The _____ supply the muscles anterior to the ear, frontal belly of the epicranial
muscle, superior part of the orbicularis oculi muscle, and corrugator supercilii muscle.

7. The _____ supply the inferior part of the orbicularis oculi muscle and zygomatic
major and minor muscles.

8. The _____ supply the muscles of the upper lip and nose and buccinator, risorius,
and orbicularis oris muscles.

9. The _____ or marginal branch supplies the muscles of the lower lip and mentalis
muscle.

10. The _____ runs inferior to the mandible to supply the platysma muscle.

cervical branch	muscles of facial expression	posterior auricular nerve
facial nerve	zygomatic branches	mandibular branch
stylohyoid nerve	temporal branches	posterior digastric nerve
buccal branches		

Reference

Chapter 8, Nervous system. In Fehrenbach MJ, Herring SW: *Illustrated anatomy of the head and
neck,* ed 4, St. Louis, 2012, Saunders.

FIGURE 9-1 Upper body lymphatics: right and left sides (frontal view)

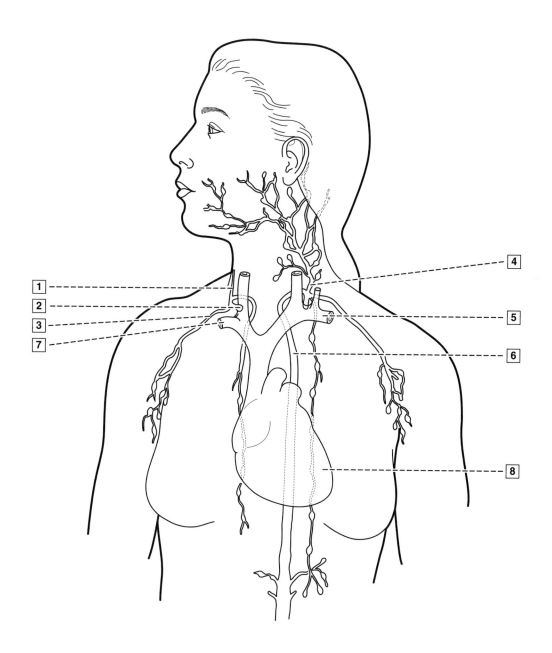

LYMPHATICS

Right side

1 Right jugular trunk

2 Right lymphatic duct

3 Right subclavian trunk

Left side

4 Left jugular trunk

5 Left subclavian trunk

6 Thoracic duct

ASSOCIATED STRUCTURES

7 Right subclavian vein

8 Heart

REVIEW QUESTIONS

Fill in the blanks by choosing the appropriate terms from the list below.

1. The _____ of the right side of the head and neck converges by way of the right jugular trunk, joining that of the right arm and thorax to form the right lymphatic duct.

2. The _____ drains into the venous system at the junction of the right subclavian and right internal jugular veins.

3. The lymphatic vessels of the left side of the head and neck converge into the _____, a short vessel, and then into the thoracic duct, which joins the venous system at the junction of the left subclavian and left internal jugular veins.

4. The lymphatic system from the left arm and thorax also joins the _____, a main duct of the lymphatic system, ascending through the thoracic cavity in front of the spinal column and discharging lymph into the blood through the left subclavian vein.

5. The thoracic duct is much larger than the right lymphatic duct, because it drains the lymph from the entire _____ of the body, both the right and left sides.

thoracic duct

lymphatic system

left jugular trunk

right lymphatic duct

lower half

Reference

Chapter 9, Lymphatic system. In Fehrenbach MJ, Herring SW: *Illustrated anatomy of the head and neck,* ed 4, St. Louis, 2012, Saunders.

FIGURE 9-2   Superficial lymph nodes of the head (lateral view)

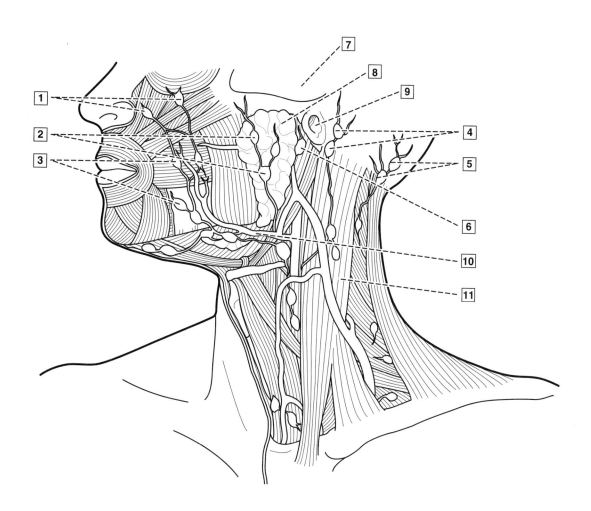

NODES

1	Facial nodes
2	Superficial parotid nodes
3	Facial nodes
4	Retroauricular nodes
5	Occipital nodes
6	Anterior auricular node

ASSOCIATED STRUCTURES

7	Zygomatic arch
8	Parotid gland
9	External acoustic meatus
10	Facial vein
11	Sternocleidomastoid muscle

REVIEW QUESTIONS

Fill in the blanks by choosing the appropriate terms from the list below.

1. The five groups of paired _____ include the occipital, retroauricular, anterior auricular, superficial parotid, and facial lymph nodes.

2. The _____ are located on the posterior base of the head in the occipital region and drain this part of the scalp.

3. The _____ are located posterior to each auricle with its external acoustic meatus, where the sternocleidomastoid muscle inserts on the mastoid process.

4. The _____ are located anterior to each auricle, and the superficial parotid lymph nodes are located just superficial to each parotid salivary gland.

5. The retroauricular, anterior auricular, and superficial parotid lymph nodes drain the external ear, lacrimal gland, and adjacent regions of the scalp and face; all of these nodes empty into the

    _____.

6. The _____ are superficial lymph nodes located along the length of the facial vein and are usually small and variable in number; these lymph nodes are further categorized into four paired subgroups: malar, nasolabial, buccal, and mandibular.

7. The lymph nodes in the infraorbital region are the _____, and the lymph nodes located along the nasolabial sulcus are the nasolabial lymph nodes.

8. The lymph nodes around the labial commissure and just superficial to the buccinator muscle are the

    _____.

9. The lymph nodes in the tissue superior to the surface of the mandible and anterior to the masseter muscle are the _____.

10. Each facial lymph node subgroup drains the skin and mucous membranes where the nodes are located; the facial lymph nodes also drain from one to the other, superior to inferior, and then finally drain together into the deep cervical lymph nodes by way of the _____.

deep cervical lymph nodes	**occipital lymph nodes**	**submandibular lymph nodes**
retroauricular lymph nodes	**anterior auricular lymph nodes**	**buccal lymph nodes**
facial lymph nodes	**malar lymph nodes**	**superficial lymph nodes of the head**
mandibular lymph nodes		

Reference

Chapter 9, Lymphatic system. In Fehrenbach MJ, Herring SW: *Illustrated anatomy of the head and neck,* ed 4, St. Louis, 2012, Saunders.

FIGURE 9-3   Deep lymph nodes of the head (lateral view)

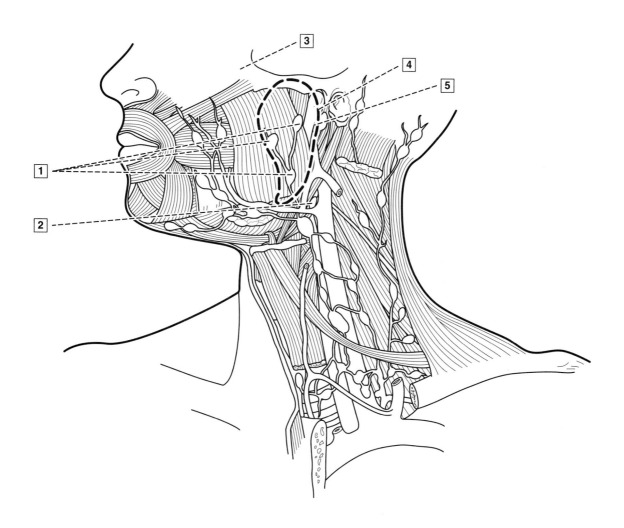

NODES

1　Deep parotid nodes

2　Retropharyngeal node

ASSOCIATED STRUCTURES

3　Zygomatic arch

4　External acoustic meatus

5　Parotid gland (outlined)

REVIEW QUESTIONS

Fill in the blanks by choosing the appropriate terms from the list below.

1. The _____ include the paired deep parotid and retropharyngeal lymph nodes.

2. The deep lymph nodes of the head drain into the _____.

3. The _____ are located deep within the parotid salivary gland and drain the middle ear, auditory tube, and parotid salivary gland.

4. Located near the deep parotid lymph nodes and at the level of the atlas, the first cervical vertebra, are the _____ of the lymphatic system.

5. The retropharyngeal lymph nodes drain and are _____ to the pharynx, palate, paranasal sinuses, and nasal cavity.

retropharyngeal lymph nodes   **deep lymph nodes of the head**

deep cervical lymph nodes   **deep parotid lymph nodes**

posterior

Reference

Chapter 9, Lymphatic system. In Fehrenbach MJ, Herring SW: *Illustrated anatomy of the head and neck,* ed 4, St. Louis, 2012, Saunders.

FIGURE 9-4 Superficial cervical lymph nodes (lateral view)

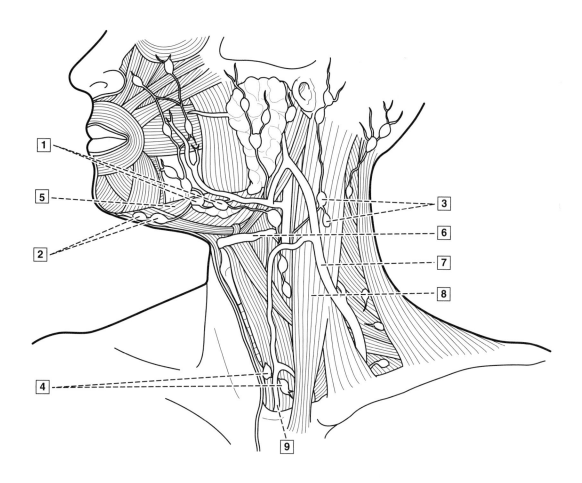

NODES		ASSOCIATED STRUCTURES	
1 Submandibular nodes		5 Mylohyoid muscle	
2 Submental nodes		6 Hyoid bone	
3 External jugular nodes		7 External jugular vein	
4 Anterior jugular nodes		8 Sternocleidomastoid muscle	
		9 Anterior jugular vein	

REVIEW QUESTIONS

Fill in the blanks by choosing the appropriate terms from the list below.

1. The four-paired groups of _____ include the submental, submandibular, external jugular, and anterior jugular lymph nodes.

2. The _____ are located inferior to the chin in the submental fascial space, near the midline inferior to the mandibular symphysis in the suprahyoid region, and also just superficial to the mylohyoid muscle.

3. The submental lymph nodes drain the lower lip, both sides of the chin, the floor of the mouth, the apex of the tongue, and the mandibular incisors and associated tissue; these nodes then empty into the submandibular nodes or directly into the _____.

4. The submandibular lymph nodes are located at the inferior border of the ramus of the mandible, just superficial to the _____, and within the submandibular fascial space.

5. The _____ drain the cheeks, upper lip, body of the tongue, anterior hard palate, and all teeth, except the mandibular incisors and maxillary third molars.

6. The submandibular lymph nodes may be _____ for the submental nodes and facial regions.

7. The lymphatic system from both the _____ and submandibular salivary gland drains into the submandibular lymph nodes; these nodes then empty into the deep cervical lymph nodes.

8. The _____ are located on each side of the neck along the external jugular vein, superficial to the sternocleidomastoid muscle.

9. The external jugular lymph nodes may be secondary nodes for the occipital, retroauricular, anterior auricular, and _____; the external jugular lymph nodes then empty into the deep cervical lymph nodes.

10. The _____ are located on each side of the neck along the length of the anterior jugular vein, anterior to the larynx, trachea, and sternocleidomastoid muscle, and drain the infrahyoid region of the neck; these nodes then empty into the deep cervical lymph nodes.

anterior jugular lymph nodes	submandibular lymph nodes	submental lymph nodes
deep cervical lymph nodes	superficial cervical lymph nodes	sublingual salivary gland
submandibular salivary gland	secondary nodes	superficial parotid lymph nodes
external jugular lymph nodes		

Reference

Chapter 9, Lymphatic system. In Fehrenbach MJ, Herring SW: *Illustrated anatomy of the head and neck,* ed 4, St. Louis, 2012, Saunders.

ANSWER KEY 1. superficial cervical lymph nodes, 2. submental lymph nodes, 3. deep cervical lymph nodes, 4. submandibular salivary gland, 5. submandibular lymph nodes, 6. secondary nodes, 7. sublingual salivary gland, 8. external jugular lymph nodes, 9. superficial parotid lymph nodes, 10. anterior jugular lymph nodes.

FIGURE 9-5 Deep cervical lymph nodes and associated cervical lymph nodes (lateral view)

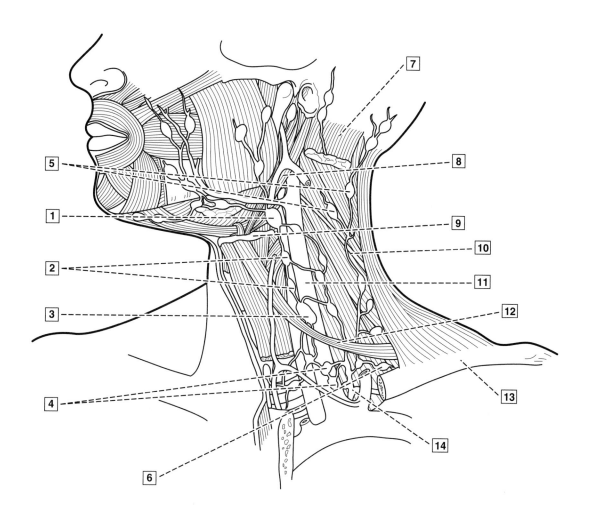

NODES

1 Jugulodigastric node
2 Superior deep cervical nodes
3 Jugulo-omohyoid node
4 Accessory nodes
5 Inferior deep cervical nodes
6 Supraclavicular node

ASSOCIATED STRUCTURES

7 Sternocleidomastoid muscle (cut)
8 Digastric muscle
9 Hyoid bone
10 Accessory nerve
11 Internal jugular vein
12 Omohyoid muscle
13 Clavicle (cut)
14 Thoracic duct

REVIEW QUESTIONS

Fill in the blanks by choosing the appropriate terms from the list below.

1. The _____ are paired groups of lymph nodes located along the length of the internal jugular vein on each side of the neck, deep to the sternocleidomastoid muscle; these nodes extend from the base of the skull to the root of the neck, adjacent to the pharynx, esophagus, and trachea and can be divided into two groups based on the vertical anatomic position of the nodes to the point where omohyoid muscle crosses the internal jugular vein: superior and inferior nodes.

2. The _____ are located deep beneath the sternocleidomastoid muscle, superior to where the omohyoid muscle crosses the internal jugular vein; these nodes are primary nodes for and drain the posterior nasal cavity, posterior hard palate, soft palate, base of the tongue, maxillary third molars and associated tissue, esophagus, trachea, and thyroid gland.

3. The superior deep cervical lymph nodes may be _____ for all other nodes of the head and neck, except inferior deep cervical lymph nodes; the superior deep cervical nodes empty into the inferior deep cervical lymph nodes or directly into the jugular trunk.

4. One possibly prominent lymph node of the superior deep cervical lymph nodes, the _____, or *tonsillar node*, is located inferior to the posterior belly of the digastric muscle and drains the tonsils.

5. The _____ are a continuation of the superior deep cervical group; these nodes are also located deep to the sternocleidomastoid muscle, but inferior to where the omohyoid muscle crosses the internal jugular vein, extending into the supraclavicular fossa, superior to each clavicle.

6. The inferior deep cervical lymph nodes are _____ for and drain the posterior part of the scalp and neck, the superficial pectoral region, and a part of the arm.

7. A possibly prominent node of the inferior deep cervical nodes, the _____, is located at the actual crossing of the omohyoid muscle and internal jugular vein; this node drains the tongue and submental region as well as associated structures and regions.

8. The inferior deep cervical lymph nodes may be secondary nodes for the superficial lymph nodes of the head and superior deep cervical lymph nodes; their efferent vessels form the _____, which is one of the tributaries of the right lymphatic duct (on the right side) and the thoracic duct (on the left).

9. The _____ are associated with the same region as the deep cervical lymph nodes and are located along the eleventh cranial nerve or accessory nerve; these nodes drain the scalp and neck regions and then drain into the supraclavicular lymph nodes.

10. The _____ are located along the clavicle and drain the lateral cervical triangles; these nodes may empty into one of the jugular trunks or directly into the right lymphatic duct or thoracic duct and are located in the final endpoint of lymphatic drainage from the entire body.

jugular trunk	**deep cervical lymph nodes**	**superior deep cervical lymph nodes**
primary nodes	**supraclavicular lymph nodes**	**jugulodigastric lymph node**
inferior deep cervical lymph nodes	**jugulo-omohyoid lymph node**	**accessory lymph nodes**
secondary nodes		

Reference

Chapter 9, Lymphatic system. In Fehrenbach MJ, Herring SW: *Illustrated anatomy of the head and neck,* ed 4, St. Louis, 2012, Saunders.

FIGURE 9-6   **Tonsils and associated structures (sagittal section)**

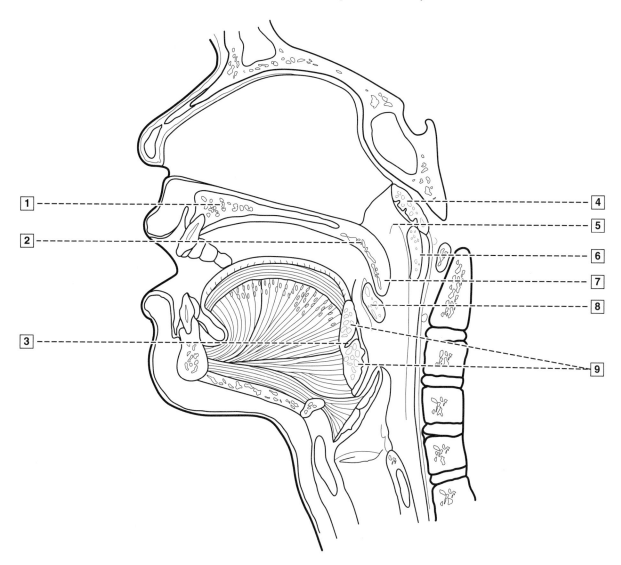

1	Hard palate	**6**	Tubal tonsil
2	Soft palate	**7**	Uvula
3	Foramen cecum	**8**	Palatine tonsil
4	Pharyngeal tonsil	**9**	Lingual tonsil
5	Opening of auditory tube		

REVIEW QUESTIONS

Fill in the blanks by choosing the appropriate terms from the list below.

1. The _____ are lymphoid tissue that drain as a group into the superior deep cervical lymph nodes, particularly affecting the jugulodigastric lymph node.

2. The _____, what most consider their *tonsils*, are two rounded masses of variable size located in the oral cavity between the anterior and posterior faucial pillars on each side of the fauces.

3. The _____ is an indistinct layer of lymphoid nodules located intraorally on the dorsal surface of the base of the tongue, posterior to the circumvallate lingual papillae; its lymphoid tissue consists of many lymphatic nodules, usually each with a germinal center and only one associated tonsillar crypt.

4. The _____, or *adenoids*, located on the midline of the posterior wall or roof of the nasopharynx behind the uvula, forms an incomplete ring of lymphoid tissue termed the *Waldeyer ring,* along with the other tonsils.

5. The _____ is also located in the nasopharynx, posterior to the openings of the eustachian or auditory tube.

tubal tonsil	**lingual tonsil**
tonsils	**pharyngeal tonsil**
palatine tonsils	

References

Chapter 9, Lymphatic system. In Fehrenbach MJ, Herring SW: *Illustrated anatomy of the head and neck,* ed 4, St. Louis, 2012, Saunders; and Chapter 11, Head and neck structures. In Bath-Balogh M, Fehrenbach MJ: *Illustrated dental embryology, histology, and anatomy,* ed 3, St. Louis, 2011, Saunders.

FIGURE 9-7 Palatine tonsil (microanatomic view)

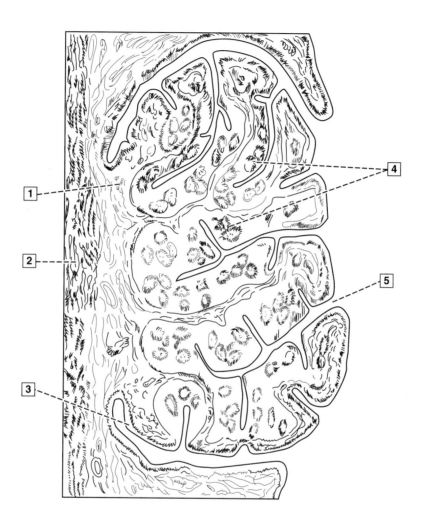

1	Connective tissue (lamina propria)
2	Skeletal muscle
3	Stratified squamous epithelium (oral epithelium)
4	Lymphatic nodules with germinal centers
5	Tonsillar crypt

REVIEW QUESTIONS

Fill in the blanks by choosing the appropriate terms from the list below.

1. Intraoral tonsillar tissue, such as the palatine tonsils, consists of nonencapsulated masses of _____ located in the lamina propria of the oral mucosa.

2. The _____ are two rounded masses of lymphoid tissue of variable size located between the anterior faucial pillar and posterior faucial pillar, with each mass containing fused-together lymphatic nodules that generally have germinal centers.

3. The intraoral tonsillar tissue, such as the palatine tonsils, is covered by stratified squamous epithelium that is continuous with the surrounding oral mucosa; like nodes, the tonsils contain _____, the white blood cells that remove toxic products and then move to the epithelial surface as they mature.

4. Each palatine tonsil also has 10 to 20 epithelial invaginations, or grooves, which penetrate deeply into the tonsil to form _____; these contain shed epithelial cells, mature lymphocytes, and oral bacteria.

5. Unlike lymph nodes, _____ such as the palatine tonsils is not located along lymphatic vessels but is situated near airway and food passages to protect the body against disease processes from the related toxic.

lymphocytes	**lymphoid tissue**
tonsillar crypts	**palatine tonsils**
intraoral tonsillar tissue	

Reference

Chapter 11, Head and neck structures. In Bath-Balogh M, Fehrenbach MJ: *Illustrated dental embryology, histology, and anatomy,* ed 3, St. Louis, 2011, Saunders.

FIGURE 10-1 Fasciae: face (frontal section)

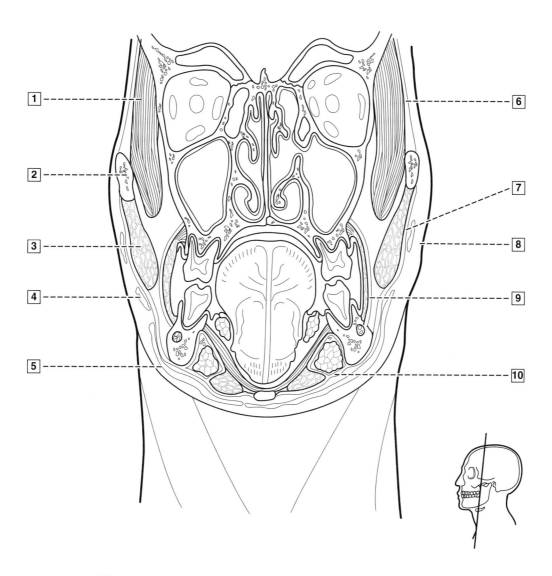

1	Temporalis muscle	**6**	Temporal fascia
2	Zygomatic bone	**7**	Masseteric-parotid fascia
3	Masseter muscle	**8**	Superficial fascia
4	Risorius muscle	**9**	Buccopharyngeal part of visceral fascia
5	Platysma muscle	**10**	Investing fascia

REVIEW QUESTIONS

Fill in the blanks by choosing the appropriate terms from the list below.

1. The _____ consists of layer upon layer of fibrous connective tissue that surrounds muscles, groups of muscles, blood vessels, and nerves; it serves to bind some structures together, while permitting others to slide smoothly over each other.

2. The fascia lies underneath the _____ and surrounds the muscles, bones, vessels, nerves, organs, and other structures.

3. Most of the fasciae can be divided into either the _____ or the deep fasciae.

4. The layers of superficial fascia are found just deep to and attached to the skin; in most cases, the layers of superficial fascia separate skin from deeper structures, allowing the skin to _____ independently of these deeper structures.

5. The layers of superficial fascia vary in thickness in different parts of the body and are composed of adipose tissue as well as irregularly arranged _____, blending with the reticular layer of the dermis.

6. The blood vessels and _____ of the skin also travel in the superficial fascia.

7. In contrast to superficial fascia, the layers of _____ cover the deeper structures of the body including the head and neck such as the bones, muscles, vessels, and nerves.

8. The layers of deep fascia consist of a dense and inelastic fibrous tissue forming _____ around the deeper structures of the body.

9. The layers of superficial fasciae of the body do not usually enclose _____, except for the superficial fasciae of the face and neck.

10. The superficial fascia of the face encloses the _____, a group of striated muscles innervated by the seventh cranial, or facial nerve, that among other things control facial expression.

deep fascia	**sheaths**	**muscles of facial expression**
nerves	**superficial fasciae**	**move**
fascia	**muscles**	**connective tissue**
skin		

Reference

Chapter 11, Fasciae and spaces. In Fehrenbach MJ, Herring SW: *Illustrated anatomy of the head and neck,* ed 4, St. Louis, 2012, Saunders.

ANSWER KEY 1. fascia, 2. skin, 3. superficial fasciae, 4. move, 5. connective tissue, 6. nerves, 7. deep fascia, 8. sheaths, 9. muscles, 10. muscles of facial expression.

FIGURE 10-2   Fasciae: face, jaws, and cervical (transverse sections)

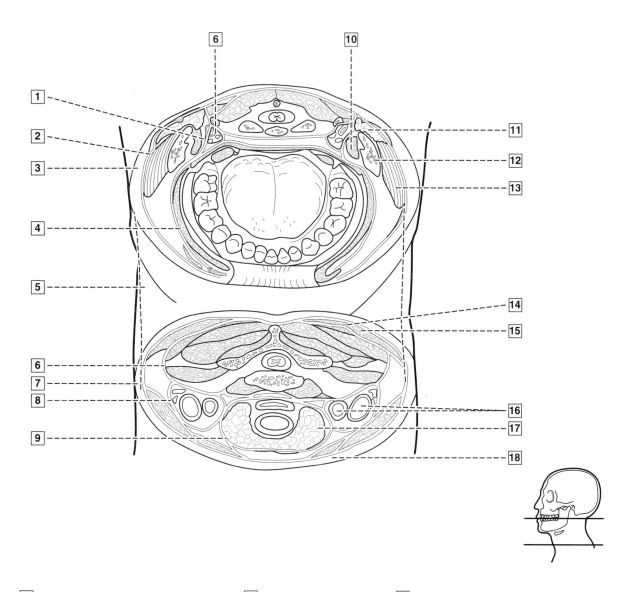

1 Pterygoid fascia	7 Investing fascia	13 Masseter muscle
2 Masseteric-parotid fascia	8 Carotid sheath	14 Trapezius muscle
3 Superficial fascia	9 Visceral fascia	15 Vertebral muscle
4 Buccopharyngeal visceral fascia	10 Medial pterygoid muscle	16 Internal carotid artery and internal jugular vein
5 Continuous layer	11 Parotid salivary gland	17 Thyroid gland
6 Vertebral fascia	12 Mandible	18 Platysma muscle

REVIEW QUESTIONS

Fill in the blanks by choosing the appropriate terms from the list below.

1. The _____ of the neck is an area of fascia that contains the platysma muscle and thus covers most of the anterior cervical triangle.

2. The layers of _____ of the face and jaws are divided into the temporal, the masseteric-parotid, and the pterygoid fasciae, which are continuous with each other and with the deep cervical fasciae.

3. The _____ of the deep fasciae of the face and jaws covers the temporalis muscle and structures superior to the zygomatic arch.

4. The _____ of the deep fasciae of the face and jaws covers the masseter muscle and structures inferior to the zygomatic arch and surrounds the parotid salivary gland.

5. The _____ of the deep fasciae of the face and jaws is located on the medial surface of the medial pterygoid muscle.

6. The layers of _____ include the investing fascia, the carotid sheath, the visceral fascia, the buccopharyngeal fascia, and the vertebral fascia.

7. The layers of the various regions of deep cervical fascia are continuous with each other and also with the deep fasciae of the _____.

8. The investing fascia is the most _____ layer of deep cervical fascia.

9. The investing fascia of deep cervical fascia surrounds the _____, continuing onto the masseteric-parotid fascia.

10. The _____ of deep cervical fascia splits around two salivary glands (submandibular and parotid) and two superficial cervical muscles (sternocleidomastoid and trapezius), enclosing them completely; the branching laminae from this fascia provide the deep fasciae that surround the infrahyoid muscles, from the hyoid bone inferiorly to the sternum.

neck	temporal fascia	superficial cervical fascia
investing fascia	face and jaws	deep fasciae
masseteric-parotid fascia	pterygoid fascia	deep cervical fasciae
external		

Reference

Chapter 11, Fasciae and spaces. In Fehrenbach MJ, Herring SW: *Illustrated anatomy of the head and neck,* ed 4, St. Louis, 2012, Saunders.

FIGURE 10-3 Fasciae: cervical (midsagittal section)

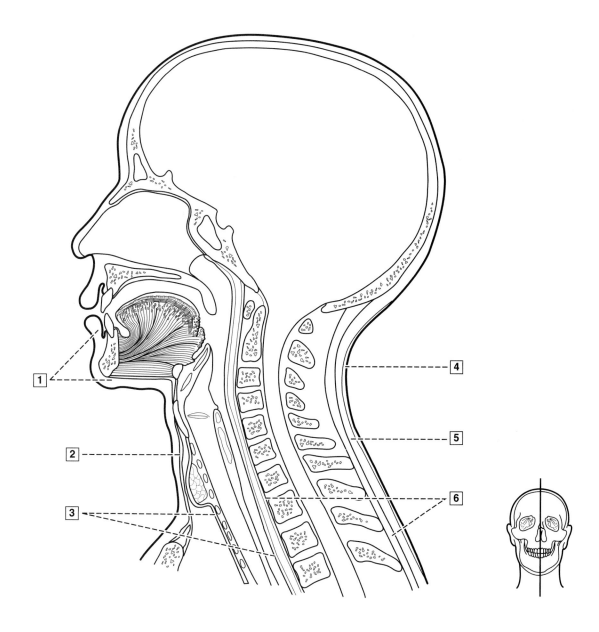

1	Superficial fascia (contains muscles of facial expression)
2	Investing fascia
3	Visceral fascia
4	Superficial fascia
5	Investing fascia
6	Vertebral fascia

REVIEW QUESTIONS

Fill in the blanks by choosing the appropriate terms from the list below.

1. The layers of _____ include the investing fascia, the carotid sheath, the visceral fascia, the buccopharyngeal fascia, and the vertebral fascia.

2. The investing fascia is the most external layer of deep cervical fascia, surrounding the neck, and continuing onto the _____.

3. The _____ also splits around two salivary glands (submandibular and parotid) and two superficial cervical muscles (sternocleidomastoid and trapezius), enclosing them completely; branching laminae from this fascia also provide the deep fasciae that surround the infrahyoid muscles from the hyoid bone inferiorly to the sternum.

4. The _____ is a tube of deep cervical fascia deep to the investing fascia and sternocleidomastoid muscle, running inferiorly along each side of the neck from the base of the skull to the thorax.

5. The carotid sheath contains the _____, the common carotid artery, and the internal jugular vein, as well as the tenth cranial, or vagus, nerve; all of these structures travel between the braincase and the thorax within the sheath.

6. Deep and parallel to the carotid sheath is the _____, or *pretracheal fascia*, which is a single, midline tube of deep cervical fascia running inferiorly along the neck.

7. The visceral fascia of the deep cervical fascia surrounds the air and food passageway including the _____, esophagus, and thyroid gland.

8. Nearer to the skull, the layer of visceral fascia located posterior and lateral to the pharynx is known as the _____.

9. The buccopharyngeal fascia of the visceral fascia encloses the entire superior part of the alimentary canal and is continuous with the fascia covering the buccinator muscle, where that muscle and the superior pharyngeal constrictor muscle come together at the _____.

10. The deepest layer of the deep cervical fascia, the _____, or *prevertebral fascia*, covers the cervical vertebrae, spinal cord, and associated vertebral muscles.

carotid sheath	vertebral fascia	pterygomandibular raphe
internal carotid artery	buccopharyngeal fascia	masseteric-parotid fascia
deep cervical fasciae	visceral fascia	investing fascia
trachea		

Reference

Chapter 11, Fasciae and spaces. In Fehrenbach MJ, Herring SW: *Illustrated anatomy of the head and neck,* ed 4, St. Louis, 2012, Saunders.

ANSWER KEY 1. deep cervical fasciae, 2. masseteric-parotid fascia, 3. Investing fascia, 4. carotid sheath, 5. internal carotid artery, 6. visceral fascia, 7. trachea, 8. buccopharyngeal fascia, 9. pterygomandibular raphe, 10. vertebral fascia.

FIGURE 10-4   Fasciae: cervical (transverse section)

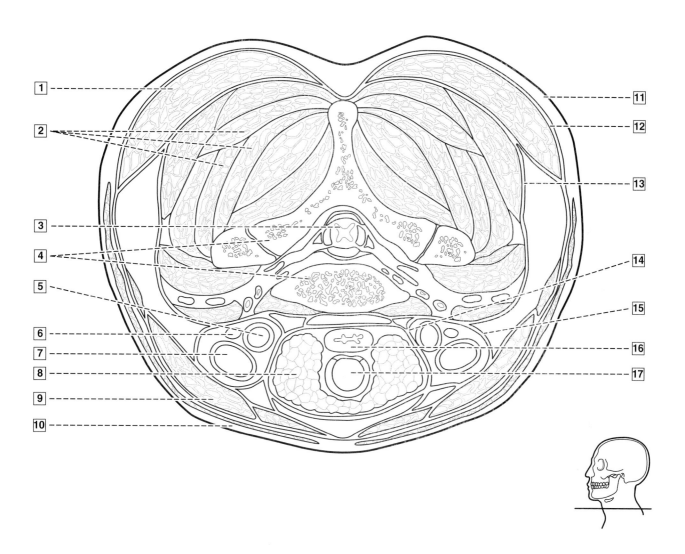

1 Trapezius muscle	**7** Internal jugular vein	**13** Vertebral fascia
2 Vertebral muscles	**8** Thyroid gland	**14** Visceral fascia
3 Spinal cord	**9** Sternocleidomastoid muscle	**15** Carotid sheath
4 Cervical vertebra	**10** Platysma muscle	**16** Esophagus
5 Common carotid artery	**11** Superficial fascia	**17** Trachea
6 Vagus nerve	**12** Investing fascia	

REVIEW QUESTIONS

Fill in the blanks by choosing the appropriate terms from the list below.

1. The carotid sheath is a tube of deep cervical fascia deep to the investing fascia and _____, a major superficial cervical muscle; this sheath runs inferiorly along each side of the neck from the base of the skull to the thorax.

2. The carotid sheath contains the internal carotid artery, the common carotid artery, and the _____, as well as the tenth cranial nerve, or vagus nerve; all of these structures travel between the braincase and the thorax within the sheath.

3. Deep and parallel to the carotid sheath is the _____, or *pretracheal fascia*, which is a single, midline tube of deep cervical fascia running inferiorly along the neck that surrounds the air and food passageway including the trachea, esophagus, and thyroid gland.

4. Nearer to the skull, the layer of visceral fascia located posterior and lateral to the pharynx is known as the _____; this deep cervical fascia encloses the entire superior part of the alimentary canal and is continuous with the fascia covering the buccinator muscle, where that muscle and the superior pharyngeal constrictor muscle come together at the pterygomandibular raphe.

5. The deepest layer of the deep cervical fascia, the _____, or *prevertebral fascia*, covers the cervical vertebrae, spinal cord, and associated vertebral muscles.

sternocleidomastoid muscle

internal jugular vein

visceral fascia

vertebral fascia

buccopharyngeal fascia

Reference

Chapter 11, Fasciae and spaces. In Fehrenbach MJ, Herring SW: *Illustrated anatomy of the head and neck,* ed 4, St. Louis, 2012, Saunders.

FIGURE 10-5 Spaces: face, jaws, and vestibular (frontal section)

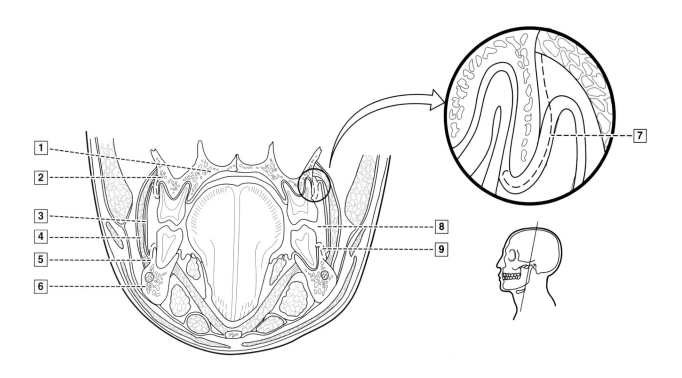

1	Palatine process of maxilla	6	Mandible
2	Alveolar process of maxilla	7	Vestibular space of maxilla
3	Oral mucosa	8	Vestibule of mouth
4	Buccinator muscle	9	Vestibular space of mandible
5	Alveolar process of mandible		

REVIEW QUESTIONS

Fill in the blanks by choosing the appropriate terms from the list below.

1. Potential spaces are created between the layers of fascia of the body because of the sheetlike nature of fasciae and are termed _____, or *fascial planes.*

2. Unlike the neck, the spaces of the face and jaws are often defined by the arrangement of _____ forming boundaries, in addition to the surrounding fasciae; thus, many of the major spaces located in the head are not strictly considered fascial spaces.

3. The spaces of the face and jaws can communicate with each other and with the adjoining _____.

4. The major spaces of the _____ include the maxilla, mandible, canine, parotid, buccal, masticator, body of the mandible, submental, submandibular, and sublingual spaces.

5. The space of the upper jaw, the _____, is located medial to the buccinator muscle and inferior to the attachment of this muscle along the alveolar process of the maxilla.

6. The vestibular space of the maxilla has its lateral wall as the _____.

7. The vestibular space of the maxilla communicates with the _____ and periodontium.

8. The space of the lower jaw, the _____, is located between the buccinator muscle and overlying oral mucosa.

9. The vestibular space of the mandible is bordered by the attachment of the buccinator muscle onto the _____.

10. The vestibular space of the mandible communicates with the _____ and periodontium, as well as the space of the body of the mandible.

oral mucosa	vestibular space of the mandible	face and jaws
muscles and bones	mandible	cervical fascial spaces
vestibular space of the maxilla	fascial spaces	mandibular teeth
maxillary molar teeth		

Reference

Chapter 11, Fasciae and spaces. In Fehrenbach MJ, Herring SW: *Illustrated anatomy of the head and neck,* ed 4, St. Louis, 2012, Saunders.

FIGURE 10-6   Spaces: canine and buccal (frontal section)

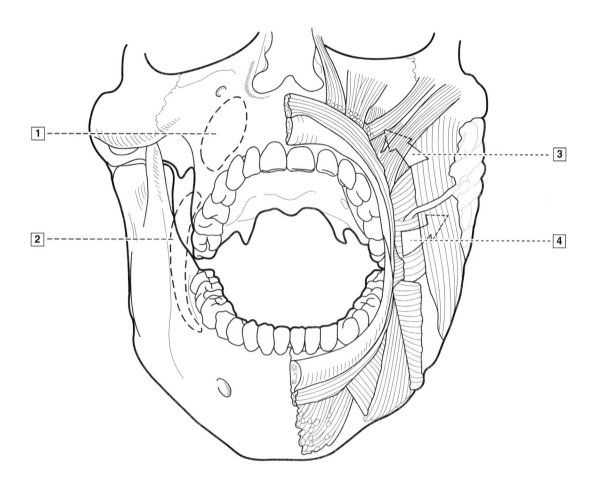

1 Canine space
2 Buccal space
3 Canine space (deep to muscles that elevate lip)
4 Buccal space (deep to masseter muscle)

REVIEW QUESTIONS

Fill in the blanks by choosing the appropriate terms from the list below.

1. The _____ as a space of the face and jaws is located superior to the upper lip and lateral to the apex of the maxillary canine, deep to the overlying skin and deeper muscles of facial expression that elevate the upper lip (levator labii superioris and zygomaticus minor).

2. The floor of the canine space is the depression of the _____ on the maxilla superior to the apex of the canine tooth, which is covered by periosteum, and is bordered anteriorly by the orbicularis oris muscle and posteriorly by the levator anguli oris muscle.

3. The _____ as a fascial space of the face and jaws is formed between the buccinator muscle (actually the buccopharyngeal fascia) and masseter muscle; therefore, it is inferior to the zygomatic arch, superior to the mandible, lateral to the buccinator muscle, and medial and anterior to the deeper masseter muscle.

4. The bilateral buccal space is partially covered by the platysma muscle, as well as by an extension of fascia from the parotid salivary gland capsule; the space contains the _____, which is composed of encapsulated adipose tissue masses in the cheek.

5. The canine space and buccal space communicate with each other, and the buccal space also communicates with the _____ and the space of the body of the mandible.

canine space   buccal space

canine fossa   buccal fat pad

pterygomandibular space

Reference

Chapter 11, Fasciae and spaces. In Fehrenbach MJ, Herring SW: *Illustrated anatomy of the head and neck,* ed 4, St. Louis, 2012, Saunders.

FIGURE 10-7 Spaces: parotid (transverse section)

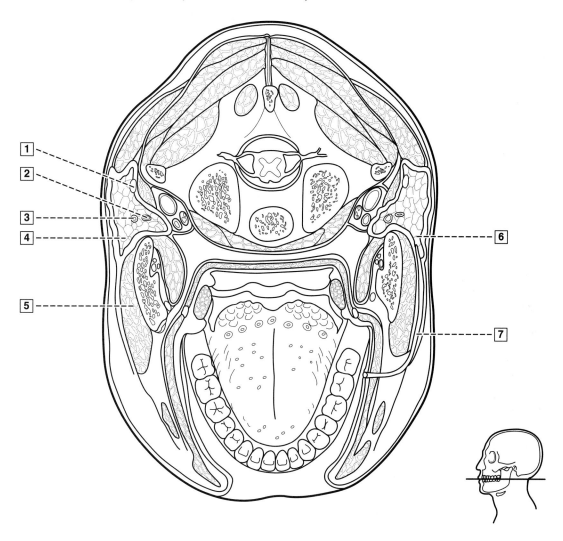

1 Facial nerve

2 Retromandibular vein

3 External carotid artery

4 Parotid salivary gland

5 Masseter muscle

6 Parotid space

7 Parotid duct

REVIEW QUESTIONS

Fill in the blanks by choosing the appropriate terms from the list below.

1. The _____ is a fascial space of the face and jaws that generally does not communicate with the other spaces of the face and jaws.

2. The parotid space is created inside the investing fascial layer of the _____ as it envelops the parotid salivary gland.

3. The parotid space contains the entire _____, the largest of the major salivary glands.

4. The parotid space contains the seventh cranial nerve, or _____, and a part of the external carotid artery and retromandibular vein.

5. The fascial _____ of the parotid space help to keep pathology associated with the parotid salivary gland (such as cancer) from spreading to other sites.

facial nerve	deep cervical fascia
parotid space	parotid salivary gland
boundaries	

Reference

Chapter 11, Fasciae and spaces. In Fehrenbach MJ, Herring SW: *Illustrated anatomy of the head and neck,* ed 4, St. Louis, 2012, Saunders.

FIGURE 10-8   Spaces: temporal and infratemporal (frontal section)

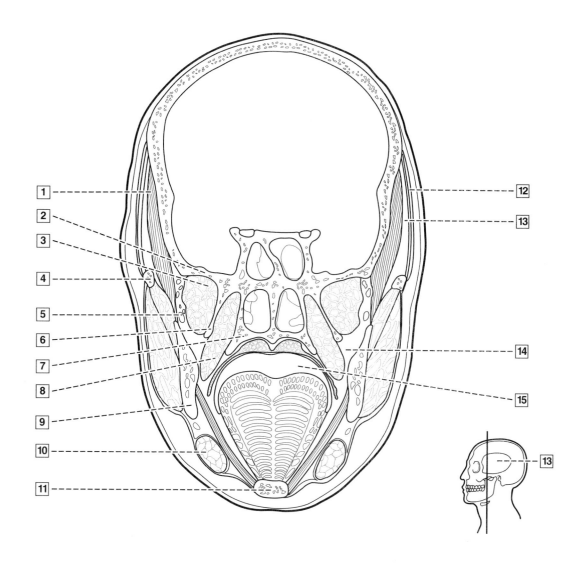

1	Temporalis muscle	**9**	Mandible
2	Infratemporal crest	**10**	Submandibular salivary gland
3	Lateral pterygoid muscle	**11**	Hyoid bone
4	Zygomatic bone	**12**	Temporal fascia
5	Maxillary artery	**13**	Temporal space
6	Lateral pterygoid plate	**14**	Infratemporal space
7	Medial pterygoid plate	**15**	Oral cavity
8	Medial pterygoid muscle		

REVIEW QUESTIONS

Fill in the blanks by choosing the appropriate terms from the list below.

1. The _____ is a general term used to include the entire area of space that includes the mandible and muscles of mastication.

2. The masticator space includes the temporal, infratemporal, and submasseteric spaces, as well as one of the muscles of mastication, the _____, and both the ramus and the body of the mandible.

3. A part of the masticator space is the _____, which is formed by the temporal fascia anterior to the temporalis muscle.

4. The temporal space is between the temporal fascia and temporalis muscle and therefore extends from the _____ inferiorly to the zygomatic arch and infratemporal crest.

5. The temporal space contains adipose tissue and communicates with the infratemporal space and the _____.

6. The infratemporal space is a part of the masticator space and occupies the _____, an area adjacent to the lateral pterygoid plate of the sphenoid bone and maxillary tuberosity of the maxilla.

7. The infratemporal space is bordered laterally by the medial surface of the _____ and the temporalis muscle, with its roof formed by the infratemporal surface of the greater wing of the sphenoid bone; medially, the space is bordered anteriorly by the lateral pterygoid plate and posteriorly by the pharynx with its visceral layer of deep fascia.

8. There is no boundary inferiorly and posteriorly for the infratemporal space, where the space is continuous with a more inferior and deep cervical fascial space, the _____.

9. The infratemporal space contains a part of the _____ as it branches to supply the deep structures of the face, the mandibular nerve and its branches, and the pterygoid plexus of veins; it also contains the medial and lateral pterygoid muscles.

10. The infratemporal space communicates with the temporal space and submasseteric space, as well as with the _____ and parapharyngeal space of the neck.

submandibular space	maxillary artery	mandible
parapharyngeal space	masseter muscle	submasseteric space
superior temporal line	masticator space	infratemporal fossa
temporal space		

Reference

Chapter 11, Fasciae and spaces. In Fehrenbach MJ, Herring SW: *Illustrated anatomy of the head and neck,* ed 4, St. Louis, 2012, Saunders.

FIGURE 10-9   Spaces: infratemporal and pterygomandibular (median section)

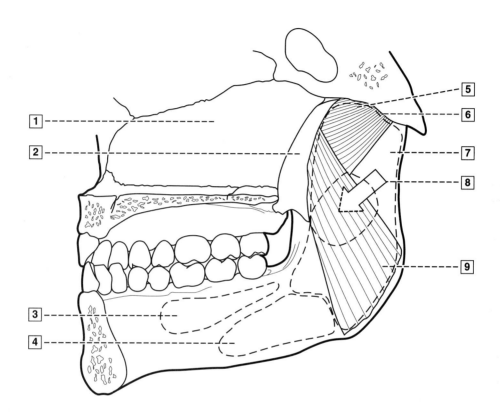

1 Vomer	**6** Infratemporal crest
2 Medial pterygoid plate	**7** Infratemporal space
3 Area of sublingual space	**8** Pterygomandibular space
4 Area of submandibular space	**9** Medial pterygoid muscle
5 Lateral pterygoid muscle	

REVIEW QUESTIONS

Fill in the blanks by choosing the appropriate terms from the list below.

1. The _____ is a space that is part of the masticator space and occupies the infratemporal fossa, an area adjacent to the lateral pterygoid plate of the sphenoid bone and maxillary tuberosity of the maxilla, bordered laterally by the medial surface of the mandible and the temporalis muscle, with its roof formed by the infratemporal surface of the greater wing of the sphenoid bone; medially, the space is bordered anteriorly by the lateral pterygoid plate and posteriorly by the pharynx with its visceral layer of deep fascia.

2. There is no boundary inferiorly and posteriorly for the infratemporal space, where the space is continuous with a more inferior and deep cervical fascial space, the _____.

3. The _____ is a space that is part of the infratemporal space, and is formed by the lateral pterygoid muscle (roof), medial pterygoid muscle (medial wall), and mandibular ramus (lateral wall).

4. The pterygomandibular space contains the _____ and blood vessels and is an important landmark for the inferior alveolar nerve block.

5. The pterygomandibular space communicates with both the _____ and the parapharyngeal space of the neck.

inferior alveolar nerve

infratemporal space

submandibular space

parapharyngeal space

pterygomandibular space

Reference

Chapter 11, Fasciae and spaces. In Fehrenbach MJ, Herring SW: *Illustrated anatomy of the head and neck,* ed 4, St. Louis, 2012, Saunders.

FIGURE 10-10 Spaces: pterygomandibular (transverse section)

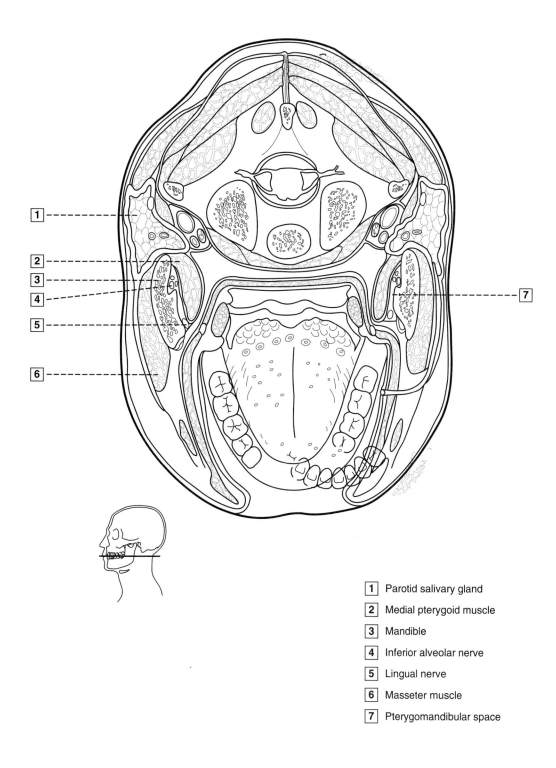

1	Parotid salivary gland
2	Medial pterygoid muscle
3	Mandible
4	Inferior alveolar nerve
5	Lingual nerve
6	Masseter muscle
7	Pterygomandibular space

REVIEW QUESTIONS

Fill in the blanks by choosing the appropriate terms from the list below.

1. The _____ is a space that is a part of the infratemporal space, which is a masticator space.

2. The pterygomandibular space has as its roof the _____, with the medial pterygoid muscle as its medial wall.

3. The pterygomandibular space has the _____ as its lateral wall.

4. The pterygomandibular space contains the _____ and blood vessels and is an important landmark for the inferior alveolar nerve block as well as the more medially placed and anterior lingual nerve and vessels.

5. The pterygomandibular space communicates with both the submandibular space and the _____ of the neck.

inferior alveolar nerve   parapharyngeal space

mandibular ramus   pterygomandibular space

lateral pterygoid muscle

Reference

Chapter 11, Fasciae and spaces. In Fehrenbach MJ, Herring SW: *Illustrated anatomy of the head and neck,* ed 4, St. Louis, 2012, Saunders.

FIGURE 10-11   Spaces: submasseteric (lateral views)

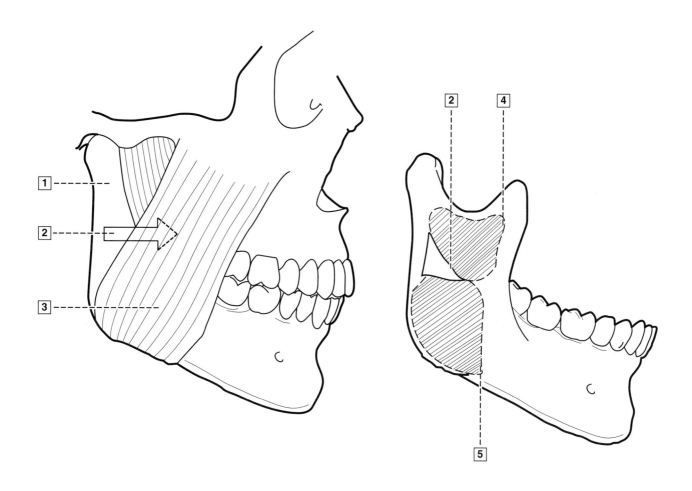

1   Ramus

2   Submasseteric space

3   Masseter muscle

4   Insertion of deep head of masseter muscle

5   Insertion of superficial head of masseter muscle

REVIEW QUESTIONS

Fill in the blanks by choosing the appropriate terms from the list below.

1. The general term of _____ is used to describe a space that includes the entire area of the mandible and muscles of mastication, which includes the masseter and temporalis muscles, as well as the medial and lateral pterygoids.

2. The masticator space includes the temporal, infratemporal, and submasseteric spaces, masseter muscle, and both ramus and body of the _____.

3. A part of the masticator space is the _____, which is anteriorly bounded by the inner surface of the masseteric fascia as it sweeps around the anterior aspect of the masseter muscle and mandibular ramus.

4. The submasseteric space is located between the _____ and the external surface of the vertical mandibular ramus.

5. The submasseteric space communicates with both the _____ and the infratemporal space.

<blockquote>

submasseteric space   **masseter muscle**

mandible   **masticator space**

temporal space

</blockquote>

Reference

Chapter 11, Fasciae and spaces. In Fehrenbach MJ, Herring SW: *Illustrated anatomy of the head and neck,* ed 4, St. Louis, 2012, Saunders.

FIGURE 10-12 Spaces: body of the mandible (frontal section)

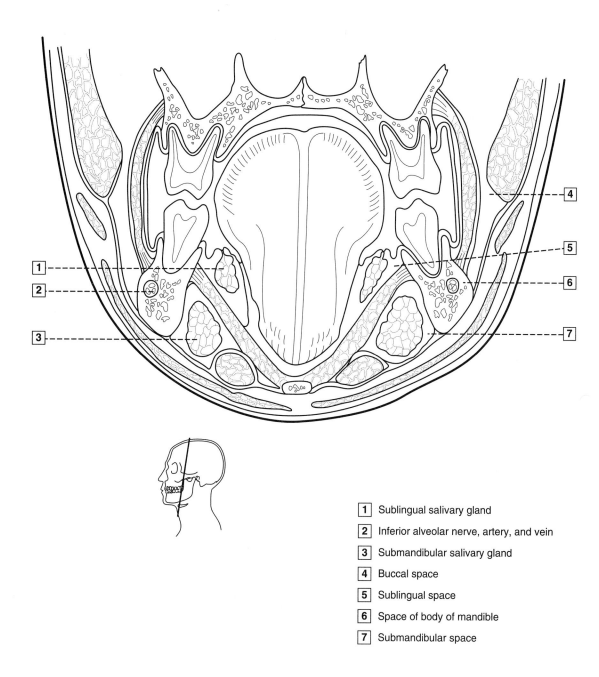

1 Sublingual salivary gland

2 Inferior alveolar nerve, artery, and vein

3 Submandibular salivary gland

4 Buccal space

5 Sublingual space

6 Space of body of mandible

7 Submandibular space

REVIEW QUESTIONS

Fill in the blanks by choosing the appropriate terms from the list below.

1. The _____ is a space formed by the periosteum covering the bony surface of the mandible, which is a specialized connective tissue membrane that lines the outer surface of all bones.

2. The space of the body of the mandible is anterior to the body of the _____ from its symphysis to the anterior borders of the masseter and medial pterygoid muscles.

3. The space of the body of the mandible contains the mandible and a part of the _____, a branch of the mandibular nerve.

4. The space of the body of the mandible contains the _____, as well as the dental and alveolar branches of these blood vessels, as well as the associated mental and incisive branches.

5. The space of the body of the mandible communicates with the _____, as well as the buccal space, submental space, submandibular space, and sublingual space.

vestibular space of the mandible	**inferior alveolar artery and vein**
inferior alveolar nerve	**space of the body of the mandible**
mandible	

Reference

Chapter 11, Fasciae and spaces. In Fehrenbach MJ, Herring SW: *Illustrated anatomy of the head and neck,* ed 4, St. Louis, 2012, Saunders.

FIGURE 10-13   Spaces: submental and submandibular (anterolateral view with the skin and platysma muscle removed)

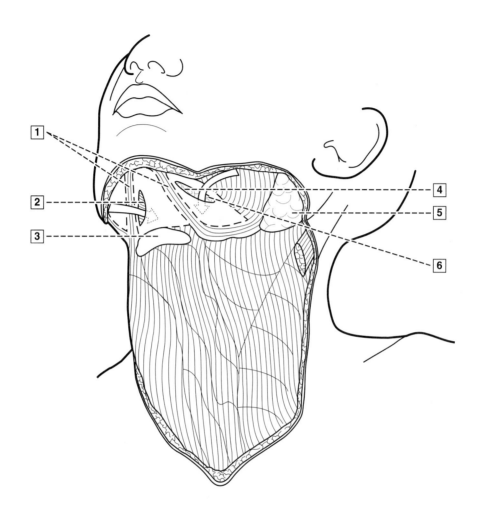

1	Anterior bellies of digastric muscle
2	Superficial cervical fascia (cut to demonstrate entrance into submental space)
3	Hyoid bone
4	Submandibular salivary gland
5	Parotid salivary gland
6	Superficial cervical fascia (cut to demonstrate entrance into submandibular space)

REVIEW QUESTIONS

Fill in the blanks by choosing the appropriate terms from the list below.

1. The _____ is a space located in the midline between the mandibular symphysis and the hyoid bone.

2. The floor of the submental space is the _____ covering the suprahyoid muscles, with the mylohyoid muscle as its roof, covered by the investing fascia.

3. Forming the lateral boundaries of the submental space are the diverging anterior bellies of the _____.

4. The submental space contains the _____ and the origin of the anterior jugular vein.

5. The submental space communicates with the _____, submandibular space, and sublingual space.

6. The _____ is a space located lateral and posterior to the submental space on each side of the jaws.

7. The cross-sectional shape of the bilateral submandibular space is triangular, with the _____ on the medial surface of the mandible being its superior boundary, which is the origin of the mylohyoid muscle.

8. The _____ forms the medial and the superior boundaries of the submandibular space, and the hyoid bone creates its medial apex.

9. The submandibular space contains the _____, most of the submandibular salivary gland, and parts of the facial artery, which is a branch of the external carotid artery that supplies structures of the superficial face.

10. The submandibular space communicates with the infratemporal space, submental space, and _____, as well as the parapharyngeal space of the neck.

submental lymph nodes	mylohyoid muscle	digastric muscles
superficial cervical fascia	submandibular lymph nodes	space of the body of the mandible
mylohyoid line	sublingual space	submandibular space
submental space		

Reference

Chapter 11, Fasciae and spaces. In Fehrenbach MJ, Herring SW: *Illustrated anatomy of the head and neck,* ed 4, St. Louis, 2012, Saunders.

FIGURE 10-14 Spaces: submandibular and sublingual (frontal section)

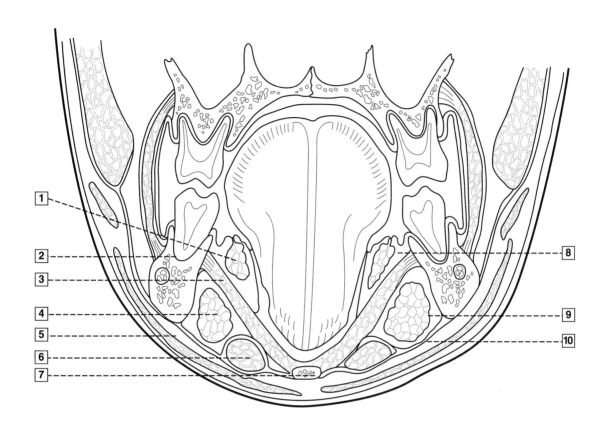

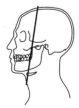

1	Sublingual salivary gland
2	Mandible
3	Mylohyoid muscle
4	Submandibular salivary gland
5	Platysma muscle
6	Digastric muscle
7	Hyoid bone
8	Sublingual space
9	Submandibular space
10	Investing fascia

REVIEW QUESTIONS

Fill in the blanks by choosing the appropriate terms from the list below.

1. The _____ is a space located lateral and posterior to the submental space on each side of the jaws.

2. The cross-sectional shape of the bilateral submandibular space is triangular, with the mylohyoid line on the medial surface of the _____ being its superior boundary, which is the origin of the mylohyoid muscle.

3. The mylohyoid muscle forms the medial, as well as the superior boundary of the submandibular space, and the _____ creates its medial apex.

4. The submandibular space contains the submandibular lymph nodes, most of the _____, and parts of the facial artery, which is a branch of the external carotid artery that supplies structures of the superficial face.

5. The submandibular space communicates with the infratemporal space, submental space, and sublingual space, as well as the _____ of the neck.

6. The sublingual space is located deep to the _____, thus making this tissue that lines the oral cavity its roof.

7. The floor of the sublingual space is the _____; thus, this muscle creates the division between the submandibular and sublingual spaces with the sublingual space superior to the more inferior submandibular space.

8. The _____ and its intrinsic muscles form the medial boundary of the sublingual space, and the mandible or lower jaw forms its lateral wall.

9. The sublingual space contains the _____ and ducts, the duct of the submandibular salivary gland, a part of the lingual nerve and artery, and the twelfth cranial nerve, or hypoglossal nerve.

10. The sublingual space communicates with the _____ and submandibular space, as well as with the space of the body of the mandible.

submental space	tongue	sublingual salivary gland
mylohyoid muscle	oral mucosa	parapharyngeal space
submandibular salivary gland	submandibular space	mandible
hyoid bone		

Reference

Chapter 11, Fasciae and spaces. In Fehrenbach MJ, Herring SW: *Illustrated anatomy of the head and neck,* ed 4, St. Louis, 2012, Saunders.

FIGURE 10-15 Spaces: retropharyngeal and parapharyngeal (transverse section)

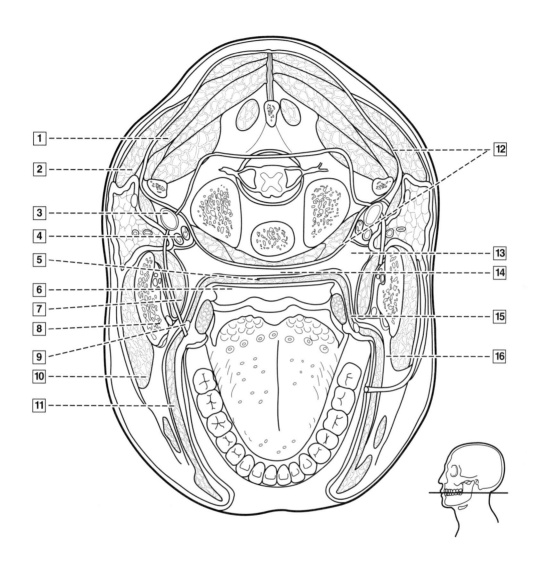

1	Vertebral muscles	9	Pterygomandibular raphe
2	Sternocleidomastoid muscle	10	Masseter muscle
3	Internal jugular vein	11	Buccinator muscle
4	Internal carotid artery	12	Vertebral fascia
5	Superior pharyngeal constrictor muscle	13	Parapharyngeal space
6	Pharynx	14	Retropharyngeal space
7	Medial pterygoid muscle	15	Buccopharyngeal fascia
8	Mandible	16	Buccal space

REVIEW QUESTIONS

Fill in the blanks by choosing the appropriate terms from the list below.

1. The _____ are spaces located in the neck that can communicate with the spaces of the face and jaws, as well as with each other.

2. The cervical spaces connect the _____ of the head with those of the thorax, which then connect to vital organs such as the heart and lungs as well as the brain.

3. The cervical spaces include the parapharyngeal space, retropharyngeal space, and

   _____.

4. The _____, or *lateral pharyngeal space,* is a fascial space lateral to the pharynx and medial to the medial pterygoid muscle, as well as parallel to the carotid sheath.

5. The bilateral parapharyngeal space in its posterior part is adjacent to the _____, which contains the internal and common carotid arteries and the internal jugular vein, as well as the tenth cranial nerve or vagus nerve.

6. The parapharyngeal space in its posterior part is adjacent to the ninth, eleventh, and twelfth _____ as they exit the cranial cavity.

7. Anteriorly, the parapharyngeal space extends to the _____, where it is continuous with the infratemporal and buccal spaces.

8. The parapharyngeal space anteriorly contains a few _____.

9. Posteriorly, the parapharyngeal space extends around the _____, where it is continuous with another cervical fascial space, the retropharyngeal space.

10. The _____, or *retrovisceral space,* is a fascial space located immediately posterior to the pharynx, between the vertebral and visceral fasciae.

pharynx	**previsceral space**	**pterygomandibular raphe**
spaces of the face and jaws	**carotid sheath**	**lymph nodes**
cranial nerves	**parapharyngeal space**	**retropharyngeal space**
cervical spaces		

Reference

Chapter 11, Fasciae and spaces. In Fehrenbach MJ, Herring SW: *Illustrated anatomy of the head and neck,* ed 4, St. Louis, 2012, Saunders.

FIGURE 10-16 Spaces: retropharyngeal and previsceral (midsagittal section)

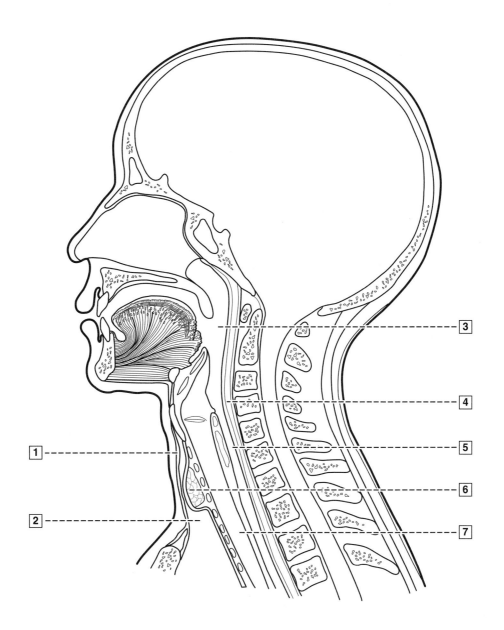

1 Investing fascia

2 Previsceral space

3 Pharynx

4 Retropharyngeal space

5 Esophagus

6 Thyroid gland

7 Trachea

REVIEW QUESTIONS

Fill in the blanks by choosing the appropriate terms from the list below.

1. The _____ are spaces in the neck that include the parapharyngeal space, retropharyngeal space, and previsceral space.

2. The _____, or *retrovisceral space,* is a fascial space located immediately posterior to the pharynx between the vertebral and visceral fasciae; the retropharyngeal space is a space bounded by the buccopharyngeal fascia anteriorly and the alar fascia posteriorly.

3. The retropharyngeal space extends from the base of the _____, where it is posterior to the superior pharyngeal constrictor muscle and inferior to the thorax; it contains the retropharyngeal lymph nodes.

4. The _____ is a space located between the visceral and investing fasciae, anterior to the trachea.

5. Both the retropharyngeal space and previsceral space communicate with the

    _____.

previsceral space   skull

parapharyngeal spaces   retropharyngeal space

cervical spaces

Reference

Chapter 11, Fasciae and spaces. In Fehrenbach MJ, Herring SW: *Illustrated anatomy of the head and neck,* ed 4, St. Louis, 2012, Saunders.

FIGURE 10-17 Spaces: retropharyngeal and previsceral (transverse section)

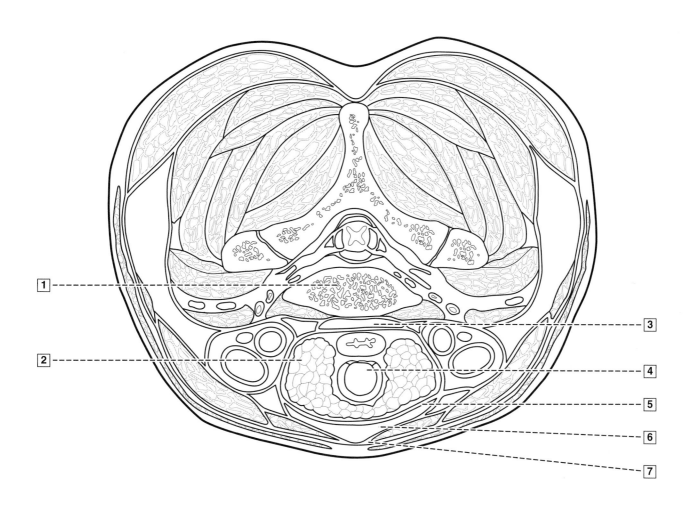

1 Cervical vertebrae

2 Thyroid gland

3 Retropharyngeal space

4 Trachea

5 Visceral fascia

6 Previsceral space

7 Investing fascia

REVIEW QUESTIONS

Fill in the blanks by choosing the appropriate terms from the list below.

1. The _____ located in the neck connect the spaces of the face and jaws with those of the thorax, which then connect to vital organs such as the heart and lungs, as well as the brain.

2. The retropharyngeal space, or *retrovisceral space,* is a fascial space located immediately posterior to the _____, between the vertebral and visceral fasciae.

3. The retropharyngeal space extends from the base of the skull, where it is posterior to the superior pharyngeal constrictor muscle, inferior to the _____.

4. The previsceral space is located between the visceral and investing fasciae, anterior to the

    _____.

5. Both the retropharyngeal space and previsceral space communicate with the

    _____.

trachea   cervical spaces

parapharyngeal spaces   thorax

pharynx

Reference

Chapter 11, Fasciae and spaces. In Fehrenbach MJ, Herring SW: *Illustrated anatomy of the head and neck,* ed 4, St. Louis, 2012, Saunders.